PERPETUITY
PUBLISHING

Light Reflections Into

THE DARKNESS OF DENIAL

... and the alcoholic mind

Light Reflections Into
THE DARKNESS OF DENIAL
...and the alcoholic mind

JOEL L. KRUGER

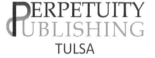

PERPETUITY
PUBLISHING
TULSA

© Copyright 2015-2024 by Joel L. Kruger

Published by:
Perpetuity Publishing
Tulsa, OK

All rights reserved. No part of this publication may be reproduced, stored in a retrieval system, or transmitted in any form or by any means—electronic, photocopy, recording, scanning, mechanical, or electronic—without the author's prior written permission.

ISBN: 978-0-9964646-2-8

Cover Design, Photography & Illustration:
Joel L. Kruger & Debra Bradley

The author and publisher have strived to ensure the information contained herein is accurate. Still, it may contain errors or omissions and should not be relied upon.

This publication should not be relied upon as a valid diagnostic or alcohol screening instrument or when deciding whether to seek *any* treatment. The author and publisher cannot provide any professional advice. Please consult the appropriate health care provider to address your concerns.

Any reference to names, characters, businesses, organizations, places, events, and incidents is fictitious or used fictitiously. Any resemblance to actual persons, living or dead, events, or locales is entirely coincidental.

Cataloging-in-publication data is on file with the Library of Congress.

First Edition
First Printing
Printed in the United States of America.

All trademarks are the property of their respective owner.

THIS BOOK IS DEDICATED
to the millions of sober alcoholics
and
the millions of suffering alcoholics
and
the tens of millions of loved ones and others
affected by alcoholics
including the silent children
caught in the crossfire without a say.

IN MEMORY
of those that went before.
Some sober and some not— including
my best buddy, Luke.

Contents

Author's Note		11
Acknowledgements		13
Introduction		15
Contact Information		**17**
Disclaimer and Explainer		21
Terms and Meanings		23

Chapter 1	Inside an Alcoholic's Mind *A True Story*		31
Chapter 2	A Description of the Alcoholic		41
Chapter 3	The Alcoholic-Craving: *A Unique Perspective*		73
	Section One—What is the Alcoholic-Craving?	76	
	Section Two—The Neuroscience of the Alcoholic-Craving	87	
	Section Three—The Importance of Recognizing the Alcoholic-Craving	93	
	Section Four—The Research	121	
Chapter 4	The Alcoholic Stigma: *A Blessing in Disguise?*		129
	Contact Information		**173**
Chapter 5	The Darkness and Lightness of Denial and the Alcoholic's Entourage		177
Chapter 6	The Periodic Alcoholic (Binge or Episodic Drinker)		221
	Contact Information		**239**
Chapter 7	Health Care, Alcoholism and the DSM *Problems and Solutions*		243
	Section One—Alcoholism and Medicine	247	
	Section Two—The Screening	266	
	Section Three—The Diagnosis	274	
	Section Four—The AUD Section of the DSM: Limitations and Improvements	279	
	Section Five—Effective Use of the DSM-5 AUD Diagnostic Criteria	298	
	Section Six—Health Care Education	327	

CHAPTER 8	THE AFFECTED:		335
	Caught in the Crossfire		
	SECTION ONE—The Endless Cycle	338	
	SECTION TWO—When the Children Became Adults	348	
	SECTION THREE—The Affected Spouse, Partner, or Parent	354	
CHAPTER 9	THE RELAPSE:		363
	Returning to the Darkness		
	CONTACT INFORMATION		**377**
CHAPTER 10	THE INTERVENTION:		381
	To Intervene or Not ...		
Chapter 11	GOD?		401
	SECTION ONE—Beliefs in God	402	
	SECTION TWO—Spirituality and Religion: A Comparison	432	
CHAPTER 12	THE HAPPILY SOBER ALCOHOLIC		443

NOTES		487
INDEX		515
	CONTACT INFORMATION	**533**

Author's Note

AS A YOUNG BOY, I tossed a stone into a pond. I listened to the sound and watched the ripples—the ripples I just made. I threw in a bigger stone, heard a deeper sound, and saw bigger ripples travel farther. The next stone was so big it took both my hands to hold, and, with all my might, I tossed it as high as I could. When it hit the water, the sound was much deeper, and I said, "Look ... Dad! I can make waves!"

He smiled, picked up a tiny flat stone, cast it into the pond, and it hit the water. And it hit the water over and over, skipping across the pond until it skipped out of sight. The pond's mirrored reflection changed into a mass of intersecting ripples traveling beyond my vision, reflecting sunlight in sparkling and memorable ways. I realized then it's not always the biggest stone that makes the most ripples.

I realize now the ripples from our actions often travel great distances to remote and unknown places. They even exist when we don't see them. We will never know for sure who has or how they have been affected by the ripples we created. I am deeply grateful to all, some known, some unknown, who created the beneficial ripples that flowed into this book.

I hope the essence of this book skips like a perfect stone cast into the silent pond of the drowning—and the ripples travel far and deep, reflecting sunlight in sparkling and memorable ways, into the darkness of denial.

Acknowledgments

"You know, I should write a book," we hear often. Rarely does that thought turn into anything that can be placed on a bookshelf. Living life interferes with writing about it, and most of us are too busy living. It's a daunting task, sometimes darkened with overwhelming discouragement, and its 'completion' is situational. I am grateful that my situation allowed me to dedicate most days to writing it over the past eight years and those who provided essential support.

Special thanks to my main editors, Phil Harriman and Pamala Sipes, who tolerated each time I handed them another revised chapter, claiming it was final as they were still editing the last revision. They patiently endured my endless and countless revisions—their talents and patience are outstanding.

Many thanks to my assistant editors, Madeline S. and Amanda Sanford.

I also want to express my enormous gratitude to my son, Aaron, for his very beneficial, thorough, and enlightening editorial assistance and to my son, Ben, who, once again, came through and shined the light of his exceptional perception on the darker portions.

And my mom, who raised me to appreciate words. Her review of chapters and gentle prodding by regularly asking, "Do you think I'll ever see these chapters in a book?" was more helpful than she'll ever know.

I sincerely appreciate the many readers and reviewers who provided invaluable feedback that helped shape this book.

I procrastinate, and like many procrastinators, I'm a perfectionist. Of course, that doesn't mean I do things perfectly; it means I waste much time trying.

All books must have an end, yet knowing when this book ended was challenging. That's because, as I finally accepted, books never end; there simply comes a time for the last page. To do that, I often reminded myself *if something is worth doing, it's worth doing imperfectly*, even though I struggled to follow that self-imposed principle.

Special thanks to all those who repeatedly asked, "Have you finished your book yet?" And I'm especially appreciative of my son, Dillon, for rolling his eyes at the perfect times as the days, weeks, months, and years passed after I would claim, "I should finish this book within the next few hours." His expressions enabled me to write the last page—eventually.

I'm eternally grateful to all who remain anonymous and collectively gave me the courage, strength, and hope to memorialize my thoughts in this written form rather than slurring them from a bar stool.

I'm also eternally grateful for my awareness of the higher purpose that enabled me to write this book and the Power within all of us.

And finally, my deep, warm-hearted appreciation, which swells more each moment, for my angelic catalyst, Debra Bradley. She endlessly reviewed revised manuscripts, listened to my nonstop jabber as this project unfolded, and collected a group of people, especially Pamala, who catapulted this project into a reality. Without her love and support, this book would not exist.

INTRODUCTION

ALTHOUGH FOR YEARS, research has shown moderate alcohol use has many health benefits, recent research reveals these past studies were flawed. According to the CDC, NIAAA, and other prominent institutions, the harm from moderate drinking outweighs the benefits.* The consensus now is no one should start drinking to obtain health benefits, and even drinking excessively° on occasion can negatively impact health and can be deadly.

That said, this book doesn't condemn alcohol or drinking for nonalcoholics. Whether one uses or abuses alcohol has little to do with alcohol. For many, drinking may serve a useful purpose, but for alcoholics, it does not.

Since nearly half of the U.S. population has been exposed to alcoholism in their family, this book has no target audience—it is for everyone. The general reader will gain insight from a different viewpoint. Healthcare providers may gain valuable knowledge from this outside perspective. Those affected by a problem drinker may benefit from the information in this book, enabling them to realize they need not continue drifting aimlessly on the dead-end road they've

---

*According to the CDC moderate drinking is having, in a day, one drink or less for women, and two drinks or less for men.

°Excessive alcohol use is 4 drinks for women, or 5 drinks for men on one occasion (binge drinking), 8 drinks for women, or 15 drinks for men within a week (heavy drinking), and any alcohol use during pregnancy.

been traveling.

And the problem drinker ... well, who knows? This book is not a manual on how to modify one's drinking or quit drinking. Nor is it a manual on how to control or outsmart the alcoholic. Any belief this can be done is an illusion.

It is said no one can tell another they're an alcoholic; only the alcoholic can make that call. Still, expressing an opinion that one has a drinking problem can be helpful. This is especially true for those whose alcoholism is apparent to everyone—everyone except the alcoholic. What problem drinkers do with that information is their decision.

In fact, telling someone they're alcoholic may accelerate a self-diagnosis. We see this when courts and others successfully intervene. Still, before alcoholics accept their alcoholism and take any meaningful action to recover, they must escape the darkness of denial. I hope this book lightens the denial with which they struggle.

IF YOU'RE SUFFERING from alcoholism or affected by another's drinking, there are many organizations and people ready to help, and receiving help is much easier than you may think.

The next, last, and several pages throughout this book provide helpful contact information. It only requires pressing 10 buttons to change your life forever.

Contact Information

SUICIDE & CRISIS LIFELINE:
Call or text **988** or chat at **988lifeline.org**

SUICIDE PREVENTION LIFELINE:
1-800-273-TALK (8255)

For confidential information about help for alcohol dependence, contact one or more of the following:

NIAAA ALCOHOL TREATMENT NAVIGATOR
"Pointing the way to evidence-based care"

A service of the U.S. federal government providing unbiased information for finding quality alcohol treatment through mutual support groups, therapists, doctors, and outpatient & inpatient care.

www.alcoholtreatment.niaaa.nih.gov

MUTUAL-SUPPORT GROUPS

(AA) Alcoholics Anonymous
www.aa.org | 212–870–3400
(or local phone directory)

Al-Anon Family Services/Alateen
For Those Affected by Another's Drinking
www.al-anon.org | 888-425-2666 for meetings

Adult Children of Alcoholics & Dysfunctional Families
www.adultchildren.org | 310–534–1815

AA Agnostica
A space for AA agnostics, atheists and freethinkers worldwide
www.aaagnostica.org | admin@aaagnostica.org.

Celebrate Recovery
A Christ-Centered Recovery Program
www.celebraterecovery.com | 800-723-3532

LifeRing
Secular (nonreligious) Recovery
www.LifeRing.org | 800-811-4142

Moderation Management
www.moderation.org | 212–871–0974

Secular Organizations for Sobriety
www.sossobriety.org | 314-353–3532

Secular Alcoholics Anonymous
AA meetings for agnostics, atheists and freethinkers
www.secularaa.org

SMART Recovery
An Alternative to AA, Al-Anon, and other 12-Step Programs
www.smartrecovery.org | 440-951-5357

Women for Sobriety
www.womenforsobriety.org | 215–536–8026

INFORMATION RESOURCES

The Alcohol and Drug Addiction Resource Center
(800) 390-4056

Alcohol and Drug Helpline
www.alcoholanddrughelpline.com | (800) 821-4357

Alcohol Hotline Support & Information
(800) 331-2900

American Council on Alcoholism (ACA)
www.recoverymonth.gov | (800) 527-5344

National Child Abuse Hotline
1-800-25-ABUSE

National Clearinghouse for Alcohol and Drug Information
www.ncadi.samhsa.gov | (800) 729–6686

Contact Information

National Council on Alcoholism & Drug Dependence, Inc.
www.ncadd.org | *HOPE LINE*: 800/NCA-CALL (24-hour)

National Domestic Abuse Hotline
1-800-799-SAFE

National Helpline
Treatment referral and information 24-7
www.samhsa.gov | 1-800-662-HELP (4357)

National Institute on Alcohol Abuse and Alcoholism
www.niaaa.nih.gov | (301) 443–3860

National Institute on Drug Abuse
www.nida.nih.gov | (301) 443–1124

National Institute of Mental Health
www.nimh.nih.gov | (866) 615–6464

DISCLAIMER AND EXPLAINER

> **CAUTION:** It could be fatal to stop drinking without medical help, so please consult the proper health care provider before attempting this.

MUCH OF THE information in this book comes from the author's empirical research, including direct and indirect observations, anecdotal evidence, personal observations, experience, interviews, professional practice, and listening to thousands of drinking and sober alcoholics discuss their experiences.

All information obtained from studies, research papers, reports, articles, books, and other publications used to collect the information contained in this book is cited. Although most sources cited were peer-reviewed, the author makes no representation regarding this.

The author provides the information in this book as a reporter, journalist, and commentator (i.e., researching, conducting interviews, and other information gathering, writing, and reporting).

Every fact stated has been extensively checked for accuracy. Still, it could contain an error or omission. As time passes, some information may not be as current or complete as when written.

The author has not subjected his theories and conclusions to experiments or testing. Much of this book's goal is to invite readers to explore the possibility that they, or someone they know, may have an issue with alcohol, suggesting further exploration and providing health care with alternative perspectives so it can better treat alcoholics.

This book is not a diagnostic or alcohol screening instrument and should not be relied upon when deciding to seek or not seek any treatment.

Nothing contained herein should be considered medical, psychological, psychiatric, or other professional advice. Nor is it a substitute for consulting with a trained professional. Please consult the appropriate professional for any related concerns.

The author and publisher disclaim any liability arising directly or indirectly from the use of this book.

—

THIS BOOK IS NOT CONNECTED WITH NOR
ENDORSES OR RECOMMENDS ANY ORGANIZATION.

Terms and Meanings

IN THE LAST several years, labels the medical establishment has assigned to people with alcohol problems have changed—inconsistently. The belief is a name change will soften the stigma—the term alcoholic is considered too harsh.

With all the words and meanings used by various sources when discussing alcoholism, we need to understand the terms used in this context.

The American Psychiatric Association (APA) now calls alcoholism mild, moderate, or severe Alcohol Use Disorder (AUD). Alcoholism is often synonymous only with physical dependence on alcohol (addiction).

The following terms have meanings contextually unique to this book and may or may not share the same meaning in another context. The definitions are the author's and are from other sources that the author considers reliable. Italicized words are terms defined elsewhere in this glossary.

—

Abstinence. Not drinking alcohol.

Abnormal Drinker. *See* **Active Alcoholic**.

Active Alcoholic, Wet Alcoholic, Practicing Alcoholic, Abnormal Drinker, and Problem Drinker. These terms are interchangeably used and mean an *alcoholic* who drinks.

Addiction. A chronic disease causing one to compulsively continue drinking despite adverse consequences. Addiction can be psychological, physical, or both. *See* **Psychologically addicted alcoholics** and **Physically addicted alcoholics**.

Affected. One who is affected by an alcoholic's drinking.

Afflicted. One who has the disease of alcoholism.

Alcohol Dependence. A medical condition characterized by the inability to control drinking due to a physical or emotional need for alcohol or both.

Alcohol Use Disorder (AUD). The American Psychiatric Association (DSM-5) uses this "more neutral term" as an alternative to alcoholism "because of its uncertain definition and its potentially negative connotation."

Alcoholic (Alcoholism). This term is broadly used and includes *any* person having *any* problems in their life related to drinking alcohol. In addition, it consists of all severity levels of *Alcohol Use Disorder (AUD)* described in the DSM-5. Many other associations and institutions define alcoholism as physical dependence on alcohol. The NIAAA defines alcohol use disorder (AUD) as a medical condition characterized by an impaired ability to stop or control alcohol use despite adverse social, occupational, or health consequences.

Alcoholic-Craving. An *unconscious* biological *progressive* brain dysfunction producing an uncontrollable, dynamic, *obsessive, compulsive,* inescapable, penetrable, persistent, and *insatiable need* to replace growing dysphoria with euphoria, usually by periodically or chronically drinking and continuing to drink alcohol or engaging in other obsessive-compulsive, self-destructive behavior. (*The author created this compound word to separate the meaning of the alcoholic's craving for alcohol as used in this book—the alcoholic-craving—and the common misunderstanding of the alcoholic's craving for alcohol.*)

Appetitive Behavior. The alcoholics' actions fueled by their focused motivation to drink, which is part of the *alcoholic-craving*.

Binge drinking. Occasionally drinking excessively. According to the CDC, four or more drinks for women and five or more drinks for men within two hours in one day.

Blackout. An alcohol-related blackout is the loss of some memory of events during intoxication caused by the brain's inability to record events. Excessive alcohol consumption causes this, and it doesn't necessarily indicate alcoholism.

Chronic Alcoholic (Daily Alcoholic). An *alcoholic* who drinks over two drinks (containing 1½ ounces of alcohol), two beers, or two five-ounce glasses of wine daily.

Comorbid (Comorbidity, Co-occurrence). An alcoholic who has a mental health disorder in addition to alcoholism. *See* **Dual Diagnosis.**

Compulsion. An uncontrollable need to drink against one's will.

Conscious. The thoughts, feelings, and memories of which the alcoholic is aware.

Dependence. *See* **Alcohol Dependence.**

Denial. A defense mechanism preventing certain information from entering the alcoholic's awareness. This information is obvious to others.

Detox, Detoxification. The body eliminating alcohol and managing the effects of withdrawal when a physically dependent alcoholic abruptly stops drinking. When medically managed, drugs are usually given to minimize withdrawal symptoms. Detoxing is lethal at times.

Dry Alcoholic (Dry Drunk). An alcoholic who doesn't drink but endures the alcoholic-craving regularly and displays behavior similar to when drinking. It can include glamorizing drinking, isolating, anxiety, discontentment, envying those who drink, feeling unfulfilled, sadness, and other negative feelings that often prompt a relapse.

Dual Diagnosis. An alcoholic who is diagnosed with *comorbidity*.

Dysfunctional. Not performing, behaving, or working normally, which includes a person or body part.

Dysphoria. A general feeling of discontentment and dissatisfaction with life and a cluster of other negative emotions.

Enabler (Enabling): A person who encourages the alcoholic's drinking with action or inaction that shields the alcoholic and the enabler from suffering consequences that might have persuaded the alcoholic to seek sobriety.

Episode (Episodic drinker). An event that happens occasionally, not regularly, such as with the *periodic alcoholic*.

Euphoria. A feeling of intense pleasure, happiness, contentment, excitement, and other positive emotions.

Functional Alcoholic. An individual who maintains a job, family, and social responsibilities while secretly suffering from alcoholism.

Grandiosity. Believing one is superior, unique, entitled to special treatment, and only understood by a few special people, none of which is based on personal capability or reality, and is often displayed by self-centeredness and condescension toward others.

Gratitude (Grateful). Feeling appreciation for a benefit received and wishing to return the benefit.

Heavy Drinker. According to the CDC, 4 or more drinks on any day or 7 or more per week for women, and 5 or more drinks on any day or 14 or more per week for men. It could be one who drinks as much or more than some *alcoholics* but is not an alcoholic.

High-Quality Sobriety. A *sober alcoholic* who prefers *sobriety* to drinking and does not endure the *alcoholic-craving*.

Insatiable. Impossible to satisfy.

Intervention. Any action that attempts to interrupt the alcoholic's drinking.

Low-Quality Sobriety. A *sober alcoholic* who prefers drinking to *sobriety* and endures the *alcoholic-craving*.

Newly Sober Alcoholic. An alcoholic who has been *abstinent* for more than 24 hours but less than one year.

Obsessive. Thinking that is intrusive, all-consuming, and unwanted causing anxiety or distress, such as the *alcoholic's* inability to think of anything other than drinking alcohol.

Periodic Alcoholic. An *alcoholic* who drinks occasionally. They may drink on weekends, once a month, or once a year, but once they start, they have little control over how much they drink.

Physically addicted alcoholics. Alcoholics who usually have an increased *tolerance* to alcohol and experience, in addition to *psychological withdrawal*, *physical withdrawal* symptoms ranging from mild to severe (fatal) when they stop drinking (e.g., tremors, headache, vomiting, sleeplessness, sweating, hallucinations, seizures, etc.).

Practicing Alcoholic. *See* **Active Alcoholic.**

Problem Drinker. *See* **Active Alcoholic.**

Progressive. A condition that gradually worsens with time, such as the progression of alcoholism.

Psychologically addicted alcoholics. Alcoholics who experience psychological, not physical withdrawal symptoms, from mild to severe when they stop drinking (e.g., anxiety, self-contempt, remorse, irritability, despair, sadness, fatigue, suicidal thoughts, etc.).

Psychosis, alcohol-induced. Psychosis caused by and present during alcohol intoxication. This psychosis may include hallucinations and delusions. It causes temporary difficulty in discerning reality.

Recovery. Treating the alcoholic to where the alcoholic no longer needs or wants alcohol to cope with life.

Relapse. An alcoholic who has abstained from drinking for a certain period returns to drinking.

Reverse Tolerance. Becoming more intoxicated when drinking less.

Signs. Signs of alcoholism are visible to others and don't need to be reported by the alcoholic to perceive (e.g., tolerance, tremors, unsteady gait, etc.) *See* **Symptoms**.

Sober Alcoholic. An alcoholic who has consumed no alcohol for over one year.

Sobriety. The state of being free from alcohol and other addictive substances.

Stereotypical Alcoholic. Drinks hard liquor daily out of a brown paper bag, is unemployed, homeless, unkempt, abandoned by friends and family, and could easily be a Skid Row resident.

Support Group (Peer or Mutual Support Group). A community of people who share their experiences and offer mutual support to other alcoholics who are either sober or seeking sobriety, such as Alcoholics Anonymous (AA).

Symptoms. Moods, feelings, and behaviors the alcoholic experiences and reports rather than observed by another (e.g., alcoholic-craving, alcohol obsession, etc.). *See* **Signs**.

Tolerance. The need to drink more to obtain the effect that drinking less once provided. *See* **Reverse Tolerance**.

Unconscious. It includes most operations of the mind that create our awareness and make us who we are. It also motivates us to satisfy instincts and compels alcoholics to drink outside the alcoholic's conscious awareness.

Wet Alcoholic. *See* **Active Alcoholic.**

Withdrawal. *See* **Physically addicted alcoholics and Psychologically addicted alcoholics.**

—

There is no significance for using gender-specific pronouns—they are used randomly. Gender-neutral singular pronouns are used where appropriate.

INSIDE AN ALCOHOLIC'S MIND
A True Story

CHAPTER 1

*You're probably an alcoholic if
when shopping for flooring, you evaluate
the pass-out comfort by placing your face on it.*

THE PEOPLE RETURN—the ones wearing flat black suits, black shirts, black ties, and short-brimmed, rounded domed, black hats. There are two—always. One is slender and tall, a little over six feet. The other is about a foot shorter but huskier. They're emotionless, speechless, faceless, and motionless. They're patiently waiting. They're not real, but they are real.

No one's around. He quietly and angrily mumbles, "Get out of here, now!" They do but return a few minutes later, a few feet away.

They don't walk but appear, disappear, and reappear in odd places. Now, he sees their figures embossed in the curtain as they stand still behind it. He considers flinging an object at their embossment, but the thought that anything he does could forever prove his condition stops him. He could jerk the curtain back, but they're fast; when and where would it end? His only choice is to put up with them . . . for now.

Taking a swig, he feels relief as the warmth comforts his thoughts, and the people disappear. Drinking keeps them away for a while. He knows they're the product of an alcohol-induced psychosis when they're gone. When they appear, he believes he's looking into another dimension. He never thinks about not drinking—it just doesn't dawn on him.

He often forgets to breathe, gasping for air. He sees the floor move closer and farther away every two or three steps. To be safe, he takes a knee.

He pauses and reflects at one of the rest stops from his living room chair to his bed. He makes it to bed. He can't imagine living his life *with* alcohol. He can't imagine living *without* alcohol. He hopes he doesn't awaken.

Morning arrives. Terror entombs him. Scheduled in an hour to attend a meeting where his signature is needed, he must stop his trembling hand. He knows a drink will help. Over time, trying to hide his shaky signature, he's simplified it.

HE GRABS A towel and two coffee cups, pours whiskey into one, and swigs it. A burning explosion erupts, shooting whiskey out his mouth and nose, stinging his eyes, nose, and ears.

He presses the towel against his face for a minute of darkness, allowing it to absorb the tears blurring his vision and the whiskey dripping from his nose and mouth. He takes a deep breath, slowly breathes out, and pauses. Telling himself it'll soon be okay, he quickly repeats it. It goes as he expected.

He has faith the third time will work. He slams it down and concentrates, gazing beyond the tile grout—it stays down. Success.

He ponders while drinking another. He glares at nothing and laments: It happened so quickly without warning. Months ago, he only drank occasionally and rarely before sunset. He had drunk this way for years.

Pouring another drink, he selects the flu from his fountain of excuses and reschedules the meeting while soothing his self-loathing with another drink.

His life is getting worse. He explores an array of solutions, which seem clustered in hopelessness. Still, he doesn't think about not drinking.

Months later, he's taken out from a local bar on a stretcher. The doctor mentions that several people seem worried about his drinking. He claims those appearing worried don't care and have ulterior motives. The doctor releases him within an hour.

TWO NIGHTS LATER, he's home, drinking nonstop. He doesn't feel drunk, so he continues drinking. Still not feeling intoxicated, he slightly staggers using his usual rest stops. He assumes his problem is blood pressure, convinced it has nothing to do with his drinking. He prefers blaming a medical condition instead of admitting a drinking problem.

Suddenly, paramedics make a surprise appearance carrying a stretcher. He refuses to go with them. As they become more persistent, he staggers to his bar and slurs that he'll go with them if they have a shot with him. They refuse—he knew they would.

He notices his two young sons, eyes wide open, watching this event etched in their minds forever. Then one son says, with tear-filled eyes, "Please go with them, Dad." He says, "Okay, let's go."

AN AMBULANCE AGAIN takes him to the emergency room. Worried the staff at the last hospital may suspect he has a drinking problem, he asks to be taken to a different hospital.

After he can't explain his symptoms (difficulty walking and breathing) yet insisting that he's only had a couple, testing begins.

A bewildered doctor quietly remarks, "I've never seen anything like this. Your blood-alcohol level is .43% . . . about six times the legal driving limit." He pauses. "Whenever I've seen a patient with these numbers, they were unconscious or dead—between .35% and .40% is fatal alcohol poisoning for most. You're beyond lethal limits but coherent and acting as sober as everyone else."

The doctor knows his tolerance reveals severe alcoholism.

The doctor is silent, looking away for a moment. Then he makes close eye contact and gently asks, "I understand you don't think you have a drinking problem?"

A long silence precedes his answer. He considers protesting and getting an independent blood test, but in a moment of clarity, he realizes it's over. With all the courage he could muster, he surrenders, catapults out of denial, and admits, "My tolerance is undeniable and speaks the truth. I've been struggling with alcohol for years."

Sounds of relief dissolve the discomfort. The doctor suggests admitting him for "observation."

"Observation or detoxification?" he asks the doctor.

The doctor raises his shoulders while awaiting a response.

"I'll agree if you excuse me for an hour."

After completing his shrug, the doctor asks, "Why?"

"I need one last drink, just one, and I promise I'll be back. You don't understand. Never having another drink for the rest of my life—"

"The rest of your life may not last an hour, especially if you drink another. And who said anything about the rest of your life? You can drink anytime you want."

"Now? How about now? One last drink. Is that asking too much? Just one last drink, forever?" His breathing is labored. He's never felt the *alcoholic-craving** so intensely. Feeling dizzy with his lips, fingertips, and toes tingling, he asks, "How about *less* than an hour?"

The doctor casually answers, "I doubt you'd survive an hour. You're dying right now. You're going into respiratory failure. And please stop removing the oxygen mask. You don't have much time. If you leave now, you've probably had your last drink... *forever*."

"You're right, I'm dying—I'm dying for a drink. Just one final drink. Just one!"

"You're dying because you've had at least *one* too many."

"If I can't even have *one* last drink, I'd rather die... Can we

---

*See Chapter 3, "The *Alcoholic-Craving*."

compromise?"

"Look, I promise we'll make you comfortable," the doctor says, raising his shoulders again.

He then thinks of his children. "Promise?"

While completing his last shrug, he smiles and says, "I promise."

"Thanks, doctor."

PEOPLE QUICKLY SURROUND HIM. They replace the oxygen mask. He smells rubbing alcohol and feels needle pricks. They attach items to his chest, which feels like they're sanding his skin. He hears a slow beeping, people whispering, mumbling, and slight metallic squealing sounds. Some whispers sound distant, and others sound clearer.

"Try to relax ...... it will soon be over ... relaxing ... come back ... we might be losing him ... talk to him ...... losing him ... inject him, now! ...Talk to him ... He's dying ...Dying? ... Dying? ... Louder! ... Hey, he can hear us; hearing is the last to go.... Can you hear me?... Did we lose him? ... Not Yet! ...Hey! Can you hear me? ... Open your eyes for me! ... Can you hear me? ... Yes! He partly opened one eye! ... You're going to be okay......I think we got it. He's improving. You're going to be all right...."

"**UH, SUE, HE'S** reaching for something."

"Hon, do you need something?" Sue, the nurse, asks.

"Yes, Sue, I do. I would like a Crown with a splash of water and two cubes, please. The doctor said I could have a drink anytime I wanted. I'm sure it's in my chart. And, not to be pushy, but if I can get that in the next few minutes, I'd appreciate it. And remember, I said *please*."

"Oh, I'm so sorry, but we're all out of that today. Is there something else I can get you?"

"Oh, well ... hold the splash and the ice cubes. I'll just take a straight shot of Crown."

"Well, that's the problem. We have the splash and the two ice cubes. It's the Crown we're out of. Sorry."

"You're kidding me! Can you quickly run to the liquor store? I'll wait —"

"Sorry again. The liquor stores closed hours ago."

"No problem. I'll just take my ticket when you have a minute and be on my way."

"You got it. Although we're a little busy now, could I get that to you within the next few days?"

"Days? I thought... overnight! Oh well... sure, that's fine. I guess I'm in no hurry. You wouldn't happen to have a cigarette, would you? Preferably non-menthol."

"No, I'm sorry, all out of those, too. Plus, cigarettes and oxygen don't mix well." Her voice becomes more upbeat, "But I'll soon have a patch for you! Meanwhile, can I get you anything else, an extra pillow... a blanket?"

"Oh, yeah! A patch, pillow, and a blanket sound like the perfect substitute for a drink and a cigarette."

"I think you'll be just fine," Sue says.

"Easy for you to say, but thanks. By the way, Sue, did I mention I think I'm falling in love with you?"

Sue smiles as she turns and sighs, "I bet you tell all the nurses that." He feels her hand grip his wrist as the ceiling tiles rush past.

THE DOCTOR ADMITS him. An intravenous cocktail of sedatives, vitamins, and hydration fluids eases his withdrawal. Still, he can't hold a jigger-sized paper cup of water without most splashing out. His parched lips prompt him to press the call button for someone to help him hold the cup. He's humiliated and frustrated.

It's all so surreal. He reflects. He's overdosing, experiencing the DTs he's heard about while wondering how this happened. He's not a skid-row, low-bottom drunk, but financially secure and high-functioning. He's well-groomed, wearing a suit most days to work, never had a DUI, never been to prison, never been homeless, and never had a blackout. He remembers every detail while in the ER. What went wrong so quickly?

He then recalls years ago when an alcoholic, claiming he'd been sober over 30 years, mumbled: "Keep drinking... it'll get worse... a lot worse, take you to places you'd never imagine—take you to a nightmare."

THOUSANDS OF LITTLE bugs, itchy little bugs, crawl on him. They're so small he can't see them. While scratching and pushing them away, they roam to unreachable places and burrow into his skin.

They chew, claw through his blood vessels, and drift in his bloodstream while touring his body. He tries everything to stop the deep and endless itching. Although he knows it's not real, he panics. They must be removed. His request for a blood transfusion and then desperate pleas for partial 'bloodletting' are refused.

The people return, standing behind the privacy curtain with less detail than usual. They suddenly disappear, only to reappear moments later. They're silent, as always. They sit on the couch. He's never seen them sit before, and they seem casual. But for the first time, they look like they're wasting their time—they almost seem bored. They become shadows.

ON THE SECOND day, the invisible bugs disappear. The people and the alcoholic-craving disappear. He closes his eyes and sleeps peacefully.

ON THE THIRD day, he awakens to the smell of latex and a needle prick.

"I'm sorry to wake you like this, but I'm almost done," claims the phlebotomist.

"Thanks," he says, watching the second glass tube turn deep red. "Today's my birthday."

"Well, happy birthday."

"Thanks. It's my mother's birthday, too. I love telling people that."

"Well, that's unusual."

"When I was a little boy, my friend had a birthday party, and I wished his mom "Happy Birthday." I guess I thought every boy had the same birthdate as his moms. That's when I learned how special it was—one out of 365. I don't know why I'm telling you this, but—"

"No, I love hearing happy stories."

"You know what else? My mom's also in the hospital. She received a kidney transplant yesterday."

"You're kidding? Well, happy birthday to both of you. But I'm sorry you're hospitalized on your birthdays."

"Don't be. These are the best birthday gifts we could ever dream of getting. She's been on the waiting list for a couple of years. Not everyone on the list gets the gift of life in time. And I read that only one out of every 20 alcoholics will ever receive the gift of sobriety. And to think, the chances of us receiving these gifts on our birthday is one out of . . . who knows. My dad would've. He was a statistician and taught a course he called 'sadistics,' but anyway—"

"Well, I'm so happy for you. You've brightened my day."

"And you have mine. By the way, you wouldn't happen to know a nurse named Sue, would you?"

AFTER THREE DAYS without a drink, his alcohol level is 0.14%. The doctor warns him not to drive because his alcohol level is twice the legal limit. Still, he's released.

He underwent an event he seldom mentions other than to say he sensed a soothing Presence.

He's amazed at how good he feels. He's not felt this good in years. He feels the euphoria that elusively escaped him when drinking. A feeling of well-being and contentment consumes him. Only now does he realize how sick he was. His vision has changed. He has changed.

THAT DAY WAS over 19 years ago. The people have never returned. Since that day, he hasn't had, needed, or wanted a drink—he drank the value out of drinking. He wouldn't drink if he could and feels neutral about alcohol. He has lived a life many see as successful. And his mother is well, too.

—

AUTHOR'S NOTE: Although I sank to a bottom that many alcoholics never experience, little about this is unique. A doctor who cared enough to spend a few extra minutes with me helped dissolve my denial. This allowed me to admit and accept my alcoholism, freeing me from my alcoholic-craving. By surrendering, I was able to emerge victoriously. I am only one among millions who have escaped from the darkness of denial.

A Description of the Alcoholic

CHAPTER 2

*You're probably an alcoholic if, after
drinking a few, you're drawn to a mirror,
suddenly convinced you're looking hotter by the
minute and alcohol helps you see the world more clearly.*

—

MILLIONS AND MILLIONS wonder if they're alcoholics. They hear this inescapable, repetitive, and relentless whisper: "You have a drinking problem." Trying to escape this, they focus on their view of the alcoholic: homeless, unemployed, unbathed, unshaved, and unkempt, in torn and tattered clothes, estranged from family and friends, swigging from a bottle wrapped with a brown paper sack, until passing out on skid row. The problem with this focus is that only nine percent of alcoholics fall into this stereotypical class.[1]

Those in denial ignore the reality that many more alcoholics are highly functioning, financially secure, have above-average incomes, and are successful in their careers and most other areas of their lives. Many own high-end cars and houses and appear well-groomed. Their family and friends love, respect, and admire them. They never drink in the morning and rarely alone. Many go days, weeks, or months without a drink or even the thought of one.

As alcoholism develops, the more apparent it becomes to even the casual observer. But for the alcoholic, denial obscures the obvious. Since problem drinkers must self-diagnose their problem before admitting and accepting it, this denial prevents most from seeking help.

If alcoholics no longer see any value in drinking—when consequences exceed benefits—the light will shine on the darkness of their denial, illuminating the path to freedom, which many will walk and, unfortunately, many will not.

Millions more, sober for years, question if they're really alcoholics. This lingering doubt is a significant symptom of alcoholism, threatening their sobriety.

They hear a different voice, quiet, patient, and taunting: "You're not an alcoholic. Have a drink and see for yourself." This voice is the *doubting* sober alcoholic's constant companion.

This voice of denial focuses on the differences between themselves and other sober alcoholics who hit a lower or different bottom. They think, "I didn't do *that* when I drank; maybe I'm not an alcoholic." They avoid comparisons to alcoholics who drank or felt the same as they did.

Observably, the more one who is sober believes they're an alcoholic, the more likely they will remain sober and enjoy sobriety.

A Comparison

AN EXCELLENT WAY to describe the alcoholic is by comparison to the nonalcoholic. The primary distinction is not how much or how often one drinks but how alcohol affects them and whether they can predict, with reasonable certainty, how much they will drink *every* time they start.

Examples of the Nonalcoholic

People without a drinking problem don't wonder whether they have a drinking problem. They don't compare their drinking to others—why would they? They don't need any excuse to drink. Average drinkers don't avoid drinking to prove they can. They've never thought or said, "I never have a problem with alcohol until I start drinking."

They don't conceal their drinking—they have nothing to hide. Nor do they think, "No one knows how much I *really* drink." They don't lie about the number of drinks they've had—they're rarely, if ever, asked. Nor do they separate liquor bottles in the trash to prevent the clatter from disclosing the truth. Their drinking isn't a secret. They don't alternate liquor stores, so clerks don't think they have a drinking problem, nor do they carry a flask—why would they? They don't try convincing others that they don't have a drinking problem.

They don't struggle to control their drinking. A drink or two satisfies; it doesn't appetize. After a couple, when feeling good, they don't drink more to feel better and rarely drink more than they intend. The more they drink, the more they feel it, so the less they want it.

They don't miss significant events because of drinking. They drink moderately and responsibly without drinking too much. When they say, "I'll have one more," they only have and want *one* more. When presented with a tray of champagne at a formal event, they only take one—not out of politeness, but because they only want one. Nor do they keep track of their drinking—drinking one or two doesn't require tracking.

Social drinkers have no problem leaving an unfinished drink behind. They don't drink rather than eat. At those rare times when they hear "last call," they don't panic.

They don't try to control their drinking; it's not out of control. Average drinkers don't make a New Year's resolution about drinking—without a problem, they don't need a solution. They don't say, "I can stop drinking anytime I want!" Nothing prompts an explanation. They don't buy alcohol rather than pay their bills.

Rarely do they suffer demoralizing consequences from drinking. They don't end nights with a foot on the floor trying to stop the room from spinning. They don't google "avoiding hangovers." When they say, "Be back in a minute," they don't return hours later, remorsefully drunk.

Regular drinkers don't capture a stranger's attention by holding them hostage while slurring ramblings about nothing, shaking hands every fifth word spoken, treating their slurred words with spit-mists because they're too drunk to swallow, and forbidding any interruption as they repeat themselves over ... and over ... and over.

They haven't been charged with a second or third DUI. If they had *one*, it was a deterrent. Seldom, if ever, do they awaken in a panic, reviewing texts sent the night before, or wake next to a stranger.

Normal drinkers aren't obsessed with alcohol. They seldom think about it. When deciding whether to attend an event, they don't wonder or ask if there will be drinking—they don't care. They rarely have a cap or other clothing imprinted with a distillery or brewery logo. If they prepare a budget, they don't decrease food and other essential expenses to allocate more for alcohol.

Regular drinkers have never endured the *alcoholic-craving*.* They may want a drink but never need one. They don't order the next one before finishing the one they're drinking to prevent an anxious moment should they have to wait.

They don't drink to improve their self-image. They drink to boost, not escape, their feelings. They won't drink if they don't like the taste. They don't feel self-loathing or hopelessly doomed when sober, counting the hours or minutes until they can drink.

They don't resent those interfering with their drinking—no one interferes. No one asks, "Haven't you had enough?" People aren't concerned about their drinking. When they switch to a nonalcoholic drink, they do so because they want to, not because anyone intervened.

Bartenders don't ask them, "Are you sure you need another one?" nor cut them off. Drinking doesn't cause problems

---

*The term *alcoholic-craving* means something different than a general craving for alcohol. Chapter 3, "The Alcoholic-Craving," discusses this in detail.

in their lives. Their boss, co-workers, family, and friends never mention their drinking.

Nonalcoholics don't boast that they can drink anyone under the table. They don't think having a higher tolerance—resulting from a brain and liver dysfunction—is anything to brag about. Over time, they don't have to drink more to produce the same effect. Typical drinkers don't survive blood/alcohol concentrations beyond standard lethal levels. They're not gradually drinking earlier each day. Nor do they try to recapture the good times when drinking.

They don't experience periods of grandiosity while drinking where they must boastfully talk about their accomplishments, skills, and talents. Drinking doesn't improve their reflection in the mirror, and they don't think they're smarter after a drink.

Social drinkers enjoy drinking with friends and don't seek praise when not drinking. They don't fantasize about drinking normally someday. They have close friends who don't drink.

Typical drinkers don't get calls from their local bar when they haven't been in for a few days.

Finally, normal drinkers don't understand abnormal drinkers.

Examples of the Alcoholic

On the other hand, alcoholics *have* wondered if they have a drinking problem. When alcoholics review their drinking, they reflexively and defensively think about those who drink more, surrounding themselves with others who drink at least as much as they do. Periodic alcoholics often say, "I'm not an alcoholic; I don't have to drink every day. It's just that I don't want to stop once I start—that's all!"

The alcoholic motto is, "If one is good, more is better." They don't *easily* leave an unfinished drink behind. After a 'couple,' they rarely say "no" to *one* more but say, "I'll have just one more, and I mean it this time!" and they do mean it every time they repeatedly say it. Alcoholics often feel a penetrating *need* for "just one more"—a need that defeats all reason. Knowing this, they insist it will be different each time they drink.

They become irritated and defensive when anyone asks how many drinks they've had. Rarely do they admit to drinking more than a couple. When they say, "I only had a *couple,*" it means from three to infinity. In the unlikely event they only had two, they will say two, not "a couple."

Their drink containers often disguise the contents. As time passes, they usually drink alone to hide their drinking to avoid arousing concern and confrontation.

Before the first drink, alcoholics may feel like hopeless failures, repulsed by their mirrored reflection. But after a few, they look in every mirror they can find with enormous self-admiration.

Alcoholics feel special and insist that everyone treats them that way. They hope people notice a drink awaits them when they frequent their neighborhood bar. They feel special when the liquor store clerk addresses them by name, although they may alternate liquor stores so clerks don't think they have a problem.

Alcoholics believe they do most things better when drinking. After a few, they can't say, "I don't know." After a few more, their minds release vast amounts of knowledge, and they feel compelled to share this flood of knowledge enthusiastically and generously with everyone. When 'everyone' fades away, they're convinced their genius intimidated those escaping.

They can't imagine living the rest of their life with or without alcohol. They need a drink more than they want one. Although they appear to enjoy the taste of alcohol, they don't. They rarely drink pretty and colorful drinks. They know where to find every liquor store within five miles.

They feel compelled to drink during and after any argument. They will create or recall resentments, enabling them to drink with less guilt. When deciding whether to drink, all memories of drinking's demoralizing consequences dissolve. They feel less overwhelmed when drinking.

They spend much of their time thinking about drinking, recovering from drinking, coping with the consequences of drinking, and drinking.

They're easy to shop for—the only gifts they want are their favorite bottles or drinking paraphernalia.

Alcoholics often apologize for their drinking-related behavior, promising it won't happen again and repeating the same apologies and promises every time it happens again.

It wouldn't be unlikely for an alcoholic attending a court-ordered alcohol assessment to drink a few to calm their nerves and then convince the evaluator they don't have a drinking problem.

They believe the people who care about them harass them unreasonably about their drinking. They can't see that those who care have no selfish agenda. Still, they resist getting help, fearing harm to their career, social, and family life if their problem becomes known.

Finally, problem drinkers don't understand normal drinkers.

It is unlikely and unnecessary that anyone relates to all the above when deciding if one has a drinking problem—*relating with just a few indicates a problem.*

THE DESCRIPTION OF AN ALCOHOLIC*

THE FOLLOWING DESCRIBES the alcoholic moving through the stages of alcoholism. Although the term alcoholic includes those who no longer drink, these pages describe the *drinking* alcoholic unless noted.

Most alcoholics have *not* experienced everything in this

---

*This description of the alcoholic is based on years of extensive research, including personal observation, anecdotal evidence, contemplation, interviews, and listening to thousands of sober alcoholics disclose their past drinking, discuss the process of seeking sobriety, and reveal how they remain sober.

chapter. If they have, they already know they have a drinking problem. Those who can identify with *anything* in this description probably have a drinking problem.

The following is my description of the alcoholic referenced in this book.

> One who is *obsessed* with the effects of alcohol and feels *compelled* to drink—either *occasionally* or daily. Trailing the first drink is *often* an automatic, *uncontrollable*, pervasive, insatiable, and compelling *need* to drink more as memories of demoralizing conduct and consequences fade, usually followed by remorse ("Why did I drink so much?"). Complicating this is a belief that drinking is *controllable* and a rigid *denial* of any alcohol-related *obsession* and *compulsion* ("I don't need to drink. I could quit if I want. I just don't want to!").

Consumption, frequency, and dependency vary among alcoholics. Some drink daily, and others drink occasionally—less than nonalcoholics. They may go days, weeks, or months without a drink or even craving one—the alcoholic-craving doesn't threaten these periods of abstinence. Yet they're no less alcoholic than chronic alcoholics who drink every day. Their drinking often results in consequences more severe than daily drinkers.[2] Those who drink occasionally are periodic, episodic, or binge drinkers. (See Chapter 6, "The Periodic Alcoholic.")

Starting with the first drink, normal drinkers tolerate alcohol differently than abnormal drinkers. Any more than a couple causes nonalcoholics discomfort, prompting them to stop, whereas the more alcoholics drink, the better they feel, and the better they feel, the better they need to feel. Often, drinking continues until their blood-alcohol concentration (BAC) reaches high levels (e.g., "She drinks until she passes out!").

Alcoholism is Progressive

NOT ONLY DOES drinking intensify, but so do the other symptoms of alcoholism. (Chapter 5, "The Darkness and Lightness of Denial," discusses the progression of *denial*.)

Few alcoholics have had all the following symptoms—two or three are enough for concern. Alcoholism doesn't progress the same for every alcoholic. The line separating each stage is not as observable as outlined here. Alcoholics don't cross a visible threshold when progressing to the next stage of their disease.

Pre-alcoholics

Although the terms "pre-alcoholic" and "pre-alcoholism" are not widely accepted medical terms, I use them for clarity and conciseness to describe those with a high risk of developing alcoholism. Their environment, genetic predisposition, and behavior suggest that developing alcoholism is probable but not inevitable.

The Pre-alcoholic Symptoms

- Although they can stop if they must or should, they have an urge to continue drinking after the first one.
- Their drinking is mildly abnormal.
- They spend more time thinking about drinking than normal drinkers, although it's not yet obsessive.
- Their symptoms are still mild and few, yet they're growing. Not all the criteria indicating alcoholism are present, and a diagnostic exam would not confirm alcoholism or alcohol use disorder (AUD).
- They find more reasons to drink than normal drinkers but don't struggle with unpleasant feelings when abstaining.

The Early Stage

In the beginning, drinking doesn't *seem* alcoholic. There

appears to be no cause for concern. Although it's challenging to identify, many signs of early alcoholism are present, and if one knew the subtle signs to look for, the alcoholic's behavior would stand out. Again, not all alcoholics show all these signs.

The Early-Stage Symptoms

- Drinking makes them feel better, have higher self-worth and self-confidence, and freely express their joy.
- After a couple of drinks, they often choose to drink more but can control their drinking and rarely appear drunk.
- They're slowly distancing themselves from those who don't drink or drink less than they do.
- They're starting to lose interest in hobbies, spending less time with friends and family, and making more time to drink.
- When drinking, they speak louder and more authoritatively about everything, even if they don't know what they're talking about.
- They may begin to have rapid mood changes.
- They affectionately refer to alcohol by nicknames such as "stiff-one, medicine, suds, sauce, liquid courage, etc."
- Their obsession with alcohol is slowly intensifying.
- They may have blackouts.

The Middle Stage

At this stage, alcoholics know they have a drinking problem, but most others don't. Still, they are unaware of its severity and contend that any comment about their drinking is an overreaction. They are more obsessed with drinking, and their compulsion to drink has increased, as well as their remorse after drinking. Alcohol now controls them more than they control it.

The Middle-Stage Symptoms

- Their new friends drink the same or more than they do.
- They're drinking more and rarely turn down a chance to drink.
- They guzzle their first couple of drinks.
- They ask if future events will include drinking.
- They talk more about drinking.
- They often "pre-drink" before going to a bar or a party.
- Their tolerance is noticeably higher—drinking more but becoming less drunk.
- They drink stronger drinks, often asking, "Could you please put some in it this time?"
- They drink to cope with life, claiming, "I just need a couple to unwind."
- Their relationships are adapting to their drinking.
- They're using less ice and only a splash of water as a mixer.
- They chronically fear running out of alcohol.
- Their drunk personality is opposite their sober one, often seen as a different person when drunk.
- They're more aggressive and say what they think—sometimes making provocative, hurtful, or degrading comments.
- They resist leaving an unfinished drink behind.
- They often want "one more" and are relentless and annoying when coaxing others to drink, such as "Come on, let's just have one more—I mean it this time—one more, and we'll call it quits."
- They are now drinking to soothe their anxiety and discomfort when not drinking. (See Chapter 3, "The Alcoholic-Craving.")
- They find less enjoyment in drinking and often drink

when they don't want to.
- They are gradually and almost unnoticeably drinking earlier in the day (7:00 pm now compared to 7:15 pm six months ago and 7:30 pm a year ago).
- They're rationalizing more and blaming others for everything, including their drinking.
- They're nursing resentments, fueling their justification to drink and diluting any guilt or remorse that would dampen their enjoyment of "a couple."
- They're more argumentative with those closest to them.
- Their blackouts may increase in duration and frequency.
- They continue drinking even though it's obviously causing problems.
- They function even when they drink excessively.
- When they don't drink, they're in a bad mood, feeling depressed, tired, irritable, and discontented.
- They know they must quit someday and may express this by claiming, "Soon, I'm going to slow down my drinking."
- They often drink at the worst times.

The Final Stage

This stage most resembles the stereotypical alcoholic. Their chances of seeking recovery are slim. If they are one of the fortunate few who become sober, their fear of returning to the misery they endured increases their chances of staying sober. Many, now sober and content in recovery, were once considered just as hopeless.

The Final-Stage Symptoms

- They're not sleeping well.
- They're drinking rather than eating.

- They're likely unemployed or close to it.
- They drink to delay the worsening feelings of the alcoholic-craving and withdrawal, which are intensifying.
- They're speaking less clearly, even when not drinking.
- They're miserable when not drinking and only a little less miserable when drinking. During those rare times they don't drink, they feel ill with headaches, shaking, sweating, nausea, and vomiting.
- They're often tired, nervous, and tense.
- It's obvious to everyone that they're alcoholics.
- Their arrest history may include public drunk, DUI, or other alcohol-related offenses.
- They resist being where alcohol isn't served.
- Their need to drink is overpowering.
- Their physical appearance reflects that their hygiene has become less important.
- They may appear malnourished.
- They can't hold a cup of coffee without half of it shaking out, so they usually prefer isolation and drinking alone.
- They drink to keep from feeling sick.
- Drinking no longer makes them feel better, so they drink and appear drunk more often.
- They're convinced they can never quit drinking.
- They've lost all self-respect, feel hopeless, and are likely suicidal.

Hey, I've Lost My Euphoria, Has Anyone Seen It?

THE EUPHORIA THAT alcoholics experience in the early drinking days is a sensation they will increasingly obsess about and feel compelled to revisit often—often for life. But they can no longer find it. Instead, they will sacrifice everything to chase it, including marriages, children, parents, friends, employment—and life.

As alcoholism progresses, this euphoria will become more elusive, gradually lessening until it's nonexistent. Even worse, alcoholics may now feel dysphoric when drinking. Despite this, they run in an endless circle, compulsively chasing the tail of euphoria for life, never catching it. It's gone forever. Many will introduce drugs into their chase—an often fatal introduction.

ALCOHOL DEPENDENCY: PSYCHOLOGICAL AND PHYSICAL

ALL ALCOHOLICS ARE psychologically dependent. About half are both psychologically *and* physically dependent (addicted).[3] If physically dependent, withdrawal symptoms will range from minor to fatal (delirium tremens[*] or DTs). In addition, some will need medical stabilization when they abruptly stop drinking to prevent a deadly withdrawal.

Alcohol withdrawal is dangerous.[4] Between 15% and 40% of alcoholics who develop DTs will die if untreated.[5] And even with treatment, 1-4% will die.[6] Surprisingly, drinking large amounts of alcohol for only one month is enough to trigger DTs during withdrawal.[7]

Another condition that can occur when withdrawing is delusional parasitosis,[8] which convinces the detoxing person that parasitic insects have infested them. They feel insects crawling on and burrowing under their skin.

In the same way, alcoholics who aren't physically dependent will still experience obsession, compulsion, craving, remorse, and hopelessness. Their suffering is no less devastating, and abstinence will cause the alcoholic-craving—a miserable feeling for any alcoholic withdrawing. (See Chapter 3, "The Alcoholic-Craving.")

---

[*]Delirium tremens (DTs) is characterized by confusion, shaking, tachycardia (an abnormally rapid heart rate), sweating, shivering, and hallucinations. In severe cases, high fever and seizures can occur, resulting in death.

Remorse → Rationalization → Resentment

THE INFINITE CYCLE of feeling remorse, then rationalizing, and then resenting is an endless rotation of thoughts and feelings alcoholics endure and use as a defense mechanism to remain in denial so they can continue drinking.

Remorse

Alcoholics prefer to express remorse, not feel it. Drinking overrides everything else, so the liquor store has become more important than the grocery store.

Drinking alcoholics may miss work, family gatherings, the birth of their children, family events, weddings, dinner engagements, and funerals. They may neglect children's school events, miss work deadlines, and lose interest in hobbies. Even plans to visit an ill relative may not be timely realized.

This behavior causes feelings that exceed mere regret. The guilt, self-loathing, anxiety, fear, and remorse suffered when missing a best friend's funeral or the first family reunion in 10 years dissolve slowly.

Most wouldn't ever miss events like these, but that's not how the alcoholic mind works. The more important the event, the more anxiety. The more anxiety, the stronger the alcoholic-craving, which explains why alcoholics often drink at the "worst" times—the most challenging times for alcoholics to cope. Although their initial intent is to relax a bit by drinking a "couple" before attending, drinking usually continues.

The alcohol obsession reveals itself and occurs in several ways. Alcoholism is time-consuming. For instance, alcoholics spend increasingly more time managing their liquor inventory, drinking, and recovering from drinking. Moreover, managing the consequences of drinking becomes even more time-consuming and triggers more remorse. These consequences include hangovers, injuries, damaged property, strained relationships, work absences, legal problems, and marital issues.

The time required to create excuses becomes substantial.

The drinker now regrets their actions, which caused debris to pile up quickly, becoming unmanageably time-consuming. Although they hide much of it well, they feel more remorseful and overwhelmed simply trying to cope.

As time slips away and after missing the event, their remorse intensifies, as does their need to drink.

Alcoholics use clever ways to deal with penetrating remorse, including creating excuses to justify their absence, which are usually never offered to anyone. If only repeated to themselves until believed, a good excuse will somewhat dilute the remorseful feelings triggered by not attending. So, reasons not to attend dominate, and rationalizations erupt.

Rationalization is the alcoholic's most favored method of manipulating remorse.

Rationalization

Rationalizing allows us to create 'explanations' for what we do. These excuses make sense on the surface, but, in reality, they obscure the truth. It's an effective way of lying to ourselves when we must believe our lies.

One technique that works well when rationalizing is to deflect blame rather than accept it. This blame could be real or imagined, justified or unjustified. It doesn't matter; skillful rationalization goes a long way.

Excuses, excuses, and more excuses. Alcoholics spend more time creating new and convincing excuses for missing these events to relieve agonizing guilt. They don't see these "explanations" as deception, further isolating them. But they view them as tools that allow them to function.

They must manage their pile of excuses with care. Repeating the same explanations to the same person loses effectiveness, so they must sprinkle them about with precision.

A flat tire, keys lost or locked in the car, the flu, and food poisoning are believable. But justifying three missed appointments with the same person within a month, claiming a flat tire each time, arouses doubt, distrust, and suspicion.

Trying to lessen this damage by claiming coincidence is as persuasive as a statistician pontificating about the *paradox of probability theory*. It doesn't help in the slightest and tends to worsen things.

Alcoholics don't sense the best times to be silent. Recalling the excuses made to each person becomes unmanageable, and those close to the alcoholic suspect a problem ... of some sort.

Alcoholics fear this suspicion as a potential threat to their armor of deception, causing them to panic. They're overwhelmed, so they pour one more drink to cope.

Alcoholism fuels false excuses. For a time, they allow the dysfunctional alcoholic to function in a world that detests alcoholic behavior. Without excuses, the consequences of drinking would erupt earlier, threatening the alcoholic with sobriety. Alcoholics habitually offer false excuses, even when the truth would work better. An honest explanation might be:

> Hey, boss, me ... again. Sorry I missed our meeting. I've been dealing with some personal problems lately, and my drinking hasn't helped. I know I need some help. It's not fair to you. I appreciate your patience. Can we reset this meeting? Just let me know when. How does that sound?

Most, alcoholic or not, will exclaim, "No, they couldn't say that!" And why? Isn't a false excuse, even if disbelieved, more acceptable than admitting alcoholism?

These false excuses result from mistakes and misfortune. No one is at fault. We tolerate reasons, even if fictional, caused by blameless, unintentional acts more than truthful excuses stemming from blameful and intentional conduct. Still, most believe admitting drunkenness is confessing the *voluntary* act of drinking and is deliberate and blameful. This belief that alcoholics drink of their own free will fuels the alcoholic stigma. (See Chapter 4, "The Alcoholic Stigma.")

Another rationalization technique used by alcoholics is

rulemaking. Alcoholics often make a rule or two to convince themselves, as well as others, that they're not alcoholics. A few common ones are:

- I only drink on weekends.
- I never drink before sunset.
- I never drink alone or at home.
- I never drink doubles or shots.
- I never keep alcohol in my house.
- I never drink more than two drinks an hour.
- I never drink before 5 pm or after 11 pm on weekdays.
- I never miss work because of drinking.
- I never drink on the job.
- I never mix my drinks with water, but I use mixers.
- I never drink before dinner.
- I never drive when drinking.
- I never drink on Monday or Tuesday.
- I never drink two days in a row.
- I never drink the hard stuff. I only drink beer or wine to help me fall asleep.

These self-imposed rules provide drinkers with a fantasy baseline reinforcing their denial. If they don't violate their chosen rule, they're not alcoholics. But this means nothing because these rules don't apply to alcoholic symptoms, yet alcoholics embrace their rule as if it does mean something.

As alcoholism progresses, they will rationalize to justify exceptions to the rule. For example, "My friend is in town, so I'll drink this time even though it's *two days in a row,*" or "I decided it's more responsible and safer *to drink at home,*" or "I heard mixing with water hydrates, is healthier, and reduces hangovers, so I now *mix my drinks with water.*" In time, alcoholics rationalize away all their rules, convinced they are too restrictive.

Alcoholics are masterful at selecting feelings that best suit them. For example, alcoholics often transform remorse into resentment, which feels better.

Resentment

Seasoned alcoholics can nurse resentments for a lifetime. And they've done it for so long with fine-honed skills that they're unaware it's occurring.

A well-nurtured resentment will fuel the alcoholic's drinking like nothing else. Resentment allows alcoholics to feel entitled. They first feel entitled to have *one* drink. Next, their resentment intensifies, sparking their right to have "*one more.*" Then, they ignore all disturbing thoughts of past demoralizing consequences—the consequences experienced almost every time they drink. Finally, they revive the fading resentment, allowing them to continue drinking guilt-free, which is more satisfying than remorseful drinking.

To bolster their resentment, they express contempt for the innocent person they blame, to anyone who will listen, and even those who won't. Repeatedly telling their fictional story to their captive listener inflates their resentment, making it more useful.

On awakening, resentments quickly soften their emerging guilt. And these resentments immediately ease the relentless truth oozing from their conscience.

Although alcoholics may escape their subtle spiraling whenever they choose, it's more challenging the closer they get to the end. Most never try. Although millions have been set free, those convinced of their uniqueness assume they're the exception. Sadly, the only relief they can imagine is a soothing drink that is no longer, and will never be, as soothing as it once was.

CHANGES IN PERSONALITY, BEHAVIOR, AND THINKING

EVERYTHING ABOUT ALCOHOLICS progressively changes the longer and more they drink. Some alcoholics have traits that progress quicker or slower than others, but all progress in time.

Personality Changes

After a couple of drinks, the nonalcoholic has a personality enhancement. When the alcoholic drinks, a different personality often emerges. Except for the typical symptoms of a staggering gait, incoordination, the odor of alcohol, bloodshot eyes, slurred speech, and others, not every alcoholic acts the same when drunk—they may be happy, sad, angry, mean, obnoxious, crazy, funny, or loving.

It's common for an alcoholic to display many moods while drinking—happy then sad, friendly then mean, serious then funny. This is called *Labile Mood,* which also includes abnormal emotional reactions. These mood swings can happen within minutes or seconds. The intensity and speed of this moodiness usually parallel their intoxication level.

The personalities of drunk alcoholics often contrast starkly with their sober ones. It's as if they're different people.

Engaging In Risky Behavior

Not all alcoholics face the following, but most experience the associated feelings.

While drinking, as inhibitions fade and impulsivities surface, many alcoholics experience courageous freedom and engage in risky behavior.

For example, they're convinced they can do most things better when drinking—including driving or operating hazardous machinery. They may feel the need for speed. Thoughts of their young, involuntary passengers or innocent bystanders elude them.[9]

Or, it may seem like the perfect time to dive off that cliff they've been talking about doing for months. Finally, they dare to do it after drinking enough 'liquid courage.' As they hike to the cliff, they don't think about those who dove before them, resulting in quadriplegia or death.

Their decision to drive to the bar or liquor store outweighs the potential harm to their passengers, themselves, and others or the risk of a DUI arrest.

Bars oust them because they're speaking everything they're thinking, provoking conflict.

Perhaps she's feeling flirtatious, compelled to display her unseen and unappreciated talents at the neighborhood bar. A chair, then a tabletop, becomes her stage. Attempts to curb her behavior and slow down her drinking fail. The audience's increasingly growing admiration fuels her raging fire. She's finally free to be her 'true self.'

Maybe she explores an admirer's invitation. Thoughts of her husband and children vanish. A risky meeting follows, threatening irreparable damage to her, her loved ones, and her marriage.

The temporary feelings during a drunk moment can result in permanent consequences. Many have dodged this type of behavior. Still, statistically, the longer one drinks, the more likely such events will occur.

Tolerance and Craving

With continued drinking, tolerance of alcohol and the alcoholic-craving increase. Alcoholics must drink increasingly more to reach the euphoric place of their obsession. After succumbing to the compulsion for "just one more," they soon realize that "just one more" doesn't provide the relief they expect as it once did. While gazing into a glass with only melting ice, the insatiable silent *craving* for "just one more" intensifies.

The feelings of despair, fear, and self-loathing become resentments toward anyone hindering their drinking.

What once was a quick couple after work is now a night of drinking. They're in disbelief when hearing "last call." Although pushed away, dinner remains on the table as a morning reminder. Due to their increased craving, tolerance, and despair, their humiliation and self-loathing rise with the morning sun.

Attempts to Control Drinking

Alcoholics obsess about controlling their drinking and try many ways of curbing their insatiable appetite to drink more. This includes eating before drinking, switching to beer or wine, pacing drinks with a companion, drinking water between drinks, or quitting. These all fail.

Drinking Continues Despite Consequences

If married, divorce is likely looming, although the alcoholic hasn't a clue. Strained relationships with friends and family are growing. Children are distancing. Longtime friends are slower to reply. So, alcoholics form new 'friendships' with people who understand and drink as much, if not more.

Problems at work are reaching a boil because no one appreciates their skills and talents. If they're students, their performance is sinking, and fear of academic probation haunts them. Legal issues may be simmering. Health symptoms nag for attention as the problem drinker shoos them away with a few drinks.

Insisting that drinking has caused none of this, they decide drinking is the solution. They rationalize and convince themselves that anyone would drink the same if enduring their misfortune. They never consider abstinence but believe drinking keeps them saner and more able to cope. While they continue drinking, their lives crumble, and the crumbs slowly entomb them.

OTHERS EXPRESS CONCERN: CONCEALMENT AND ISOLATION

ALCOHOLICS ARE OFTEN offended by the concerns expressed by others, believing them to be misguided. So, they become defensive and ignore these concerns as a nuisance. If they considered these concerns that they drink alcoholically, they would have to ponder abstinence—a terrorizing ponderation.

Denial creates thinking that distorts logic. They don't see that they likely have a problem if others see one. They don't ask, "What motive could anyone have to express their concern other than concern?"

Alcoholics Must Conceal Drinking

As more people worry about their drinking, they feel the need to hide it and hopefully prevent those who are worried from planning an intervention. As alcoholism progresses, they will even hide their drinking from those unconcerned, such as sanitary workers, liquor store clerks, neighbors, and postal workers.

The need to hide their alcoholic behavior involves doing anything to disguise the truth, which includes paying cash at alternating liquor stores, acting sober, secretly drinking, trying to mask the smell of alcohol, minimizing the consequences of drinking, and hiding everything about their drinking. (See Chapter 5, "The Darkness and Lightness of Denial," for more detailed information on concealment.)

Denial prevents alcoholics from realizing others know more about their drinking problem than they thought.

Isolation

Alcoholics may think their isolation prevents others from discovering the truth, but it doesn't take much time with a drinking alcoholic to see a problem.

Alcoholics suspect most are judgmentally watching them and are close to uncovering their 'secret.' They're sure people are talking about them. As their guilt and shame consume them, they scramble to hide from those who, they believe, pity and condemn them.

They frantically chase relief by secluding. Their need to insulate their feelings surges, reinforcing their need to disguise their drinking as they find brief solace in solitude. Now alone, the compulsion to drink overtakes them.

As drinking continues, the time and energy used to hide it take much more effort. So, alcoholics seek the path of least resistance. They isolate since they're unwilling or unable to disguise or change their drinking pattern, which further reveals their worsening condition.

This isolation is a self-imposed life sentence of solitary confinement pardoned only by sobriety.

However, the ignored concerns of others slowly seep into the alcoholic's mind. And when a moment of reasoned clarity arrives, the voice of truth echoes, and the echoes never end—not until light shines on their denial.

Demographics of the 'Typical' Alcoholic

THE TYPICAL ALCOHOLIC doesn't exist. Many alcoholics and nonalcoholics embrace the misconception that alcoholics are homeless residents of Skid Row. This stereotyping fuels denial.

Alcoholism Does Not Discriminate

Alcoholism does not discriminate nor emancipate. It casts its shackles on those of all socioeconomic levels, races, religions, genders, and ages. Any doctor, lawyer, CPA, or minister could be an alcoholic.

Of the professions with the highest rate of alcoholism, lawyers rank highest, with 20% afflicted—twice the national average,[10] while doctors, nurses, and surgeons rank at 15%.[11] Additionally, bartenders ranked 11.8%, and education ranked 4.7%.[12]

In contrast to the stereotype, the wealthy drink more than the poor by 27.4%, and college graduates drink twice as much as high school dropouts.[13]

In other words, no one can be too rich, too poor, too intelligent, too young, too old, or too anything to be an alcoholic.

Research of the Alcoholic Stereotype

A report by the National Institute on Alcohol Abuse and Alcoholism (NIAAA) shattered the stereotype of alcoholics. This report identified subtypes of alcoholics:[14]

- Twenty percent are highly functional, well-educated, and middle-aged, with good incomes, stable jobs, and intact families. As discussed below, they are the most ignored subtype, and very few seek treatment.
- Thirty-two percent are the "young adult" type, rarely addicted to other substances or diagnosed with other disorders, and seldom seek help with drinking.
- Twenty-one percent are the "young antisocial" type, usually with other diagnosed disorders (i.e., bipolar, depression, etc.) and often addicted to other substances. More than one-third have received treatment.
- Nineteen percent are the "intermediate family subtype." They are middle-aged, with half suffering from depression. Twenty percent have bipolar disorder and problems with cocaine and marijuana use. About 25% have sought treatment for drinking.
- Only nine percent are the "chronic severe" type, which fits the stereotype. They have high rates of antisocial personality disorder and criminality. They have more psychiatric disorders and other substance abuse. Two-thirds seek treatment, and they represent a majority of recovering alcoholics.

The Neglect of the High-Functioning Alcoholic

How can a sophisticated society have such a skewed perception of alcoholics? How do the homeless see, receive, and clutch the life preserver while those more successful remain under the radar, escaping detection, so the life preserver isn't cast their way? I speculate that poor, low-bottom alcoholics seek treatment at a much higher rate because they no longer care what people think—it can't be worse than they feel about themselves. They've got nothing to lose.

Conversely, the high-functioning alcoholic of a higher socioeconomic class focuses on status; their self-image reflects how others view them. They measure their self-worth by their net worth. Their suffering remains a secret. They can't admit their alcohol problem and risk someone thinking less of them than they already think of themselves. They don't see that addressing their drinking will cause those who matter to think more of them. Further, if they considered sobriety, it would, at least, lessen the anxiety of those who love them.

Another likely reason is that the high-functioning alcoholic still has 'everything.' They have above-average incomes, high-end homes and cars, and a surplus of most things. Their family *appears* intact. They *seem* to manage their lives well. Their ruddy complexion suggests more time playing golf rather than Rosacea.* Finally, the stereotypical perception prevents suspecting that the high-functioning alcoholic has a problem. (See Chapters 5 & 7.)

GENETICS AND ENVIRONMENT

THE CONSENSUS IS that genetics and environment play a significant role in predicting alcoholism; however, the extent of this significance is inconclusive. Whether one becomes an alcoholic is half hereditary and half environmental.[15,16] While children of alcoholic parents are more likely to be alcoholics, nearly half of their ancestry has no trace of alcoholism, and many nonalcoholics have alcoholic parents.[17]

Despite the accepted view that environment plays a significant factor in activating alcoholism, many alcoholics and nonalcoholics have similar backgrounds.

Nevertheless, the DSM-5, the National Association for Children of Alcoholics, and other researchers state that children who grew up in an alcoholic family are three to four times

---

*A medical condition triggered by excessive drinking, causing redness and spider veins in the cheeks.

more likely to develop alcoholism.[18] This is true even if they were removed from the family when they were young.[19]

Several studies suggest that sons of alcoholic fathers are 11 times more likely to develop alcoholism. While this doesn't mean this high-risk population should resign to alcoholism, it suggests caution. Yet, exercising caution means restraint or abstinence, which is unlikely in this group, who are convinced they will never be like mom or dad—until they are.

Still, it's useless for alcoholics to blame heredity or the environment for their affliction. Although it's relevant to research that is studying treatment, prevention, and propensity, blaming doesn't excuse or prevent one from seeking sobriety and staying sober.

THE DANGERS OF BRAIN DAMAGE

ALCOHOLICS ENDURE INCREASING brain damage as their condition progresses. Although much is temporary, some may be permanent.

Research conducted at Harvard Medical School in 2014 found that chronic alcoholism damages the part of the brain that, ironically, affects self-control and recovery from alcoholism.[20]*

Neuroimaging that compared alcoholic brains to the brains of light drinkers showed alcoholic brains had noticeable shrinkage of the part that rewards pleasure, which results in life feeling dull.°

As suspected, the study also found that longer and heavier alcohol abuse correlates with greater impairment.

Early results suggest that abstinence may eventually reverse some of this damage, but it's inconclusive.

---

*This is the pre-frontal cortex, essential for controlling impulsive behavior and abstinence.
°This brain damage includes the pathways associated with the amygdala, hippocampus, nucleus accumbens, etc.—the brain's reward system.

The Liver and Brain

Research also reflects that because of the close relationship between the liver and the brain, a dysfunctional liver can cause brain damage.[21] A healthy liver detoxifies alcohol, filtering out toxins before reaching the brain.[22] However, liver disease prevents the liver from protecting the brain and other organs. Beyond that, even without alcohol, a damaged liver produces toxic chemicals that alone can cause brain injury.[23]

Thiamine (Vitamin B1) Deficiency

Alcohol thwarts thiamine absorption, and alcoholics often have poor eating habits, contributing to this deficiency. An alcohol-induced thiamine (vitamin B1) deficiency causes other damage to the brain, such as Wernicke-Korsakoff syndrome. This syndrome consists of Wernicke's encephalopathy and Korsakoff's psychosis.

Wernicke's encephalopathy is short-lived but life-threatening, with symptoms of mental confusion, eye immobility, and incoordination. Those with this condition may be unable to walk or too confused to find the exit door in a house.

A high percentage with Wernicke's encephalopathy develops Korsakoff's psychosis. This long-lasting condition causes abnormal behavior and problems with memory.

A more common condition caused by thiamine deficiency is Cerebellar Degeneration, usually after 10 or more years of heavy drinking. Forty percent show this condition, characterized by shrinkage of the brain regions related to muscle coordination and cognitive and sensory functioning.

A few alcoholics with inadequate thiamine have worse brain damage, including alcohol amnestic disorder (impairment in short-term and long-term memory, disorientation, confabulation,* and unawareness of their memory deficit) and

---

*Confabulation is a symptom of several brain disorders in which false information fills gaps in memory without any intent to deceive and unawareness the information is false. Confabulation can be coherent, internally consistent, and relatively normal.

alcohol-induced persisting dementia. This can also contribute to dysarthria, characterized by the sober alcoholic slurring speech and sounding intoxicated.

Studies have shown that adequate thiamine intake may reverse much of this damage.

Symptoms of Other Brain Damage

Other alcohol-related brain damage reveals itself in several ways. An alcohol-induced psychosis or other disorders may surface, causing some alcoholics to experience hallucinations and lack logical reasoning. Their intensifying obsession with keeping everyone in the dark about their drinking, including those unknown, reveals this distorted thinking. With continued drinking, the alcoholic's denial surges as further brain damage occurs.

Studies reveal that long-time chronic alcoholics may have trouble "reading" others. Since most communication is nonverbal, this matters. For example, the alcoholic may *sense* a hostile facial expression when talking with someone sad.[24] Another area of the brain that is often affected hinders humor.[25]

None of this is new. For years, we've heard insulting references to the alcoholic's brain (e.g., wet brain, pickled brain, etc.).

The American Society of Addiction Medicine (ASAM) and the World Health Organization list "distortions in thinking" as a characteristic of alcoholism. ASAM defines alcoholism as a "brain disease affecting one physically, emotionally, socially, and spiritually."

The inconclusive and vague consensus is that it's possible to reverse various brain damage at different severities to an extent.

Alcohol-Induced Temporary Damage

The alcoholic blackout is "a form of amnesia in which a drinker has no memory of what occurred during heavy drinking."[26] Although many alcoholics and nonalcoholics have had blackouts, many have not (that they can recall). Having blackouts doesn't confirm alcoholism, yet it reveals excessive drinking.

Fragmentary blackouts (also known as "brownouts") are more common. This occurs when the drinker can't recall portions of a drinking period unless prompted by a simple reminder, which refreshes recollection, filling in the memory gaps.

The embarrassment from a random or assisted recall of drunken behavior demoralizes and blankets alcoholics with pervasive shame and despair.

Brain Damage and Suicidal Ideation

Suicidal ideation ranges from mild to severe—from not wanting to live to considering specific methods of dying. Alcoholics die by suicide 10 times more than the general public.[27]

In the final stages, alcohol is no longer providing the relief it once did, and most alcoholics finally realize it never will.*

They're preoccupied with suicidal thoughts. Although they've been slowly shaving time off their lives with each drink, they now stagger in consuming misery, causing them to consider specific methods of suicide, often leading to a completed suicide.

SOME FACTS ABOUT
THE DISEASE CALLED ALCOHOLISM

ALCOHOLISM IS DEADLY. Each year, about 178,000 alcohol-related deaths occur in the United States.[28] It's the third-leading preventable cause of death. According to the Department of Justice, 40% of all violent crimes involve alcohol, and 37% of offenders are drinking when arrested.[29] The Bureau of Justice Statistics reports that 75% of spousal victims involved a drinking offender.[30]

---

*This is usually the best time for an intervention.

About 29.5 million adults in the United States had an Alcohol Use Disorder (AUD) in 2022, yet the evidence suggests this number is much greater.[31] This figure excludes millions of alcoholics who didn't drink within the past year or didn't disclose their alcohol use.

Over 401,000 children aged 12-17 were current alcohol users in 2019, with 94,000 of them having an alcohol use disorder—nearly 55,000 received treatment in 2014.[32]

More startlingly, less than 10% of all alcoholics will ever seek treatment, and only half of those will stay sober for more than a year.

Questions for Discussion

1. How would this chapter help if a loved one's drinking concerned you?
2. How has this chapter affected you?
3. Has this chapter altered the way you viewed alcoholics?
4. Do you identify with any of the characteristics listed in the alcoholic description in this chapter? If so, which ones?
5. If you're a sober alcoholic, what stage of alcoholism did you reach before sobriety?
6. Did you have any alcoholic rules like the ones in this chapter?
7. Were you surprised that only nine percent of alcoholics fit the "stereotypical" alcoholic? Why?
8. Did this chapter persuade or dissuade you from thinking alcoholism is more physiological than behavioral? (i.e., more of disease than poor character?)
9. Do you believe the comparison between alcoholics and nonalcoholics was helpful? If so, explain.
10. Do you strongly agree or disagree with anything in this chapter? If so, what? Why?
11. Have you learned anything from this chapter? If yes, discuss.

THE ALCOHOLIC-CRAVING
A Unique Perspective

CHAPTER 3

*You're probably an alcoholic if after
drinking a few, you're feeling so good
you quickly drink more to feel even better!*
—

CONTRARY TO POPULAR myth, an alcoholic craving alcohol is not the same as a nonalcoholic craving a cold, frothy beer on a hot summer afternoon. That's simply a craving for a beer. The *alcoholic-craving** is a *compelling* and *insatiable need* to artificially change feelings, *usually, but not always*, with alcohol.

The normal drinker satisfies the craving for a cold, frothy beer by drinking one. But not the alcoholic. Although alcoholics may briefly pacify the alcoholic-craving, they never satisfy it. Not even when they think they have.

The alcoholic-craving compels self-medication—trying to 'treat' a cluster of unbearable feelings away.

The difference between the alcoholic and the average drinker hinges on the alcoholic-craving. The nonalcoholic drinks to boost feelings of contentment—it's icing on the cake. The alcoholic drinks to escape discontentment—it's icing without the cake. The persistent alcoholic-craving fuels repeated attempts to spread icing on a cake that doesn't exist.

---

*I have created this compound word to separate the meaning of the alcoholic's craving for alcohol as used in this book (*alcoholic-craving*) and the common misunderstanding of the alcoholic's craving for alcohol.

Alcohol could be the perfect drug to treat the suffering alcoholic, except for the side effects of intoxication and increasing tolerance (drinking more with less effect).

The normal drinker flies through life, correcting course, avoiding most turbulence, refueling long before empty, and enjoying the overall journey.

The alcoholic also flies through life but with a flutter, unable to alter course and avoid turbulence, making frequent emergency landings to refuel when on empty, and suffering through much of the journey.

Now, the alcoholic's flight is stalling, and the alcoholic-craving hides the warning. So, unaware the flight is diving, the alcoholic doesn't try recovering from the stall. Soon, it will spiral out of control.

Still, if the alcoholic chooses sobriety, the chance of surviving is good. But most don't see this choice, or they ignore it and live the rest of their shortened lives hopeless and helpless while rudderless and adrift. So, while falling faster and deeper into the darkness, they can't see the terrorizing end, but they can sense it.

—

I have divided this chapter into four sections.

SECTION ONE — WHAT IS THE ALCOHOLIC-CRAVING exposes the expert's common misunderstanding of the alcoholic's "craving" for alcohol and provides a detailed description and exploration of the alcoholic-craving by contrasting the nonalcoholic's simple *desire* for a drink to the alcoholic's intense, insatiable *need* for alcohol.

SECTION TWO — THE NEUROSCIENCE OF THE ALCOHOLIC-CRAVING delves into the neurobiology behind craving by explaining, in standard terms, how alcohol affects the brain's reward network and alters its structure and function, creating the obsession and compulsion to drink. It also discusses how this understanding will diminish the unreasonable part of the stigma, inviting more alcoholics to seek help.

SECTION THREE — THE IMPORTANCE OF RECOGNIZING THE OFTEN UNRECOGNIZED ALCOHOLIC-CRAVING AND ITS TYPES emphasizes that understanding the alcoholic-craving and its types is crucial for recognizing alcoholism and how withdrawal and tolerance relate to the alcoholic-craving, which prevents many alcoholics from seeking recovery. It also provides information that will help reveal if one has a drinking problem.

SECTION FOUR — THE RESEARCH touches on how, until recently, researchers have largely ignored the alcoholic-craving. It discloses research findings that reveal alcoholism is more a lifelong biological brain disorder than a behavioral disorder. It also discusses research findings about the effectiveness of treating the alcoholic-craving with drugs and other techniques.

SECTION ONE

WHAT IS THE ALCOHOLIC-CRAVING

IT WOULD HELP if one could explain the alcoholic-craving with a collection of words, selected and arranged, creating a vibrant description so everyone understood it.

Searching for a satisfactory definition, description, or explanation of the alcoholic-craving only yields methods of coping with the common misconception of 'craving.'

Ironically, even many drinking and sober alcoholics can't describe or recognize the alcoholic-craving—they think they've never had it. This chapter invites reconsideration.

COMMON MISUNDERSTANDINGS OF THE ALCOHOLIC'S CRAVING FOR ALCOHOL

The Experts' Definition of Craving

Several years ago, the National Institute on Alcohol Abuse and Alcoholism (NIAAA) published a paper called "What is Craving?"[1] The researchers answered, "Understanding the exact nature of craving has been difficult. Craving is very complicated."[2] Researchers now accept that craving is essential to understand but "difficult to describe."[3] Despite this difficulty, their paper defines craving as "a powerful *urge* to drink ... [with] intense thoughts about alcohol."[4]

Merriam-Webster defines craving as "an intense, urgent, or abnormal *desire* or longing [for alcohol]."

The International Classification of Diseases (ICD–10) defines craving as "a strong *desire* or sense of compulsion to [drink alcohol]."[5]

The American Psychiatric Association defines craving as "a strong *desire* or *urge* to use alcohol."[6]

The World Health Organization defines craving as "a very strong *desire* or sense of compulsion to [drink]."[7]

McGraw-Hill Concise Dictionary of Modern Medicine

defines craving as "a strong *desire* to consume ... [alcohol]; craving is a major factor in relapse and continued use after withdrawal ... and is both imprecisely defined and difficult to measure."[8]

The *Surgeon General's Report* explains craving as "an intense *desire* for ... [alcohol]" and a preoccupation with drinking.[9]

These are simply the generic definitions of "craving" in Merriam-Webster with the word "alcohol" added. The terms *compulsion, longing, yearning,* and *urge* are synonyms for craving—they don't define craving. Instead, these definitions are circular—they include a synonym for the defined word as part of the definition.

For example, the *circular* definition of a grateful person is "a person who is thankful." The word "thankful" is a synonym for "grateful." However, a more accurate and helpful definition of a grateful person is "one who feels appreciation for a benefit received and wishes to return the benefit."[10]

The DSM-5 states, "*Craving for alcohol* is indicated by a strong *desire* to drink that makes it difficult to think of anything else, and that often results in the onset of drinking."[11]

This bland definition misses the mark. It defines obsession more than craving. Again, a "craving for alcohol" is not the issue—the alcoholic-craving is. Further, "difficult to think of anything else" is an obsession. So, the DSM-5 implies the craving for alcohol is a strong *obsessive* desire to drink.

However, a simple craving for anything could be similarly defined by substituting any word for "alcohol." For example, *a craving for chocolate milk is indicated by a strong desire to drink chocolate milk that makes it difficult to think of anything else, and that often results in the onset of drinking chocolate milk.* Yet unlike the alcoholic drinking alcohol, drinking enough chocolate milk *will* satisfy the craving for it.

In the 1950s, the World Health Organization defined craving as an "urgent and overpowering *desire* or irresistible impulse." Although lacking, "irresistible impulse" is more accurate than the definitions that followed.

The first problem is that these flawed definitions recognize desire instead of need. They use an adjective to modify and strengthen desire. But no modifier will change a strong, urgent, abnormal, eager, intense, or overpowering desire, or even an intense and strong urge, into a need. The second problem is that these prominent definitions fail to recognize the alcoholics' lack of satiety when drinking. Both are critical errors.

Desire or Need, So What?

When we desire something, we want it—it's our choice. But, when we need something, we must have it—it's essential—necessary, indispensable, a requirement.

Although we're disappointed if we don't get the new car we want, it won't kill us. However, not getting something we need, like food, water, or air, *will* kill us.

We often need something we don't desire, such as surgery. The cost of something we need, like emergency lifesaving surgery, won't stop us from getting it. We've heard, "Whatever it costs, we'll pay it. We need it!" But if it's something we desire, like elective cosmetic surgery, the cost is more relevant.*

A desire withstands patience; a need doesn't.

Desire often prompts pleasure, but need usually feels unpleasant. So, wanting a new car feels better than needing food.

Desire and *need* aren't related or interchangeable. A desire doesn't become a need merely because it intensifies. Our desire for a new car will never become a need just because we want it more each day. Conversely, when we no longer have a need, it's not reduced to a desire.

Although generally unknown, *most alcoholics dislike alcohol. Many drink when they don't want to.* It's not the *desire* or *choice* to drink that precedes drinking. It's the *need* to feel

---

*That is why government regulates the cost charged by utilities for certain monopolized services considered a need (e.g., electricity, water, gas, etc.).

different and obey unconscious commands from a dysfunctional brain that triggers drinking. Late-stage chronic alcoholics *desire* sobriety. They drink because of a compelling need.

Who would give up everything, including dignity, to satisfy a mere desire?

An alcoholic refusing an intensely craved drink is like a person stranded in the desert for three days refusing water.

Self-deprivation of something we desire or want is exercising our willpower. If we don't resist that desire, we're seen as undisciplined—lacking self-control—it's a character flaw. But getting something we need, like air, food, or water, is survival and unrelated to character.

It's like our need for sleep. Our willpower can avoid the craving to sleep for a time. But, eventually, the need to sleep will overpower our desire to resist it, and our brain will force us to sleep.

Information in dictionaries, encyclopedias, medical school textbooks, and peer-reviewed papers is reliable, or so we think. Defining the alcoholic-craving as a *desire* rather than a *need* for alcohol is unreliable and spreads false information. These references suggest the alcoholic *chooses* to drink out of deliberate recklessness and self-absorption. It implies willful misconduct.

How can healthcare professionals adequately treat and others understand a condition when they learn it is something it is not? These past explanations of the alcoholic-craving are false, and they support the alcoholic stereotype. They boost ignorance, not knowledge.

The Satiation System and the Alcoholic-craving

We know when we've had enough food, water, and sex. Our brain tells us we're satisfied. Most have felt the discomfort of overeating. Our eyes are sometimes bigger than our stomachs.

To illustrate, we may crave doughnuts. We can't think of anything else. We're sure we can eat half a dozen. But as we struggle to finish the second one, our craving for doughnuts is abruptly interrupted by feeling satisfied—we've had enough. When the brain senses we've eaten too many, we are beyond satisfied. We feel uncomfortably full. This is our biology working normally.

When normal drinkers have one or two, their brain tells them they've had enough—they're satisfied. But this satiation system is missing when alcoholics drink. So, the signaling that the alcoholic has had enough to drink doesn't come. And while other cravings motivate 'getting it' followed by the sensation of 'got it' (like nicotine, heroin, and other drugs), the alcoholic-craving only produces the need to 'get it,' and the 'got it' never comes.[12] So, unsatisfied, drinking continues.

Moreover, the simple craving for a doughnut will not cause us to lose jobs, friends, or family and sacrifice other essentials. Nor will eating a doughnut provide us with feelings of well-being, self-confidence, purpose, courage, and other euphoric feelings alcoholics seek when drinking.

In short, the insatiable alcoholic-craving is never a simple "desire."

THE ALCOHOLIC-CRAVING

THE ALCOHOLIC-CRAVING ISN'T easy to explain, especially to one who has never had it. It's like explaining the feelings of loneliness to one who has never been lonely. We can't. We can only talk about the actions and thoughts produced when feeling lonely. It's the same with the alcoholic-craving. One who has endured it will understand it more.

Although similar, no alcoholic experiences the alcoholic-craving precisely the same. As alcoholism progresses, so does the alcoholic-craving.

Within the limits of explaining the abstract, I suggest the following description.

> **THE ALCOHOLIC-CRAVING**
> An unconscious biological progressive brain dysfunction producing an uncontrollable, dynamic, obsessive, compulsive, inescapable, penetrable, persistent, and *insatiable need* to replace growing dysphoria with euphoria, usually by periodically or chronically drinking and continuing to drink alcohol or engaging in other obsessive-compulsive, self-destructive behavior.

The Components of the Alcoholic-craving

- The *unconsciously* produced alcoholic-craving and the *need* to drink slowly intensifies, like the need to eat.
- It can be so powerful and *uncontrollable* that nothing can tame it.
- It's *dynamic*—more and less intense at times.*
- It's *insatiable*—never satisfied, always needing more.
- It's so *penetrable* it pierces through memories of consequences and reasons not to drink.
- Its *persistence* is *inescapable*. The demands for a drink don't stop, and the alcoholic feels imprisoned by these demands, unable to avoid them.
- It's not merely a want, desire, longing, yearning, or urge to drink, but it's a *need* so irresistible that one will sacrifice everything to drink. This need often eclipses instincts for water, food, sleep, and sex.
- The *intensifying dysphoria,* when abstinent, is the growth of negative feelings, such as misery, guilt, sadness, hopelessness, irritability, anger, loneliness, self-hatred, obsession, compulsion, and fear, so entombed in the alcoholic's essence that death often appears more

---

*One way of coping with it is realizing relief is near, and it won't last forever.

attractive than life.

- The *euphoria* sought includes intense feelings of well-being, happiness, pleasure, excitement, courage, trust, exhilaration, self-confidence, purpose, gratitude, and hopefulness.
- It is *often periodic*. For those alcoholics who don't drink daily, the alcoholic-craving only strikes occasionally. But when it strikes, it's usually more robust for the periodic drinker than the daily drinker.
- Drinking doesn't always result from the alcoholic-craving. Although drinking alcoholics prefer it, those sober long-term *usually* select other ways to satisfy their alcoholic-craving.
- When alcoholics don't drink to soothe their alcoholic-craving, they often seek other ways to change their feelings. For example, many sober alcoholics try satisfying the alcoholic-craving with *obsessive, compulsive, addictive, and self-destructive activity*. The alcoholic brain reinforces this behavior with pleasure.

   These activities aren't easy to stop, often harming the sober alcoholic and others. These activities may include *excessively* engaging in shopping, working, writing, overeating, spending, gambling, online gaming, exercising, hoarding, seeking power, playing or watching sports, seeking endless amounts of money, and chasing constant approval and admiration. Others engage in hypersexuality or co-dependency. Some will abuse drugs. It's not unheard of for a suffering alcoholic, many years sober, to select death over alcohol.

—

If the alcoholic is sober and in a recovery program, healthy action will usually expel or lessen the alcoholic-craving, creating contentment and joyful feelings. (See Chapter 12, "The Happily Sober Alcoholic.")

Once sober, the alcoholic-craving disappears—for some

quicker than others. But this disappearance doesn't mean it's gone forever. It can make a surprised reappearance months or years later, although its duration and intensity are usually much less.

When periodic or chronic alcoholics resist drinking, their anxiety, stress, and despair deepen. Usually, the most compassionate act one can do for the alcoholic not ready to explore sobriety but enduring the alcoholic-craving is to give them a bottle.

In short, an alcoholic could be defined as *one who has had the* alcoholic-craving—*whether they knew it or not*. One certain fact is the average drinker may crave a drink but has *never* had the alcoholic-craving.

THE NEIGHBORS: A STUDY
Joe's alcoholic-craving contrasted with Steve's normal craving for alcohol

STEVE IS A typical drinker who doesn't behave the same as Joe, who is troubled by the *alcoholic-craving*. Steve likes routine. The unfamiliar yields discomfort. If he could, he would sacrifice the thrill of the unknown future in exchange for knowing every detail that will unfold in his life. He could never be the life of the party. His rigid routine feeds him with contentment and control. His habitual activity massages away lurking anxiety.

Steve's routine is so compelling that he calls the same three people every Sunday strictly at 5:00, 5:15, and 5:30 p.m. He mows every Saturday afternoon at three unless, after reviewing the radar, he expects rain. If so, he adjusts the scheduled mowing time precisely. His yard looks perfect.

Then there's Joe, a drinking alcoholic who has been Steve's neighbor for over twenty years. Joe insists he *is* the life of the party because wherever he goes, so does the party (unless he's mowing). Joe makes Steve look good.

They catch a fleeting glance of each other almost daily but never say more than a word or two. At most, they may mumble a comment here and there.

Joe appears far more relaxed than Steve. He knows it's time to mow when Steve mows. Joe avoids the same rut he sees Steve stuck in but doesn't mind benefiting from it.

For example, Joe considers a scheduled time a guideline. Yet he's intolerant if he must wait on anyone, and he's not shy about expressing it. He insists arriving early is rude—it's an intrusion, not a visit.

Consistency governs Steve's life—chaos rules Joe.

WHILE MOWING ON a hot Saturday afternoon, Steve imagines a cold, frothy beer foaming slightly over a frosty mug. As he removes the foggy, steamy, cold mug from the ice, he hears it clank. As he pours it, he hears ale escaping, sounding a bubbly melody while watching foam fizzing, bubbles vaporizing.

He raises the brew to his parted and parched lips, smells the aroma of cascade hops, and then fills his mouth with perfection. After pausing, he swallows with an approving hum and whispers, "Ah, ... good beer." After licking foam from his upper lip, he ends his daydream and finishes mowing.

After Steve finishes mowing, he rewards himself by slowly swinging in his hammock chair like a monotonous metronome, drinking cold beer from his frosty mug, admiring his work, smelling freshly cut grass, and watching Joe struggling to start his mower. After drinking *most* of the mug, he has satisfied his craving for a beer and is content. He won't think of a beer until the next time he mows.

JOE FINALLY STARTS his mower, using a twig to override the safety switch. While mowing, thoughts of Steve and a cold beer distract him. He thinks of good reasons to take a break to drink one, such as doubting he can finish before dark, the grass isn't cutting right, the blade needs sharpening, there's probably not enough gas to finish, he didn't check the oil, and Steve irritating him by taking so long to drink one beer.

He then wonders if he set the mower at the best height. He usually cuts it short, hoping he won't need to mow it as often as Steve does. But Steve's lawn is green, smooth, soft, and so inviting a baby could roll in it. Joe's grass appears scalped and mostly brown; the green spots are prickly, weedy patches.

Joe sees Steve still drinking the same beer, and his swinging is becoming more annoying. He wonders how Steve does it—drinking so slowly. Then, feeling more frustration and resentment brewing, he focuses on drinking.

Joe's restlessness and irritation are also growing, a characteristic of the alcoholic-craving. Steve's swinging and drinking the same cold one isn't helping.

He thinks he feels raindrops and again ponders a beer. Maybe the grass is too wet—it's probably better to finish tomorrow. Although he's a little down and doesn't want to mow, he decides to finish the front.

After almost finishing the front, he decides to take a break and figure out the best way of managing his mowing problems while drinking a beer. He feels better just knowing he'll soon be drinking.

HE OPENS THE cooler and sees he forgot the ice. Oh well, warm beer brings out the taste and aroma of hops, he tells himself. He pops open a can—half fizzes out while he slugs down the leftover suds. Since he only had half a beer, he figures it doesn't count. So he carefully opens another, holding it closer to his mouth to capture any escaping fizz. He feels better. And the relentless thoughts twisting in his mind about ways to damage Steve's grass and cut the rope suspending his swinging chair, begin to fade.

HE SCANS THE section he mowed with a smile. After finishing the second beer, he feels slightly down and persuades himself to delay mowing. While drinking the third one, he feels better.

He drains the third can but soon feels dissatisfied, so he gives in to drinking one more. While opening the fourth one, he feels content, convinced it's Steve's fault he didn't finish mowing. He drinks it.

Although he can't satisfy his craving, he will briefly soothe it by drinking. In the unlikely event he continues mowing, his mind will increasingly focus on drinking another beer. He will feel more dissatisfied, irritable, and uncomfortable until he resumes drinking.

—

THIS PEEK INSIDE the minds of two fictional characters shows the power and complexities of the alcoholic-craving compared with a simple craving for a beer. Joe unconsciously decided to stop mowing and drink a beer when he saw Steve drinking one.

Joe felt guilt and remorse. To ease these feelings, he created and nurtured thoughts that led to frustration, anger, and resentment. He used these feelings to support his 'right' to drink. He talked himself into believing it made sense to stop mowing and drink a beer. That's an example of the time-consuming rationalizations spawned by the alcoholic-craving.

It also shows how drinking is just one symptom of alcoholism seeping into the alcoholic's unmanageable life. If the alcoholic-craving interferes with the mundane task of mowing, it affects his entire life. Yet denial stops Joe from seeing this.

SECTION TWO
THE NEUROSCIENCE OF CRAVING
(It's all in our head)

IT'S UNIMAGINABLE THAT any discussion about alcoholism, especially the alcoholic-craving, can be meaningful without reviewing the brain.

Neuroscientists have made great strides as they explore the brain. This alluring science gives us a better view and understanding of the alcoholic-craving. Still, they've barely scratched the surface of the well-locked vault holding this knowledge.

Despite this, science has proven alcoholism is an incurable brain disease and doesn't flow from a character flaw. One benefit of recognizing it as a disease is that primary and emergency doctors, the ones alcoholics usually see first, are now responsible for alcohol screening. So, it's no longer the *sole* responsibility of mental health professionals to screen for, diagnose, and treat alcoholism.

Much of this science is complex, and the research is often conflicting and uncertain. However, widely accepted findings support the following summary of how our brain creates the alcoholic-craving.

Neuroimaging

For several years, scientists have been using neuroimaging to scan images of our brains. This imaging uses colors to show the stimulated parts of our brain—bright and rich colors show high stimulation. We finally have visual proof the alcoholic brain differs from the nonalcoholic brain.[13] This imaging supports the notion that alcohol uniquely changes the alcoholic brain.

Remarkably, these images also reveal that the size and shape of the brain change. This is called *neuroplasticity*.[14,15] Our brains are not permanently hard-wired one way like we once thought. The pathways that route messages change as the brain makes new pathways.[16]

For example, the parts of the brain that receive pleasure (*dopamine receptors*) aren't as colorful nor as many in the alcoholic brain as in the nonalcoholic brain.[17] Drinking changes the part of the brain that makes decisions, forms beliefs, controls our impulses, and determines whether we should drink, quit drinking, or drink more (*prefrontal cortex*).[18] Fortunately, these alcohol-induced changes return closer to normal the longer alcoholics stay sober. Still, it takes time.*[19,20]

The younger brain is more 'plastic' than the older brain. That's why children and teens learn faster and have better memories. It also explains why beliefs we adopted as children are nearly impossible to entirely disbelieve as adults, even when we know they're wrong. *And it explains why teenage drinking significantly increases the chances of developing a drinking problem.*[21]

These neuroimages also reveal that meditation and mind-body relaxation increase the size of various structures, including the 'judgment center' (*prefrontal cortex*). This change improves the executive tasks mentioned above, including focusing and controlling our behavior and impulse to drink.[22] Meditation reduces worry, sadness, fear, and anger.[23] It also promotes self-healing and empathy, weakening the alcoholic-craving.[24] So meditation lessens relapses, nurtures sobriety, and is widely used to treat alcoholics.

The Neuroanatomy of the Reward Network

Our brain aims to keep us alive and reproduce to prevent human extinction. The part of our brain that targets this aim by influencing our behavior is the reward network (*mesolimbic circuit*).[25] This network rewards us with pleasure when we take life-preserving actions such as eating, drinking water,

---

*This is the theory behind the proliferation of brain exercises sold as games, puzzles, and teasers. Also, aerobic workouts are widely accepted as the best and fastest way to create vast quantities of neurons in the brain, which accelerates this process.[19]

sleeping, reproducing, and protecting ourselves and our children.[26] These rewards keep us coming back for more.

Although this reward network includes many parts,[27] the following five are the most basic to the alcoholic-craving. (*I've given these descriptive names and parenthetically noted their scientific names.*)

> 1. **Assessment center** (*ventral tegmental area*): Packed with pleasure-seeking dopamine, this center is ready to release it. It *unconsciously* works while sensing and responding to triggers and evaluating how satisfied our needs are. It then sends a chemical message to the pleasure center (*nucleus accumbens*) and other centers, reporting how well we are meeting our survival needs. For example, the alcoholic brain receives the message that "Drinking is essential. Remember how to do it again." In time, the mere anticipation of drinking produces more pleasure than actually drinking.[28] This results in an irresistible motivation to drink—the alcoholic-craving.
>
> 2. **Pleasure center** (*nucleus accumbens*): This center *unconsciously* processes information from other brain structures, decides drinking is necessary, motivates drinking, and chooses the quickest way to drink. It sends a message to different parts of the brain, which compels drinking. This center produces pleasure while drinking and even more pleasure when expecting to drink, causing the alcoholic-craving.[29]
>
> 3. **Emotional center** (*amygdala*): This center, commonly called the fear center, regulates how we respond to external stimuli (fight or flight response). It *unconsciously* learns with the memory center which actions are safe or dangerous, pleasant or unpleasant. It connects drinking to a positive reward and creates negative emotions when the alcoholic doesn't drink. These emotions include stress, anxiety, irritability, and other negative feelings. It rewards pleasure when sensing anything that prompts drinking,

such as a particular song or the sight of a drink, known as relapse triggers. This reward promotes the alcoholic-craving and relapses.[30]

4. Memory center (*hippocampus*): Without the memory center, we wouldn't feel hunger, thirst, or sexual arousal. And if we did, we wouldn't remember how to satisfy them, and humans would perish. This center *unconsciously* memorizes how to get a drink.* It does this with help from the emotional center (*amygdala*). It also contributes to the *advanced* pleasure rewarded when the alcoholic *plans* to drink. The memory center intensifies the alcoholic-craving.

5. Judgment center (*prefrontal cortex*): This is the only *conscious* center of the reward network. Its job is to exercise judgment, control our emotions and impulses,° make decisions and plans, and focus our attention. It's always talking with our unconscious parts, although we're unaware. It decides whether we should drink now, delay drinking, or never drink again. If it decides to drink now, it causes the alcoholic to get a drink. But eventually, drinking disrupts the judgment center, causing the alcoholic-craving, drinking, and relapses.

These centers communicate through about 60 chemical neurotransmitters traveling the brain's pathways, including dopamine and serotonin.[31]

The alcoholic's drinking disturbs the reward network.[32] This disturbance causes complex rationalizations, which result in self-destructive choices and loss of control. It also raises alcohol tolerance and lowers impulse control by replacing negative emotions with positive ones.[33] This causes a persistent and irresistible need to drink: The alcoholic-craving.[34]

---

*Declaratory memory is stored here, which can be consciously retrieved.
°Impulse control is the ability to resist urges, delay instant gratification, and consider consequences and long-term goals over immediate rewards.

The Pleasure of It All

Both alcoholic and nonalcoholic brains record pleasure-producing activity the same.

Our brains naturally reward us with pleasure when we act to survive. But if we're not meeting our essential needs, like food, water, or sex, the pleasure center announces this to the other centers. And the longer we go without meeting these survival needs, the more displeasure we'll feel. So, this growing displeasure motivates us to satisfy these needs quickly by craving them. The memory center (*hippocampus*) stores the details required to satisfy these cravings, with help from the emotional memory center (*amygdala*). It then sends an alarm call to other brain structures, motivating us to get what we need (*appetitive behavior*).

Alcohol Takes a Shortcut

It takes time and effort for natural survival action to pleasure us. We get water more easily and faster than food. Sex takes more time and effort, but the reward is usually better.

Because alcohol shortcuts this time and effort by cutting in at the front of the line, it tricks the alcoholic brain into thinking survival action has occurred. This suddenly floods the alcoholic with pleasure, taking less effort and time than getting it naturally with food, water, or sex.* So drinking, quickly and mistakenly, rewards us with temporary and unearned pleasure.

The Neurobiology of the Alcoholic-Craving

The alcoholic-craving can occur while sober or drinking. The reward network learns and believes the alcoholic *needs* alcohol to survive, which motivates drinking. This motivation hijacks the judgment center, ignores logical reasons not to

---

*As quickly as alcohol does this, other drugs do it much faster with much more reward. According to the DSM-5 (p. 486) and other research, the faster the effect and more rewarding the drug, the more addictive it is (e.g., intravenous versus tablet).

drink, and reduces impulse control, which compels drinking.

Although the alcoholic rarely senses or recognizes it, this is the alcoholic-craving controlling thoughts, feelings, and actions.

Section Three

The Importance of Recognizing the Often Unrecognized Alcoholic-Craving and its Types

THE ALCOHOLIC-CRAVING OFTEN exists without the drinker ever knowing it. It's like breathing. We don't *decide* to breathe or even think about breathing before each breath . . . unless we interrupt our breathing.* If we hold our breath, we'll soon sense a *need* or a craving to breathe, which will intensify until we breathe. Like breathing, alcoholics won't feel the alcoholic-craving unless they're sober or their drinking is interrupted.

Three main reasons many alcoholics, drinking or sober, question whether they've had the alcoholic-craving are:

1. The alcoholic-craving is primarily fueled unconsciously, so they're usually unaware of it.

2. They unknowingly and quickly surrender to the alcoholic-craving by drinking before they notice it.

3. When dry, they have no idea the alcoholic-craving is prompting their sulking mood.

The Importance of Recognizing the Alcoholic-craving

The alcoholic-craving propels alcoholism. Without it, relapses wouldn't occur—alcoholism wouldn't exist. So, it's essential to recognize the alcoholic-craving for many reasons.

- Since the alcoholic-craving is a primary symptom of alcoholism, the more we understand it, the more we'll understand the disease, which will enhance recovery.

- It will dilute stereotypical beliefs, reduce the stigma,

---

*An exception is those with *Dysautonomia,* which refers to a wide range of conditions that affect the autonomic nervous system and can cause problems with autonomic breathing.

and increase the recovery rate.
- It will improve health care's ability to recognize alcoholism in patients complaining of hypertension, fatigue, gastritis, and other alcohol-related symptoms.
- It will lessen the high rate of misdiagnoses.
- It will allow those affected by the drinker to gain a new perspective, allowing them to make rational decisions instead of automatically reacting emotionally.
- Alcoholics who know that the alcoholic-craving is an alcoholic symptom but believe they've never had it won't have a 'logical' reason to deny their alcoholism.
- If sober alcoholics realize the alcoholic-craving has fueled most of their actions, this will likely prevent them from feeling unique—a feeling that nurtures relapses.
- If alcoholics know the temporary alcoholic-craving will not last forever, it will be easier to avoid a relapse.

THE FOUR TYPES OF THE ALCOHOLIC-CRAVING

ALTHOUGH ALCOHOLICS EXPERIENCE them differently, all alcoholic-cravings fuel a compelling need to avoid unpleasant feelings, which intensify when struggling not to drink.

The brain's reward network insists it needs alcohol to survive and motivates drinking by rewarding pleasure.

I've observed four types of alcoholic-cravings and have classified them according to when they arise and their effect:

1) *The Type I Triggered Craving*;
2) *The Type II Sober Craving*;
3) *The Type III Silent Craving*; and
4) *The Type IV Dysphoric Craving*.

Why Classify the Alcoholic-craving Types

This chapter shows that the alcoholic-craving is much more

complicated than the prevailing definition of a mere *desire for alcohol*. Most agree that the alcoholic-craving hasn't received the attention it deserves. Classifying it gives it some of that missed attention.

Classifying signs and symptoms helps us understand and communicate about them.[35] It also allows us to identify symptoms, and the alcoholic-craving standing alone is a decisive symptom.[36] The nonalcoholic will never have it.

The Diagnostic and Statistical Manual of Mental Disorders (DSM) is the most trusted mental health guide in the United States. It organizes mental disorders and their symptoms to help with diagnoses and research. The DSM is the source used for creating most alcohol screenings. Still, it has serious flaws. (See Chapter 7, "Health Care, Alcoholism, and the DSM.")

Incredibly, the DSM-IV, the primary source used to diagnose alcoholics for 19 years, from 1994 until 2013, unfortunately omitted craving. This omission sent the message that the alcoholic-craving symptom is irrelevant when diagnosing alcoholism.

Before now, the main craving discussed was the loss of control that compelled drinking after the first drink (*Type III Silent Craving*). Many insist there's no other type of craving. Most alcoholics in denial would excuse their triggered reaction to this craving type as "just having a good time" or "I drank more than I planned—got a little carried away." However, the detailed labeling of the other three types lists many more traits, which can reduce denial if one is aware of them. So, it increases the chances of alcoholics escaping denial and accepting their alcoholism.

For example, recognizing *Type I Triggered Craving* alerts the alcoholic, sober for years, to be on guard if the alcoholic-craving strikes. *Type II Sober Craving* produces the alcoholic's dysphoric mood, which prompts the alcoholic to pick up the *first* drink. *Type IV Dysphoric Craving* shows the dreadful feelings the alcoholic endures after a drinking episode.

So, responding to these four cravings by drinking doesn't simply take the edge off some random feelings that emerge from nowhere. Instead, the alcoholic-cravings create feelings the alcoholic scrambles to avoid. Moreover, when trying to identify alcoholism, it's necessary to know that drinking, compelled by the alcoholic-craving, is not just a "desire" to drink—it's a need to survive.

Classifying the four types of alcoholic-craving and their elements benefits clinicians, alcoholics, and researchers. The clinician has more signs to choose from, supporting a more accurate diagnosis. More signs plant more seeds that grow and may fuel the alcoholic's flight from denial, resulting in a self-diagnosis. Also, these added symptoms aid researchers in forming more relevant hypotheses and treatment plans.

For example, by revealing the elements of the *Type II Sober Craving,* instead of asking the alcoholic the general question, *"How intense is your craving for a drink?"* a clinician may now ask a specific question about any of the 33 signs under *Type II Sober Craving,* such as: "Do you think those concerned about your drinking are overreacting?" or "What are your thoughts before you start drinking?" or "Have you ever been unable to find a bottle you hid?" or "Do you ever drink to take the edge off bad feelings and not merely to enjoy a drink?"

The alcoholic-craving is hardly noticed when it compels drinking. It's much more subtle as it creates and strengthens negative thoughts and feelings. The alcoholic *believes* the only way to escape these feelings is to drink.

This craving classification allows drinkers to reduce their denial, which promotes recognizing their alcoholism.

Reliable research also supports this, although it doesn't classify the four types of cravings as here. For example, classifying the alcoholic-craving can reduce stigmatizing stereotypical beliefs, persuading more toward sobriety. Also, understanding these craving types leads to a better understanding of alcoholism and the alcoholic. Finally, this knowledge promotes discovering more effective methods of treatment.

Type I Triggered Craving

> An unexpected, penetrating, and compulsive need to drink, triggered unconsciously by a stimulus. It causes at least a brief expectation of drinking, and alcoholics often feel worse than before the trigger if they don't drink.

This *Type I Triggered Craving* may pop up occasionally and unexpectedly, or never. Anything reminding the alcoholic of drinking can trigger it and could happen to one who's been sober for years.

The Pleasurable Anticipation

Studies show that merely *expecting* to eat when hungry, drink water when thirsty, or have sex when aroused rewards us with an advance of pleasure.[37]

But our reward network withdraws this advance if we don't get something it had advanced us pleasure to get.[38] This leaves us with a negative balance of only unpleasant feelings.[39]

Suppose we're looking forward to a vacation. If we must cancel it, we'll feel worse than before we planned it. And the longer we planned it, the worse we'll feel. Or, if frozen fish sticks cover our plate when we've been expecting lobster with butter sizzling over a flame, we'll feel worse than before we expected the lobster dinner.

Alcoholics experience this anticipatory pleasure or relief when simply planning to drink. Drinking has trained the alcoholics' reward network. When sensing a trigger, such as seeing a frothy cold beer, hearing a suggestive song, smelling an evocative scent, tasting alcohol, or anything else associated with drinking, the reward network *foresees* 'survival' action.[40] This foresight causes the assessment center to release a teasing dose of pleasure (*dopamine*), motivating the alcoholic to follow through and seek what the brain believes it needs (*appetitive behavior*).[41]

Further, the alcoholic will feel even worse than before the craving struck. The alcoholic-craving will intensify as the emotional center casts more feelings of stress and anxiety.[42] Those sober in recovery have various tools to defeat this. These tools include support for knowing these feelings will soon pass rather than giving in to the moment and drinking.

Possible Triggers of Type I Triggered Craving

The following are possible triggers, also called environmental cues, which cause dysphoria when the *Type I Triggered Craving* strikes the alcoholic who quit drinking. Knowing what to be alerted to will help the alcoholic avoid relapsing.

- The scent of beer, liquor, freshly cut grass, suntan lotion, perfume, or cologne.
- Passing a liquor store or bar once patronized or seeing a liquor, beer, or wine bottle.
- Hearing a song that recalls a past enjoyable drinking event.
- Tasting alcohol in food or mouthwash.
- Seeing a former drinking companion.
- Feeling resentment, anger, fear, loneliness, or sadness.
- Feeling happiness, enjoyment, excitement, love, or success.
- Feeling grief from a divorce, the death of a loved one, a romantic breakup, or losing a job.
- Receiving a promotion, winning the lottery, or any other celebratory event.
- Any other cue linked with the 'good times' when drinking.

Type II Sober Craving

> When sober, this unconsciously produced craving is a recurring, insatiable, uncontrollable, obsessive, compulsive **need,** often periodic, to end intense dysphoria with alcohol.

This *Type II Sober Craving* is the expanding dysphoria *before* the first drink. This craving is not merely an impulse to drink; it intensifies dysphoria, compelling the alcoholic to artificially change their feelings, *usually* with alcohol.

At first, the alcoholic senses the alcoholic-craving as feeling edgy and intolerant. He's easily annoyed when merely asked for the time. He briefly thinks about a drink. Soon, these feelings intensify, and he increasingly thinks about drinking if he has held out, overshadowing all other thoughts. This nagging reminder is now an obsession.

Suppose his environment prevents him from immediately drinking. In that case, he will *plan* to drink, temporarily giving him an anticipatory 'pleasure boost,' briefly reducing the alcoholic-craving until he's had time to get a drink. But, if he doesn't get one soon, his obsession and misery will return and worsen.

At this point, the alcoholic-craving might manifest as moodiness. He seems pensive but is brooding. He doesn't feel like doing anything he needs to do. His blurred attention prevents him from focusing on any task.

He's feeling increasingly anxious. The thought of people irritates him. He even irritates himself. He may decide he needs alone time, and those around him agree. He's feeling more dissatisfied. Everything seems gloomy.

He's unaware of the alcoholic-craving lurking behind the scenes. Whether he assumes he's just in a bad mood or having one of those days, he knows a drink will lift his spirits, and he's right.

If he drinks now, he's sure he drank because he's feeling down, never thinking he surrendered to the *Type II Sober*

Craving. If he admitted the craving fueled his drinking, he would be admitting alcohol dependence—an unlikely admission—unless he's ready to quit drinking.

Dr. Silkworth and the "Phenomenon Of Craving"

One often hears: "Just don't take the first drink," which suggests that refusing the first drink when in the depths of the alcoholic-craving merely requires willpower and self-control. However, this ignores science and supports the alcoholic stigma.

William D. Silkworth, MD, a "neuro-psychiatrist," had years of experience during the 1930s as director of the busy Charles B. Towns Hospital for Drug and Alcohol Addictions in New York City. He treated over 40,000 severe alcoholics and addicts.* Bill Wilson, the co-founder of Alcoholics Anonymous (AA), was one of his patients.

Dr. Silkworth, best known for coining *"the phenomenon of craving,"* was the first doctor known to opine the compulsion to continue drinking after the first drink is a physical reaction to alcohol. He wrote a letter published in the book *Alcoholics Anonymous* (called *"The Big Book"* by AA members), which propelled his theory.[43]

Dr. Silkworth describes the symptoms of the *alcoholic-craving* during times of abstinence in another paper he wrote dated March 17, 1937, of which most are unaware. He entitled it *Alcoholism as a Manifestation of Allergy*.[44] And although he claims it's not the craving, it describes the *Type II Sober Craving*:

---

*William Duncan Silkworth (1873-1951) was a physician and specialist in the treatment of alcoholism. He was a neurologist with an emphasis in psychiatry. He was a member of the psychiatric staff at the US. Army Hospital in Plattsburgh, New York, for two years (1917-1919). Ernest Kurtz referred to him as a "neuro-psychiatrist" in his book *Not-God* (Hazelden 1979). He was and is affectionately known as "the little doctor who loved drunks."

> [D]uring periods of partial or complete sobriety, [the alcoholic] develops a state of anxiety amounting to a vague fear, then depression and lack of concentration, with gradually growing indifference or complete apathy toward his former interests. Unreliability, changes in personality, loss of appetite, insomnia, and tachycardia follow. He is under such tension in the effort to control himself that he has to have a drink ... to hold himself together. *At the same time, and we have observed few exceptions to this, these individuals will tell you that they ... [dislike] liquor [and] ... dread to take it*; and, to anyone who has watched such a person, it is obvious that this is true. But he believes he must have it, even though he realizes that, in his particular case, a single drink will plunge him into such a condition that a prolonged spree will be the inevitable result. *After the first drink, and only then, does he experience the physical phenomenon of craving.* [Emphasis added]

The doctor describes the physical feelings and emotions *before* the first drink, which sound much like withdrawal and the alcoholic-craving. Yet *again,* he focuses on the *physical* craving *after* the first drink, as the "only" time craving is present.

—

A few excerpts of thoughts and behaviors alcoholics had just before their first drink from the main text of the *"Big Book"* follow. I have italicized the parts showing it was the *compulsion* to drink, not just a mere *desire* or obsession to drink, that spawned the alcoholic-craving.

- There was *little ... thought ... of* what the terrific *consequences* might be.[45]

- The *curious mental phenomenon ... insanely trivial excuse* for taking the first drink. *Our sound reasoning failed... The insane idea won...* We would ask ourselves ... *how it could have happened.*[46]
- I saw that will power and self-knowledge would not help in those *strange mental blank spots.*[47]
- *What* sort of *thinking dominates* an alcoholic who repeats ... the *desperate experiment of the first drink?*[48]
- *Not only had I been off guard, I had made no fight whatever against the first drink... I had not thought of the consequences at all.*[49] [Italics original]
- The alcoholic at ... times has *no ... mental defense* against the first drink.[50]
- Our behavior is *absurd* and *incomprehensible* with respect to the first drink.[51]
- Where alcohol has been involved, we have been *strangely insane.*[52]
- *Alcoholics, for reasons yet obscure, have lost the power of choice in drink. Our so-called will power becomes practically nonexistent. We are unable, at certain times, to bring into our consciousness with sufficient force the memory of the suffering and humiliation of even a week or a month ago. We are without defense against the first drink.*[53] [Italics original]
- *No ... idea why he took that first drink...*[54]

Clearly, the "thinking" and "thought" before the first drink is anything but thinking. It's a mind that ignores probable consequences and is *"desperate, absurd, incomprehensible, and insane."* This mind has *"no mental defense, no idea,"* is *"off guard,"* and has *"no fight against drinking."* So, isn't this an unconscious, impulsive, compulsive need? These all describe the Type II Sober Craving *before* the first drink, revealing it's more than just a *desire*.

The book also references the sober alcoholic, stating "that occasionally in the night a vague *craving* arose," and later mentions the possible need for "physical treatment" for the alcoholic so he "no longer *craves* alcohol."[55] [Italics added]

Further along in the *"Big Book,"* Robert Smith, MD, cofounder of AA (fondly called Dr. Bob), discusses the alcoholic-craving.[56] He reveals:

> ### Before Sobriety
> "I did not take the morning drink which I *craved* so badly... Occasionally, I would yield to the morning *craving*..."
> ### During Sobriety
> "Unlike most of our crowd, I did not get over my *craving* for liquor much during the first two and one-half years of abstinence. It was almost always with me." [Italics added]

Dr. Bob recognized that the alcoholic-craving occurs after *and* before the first drink. No alcohol consumption is needed to spark it.

Yet, Dr. Silkworth insisted that only one type of alcoholic craving occurs, and that's *only* after the first drink. However, in his published letter ("The Doctor's Opinion"), he refers to the state of mind before the first drink as "the desire" followed by the *phenomenon of craving* (the uncontrollable drinking of one after another).

Nevertheless, he seems to recognize the Type II Craving when he discusses the alcoholic detoxifying with the intention that he be "freed from his *craving* for liquor." [Italics added] He further describes these dry alcoholics as "restless, irritable, and discontented unless they can experience the sense of ease and comfort which comes at once by taking a few drinks..."

The *Type II Sober Craving* has not received the attention it deserves, even though a relapse can't occur without it. To re-emphasize, it's not the "allergy" or the "phenomenon of craving" the second, third, or fourth drink that causes the relapse. *The relapse occurs with the first drink* (Type I and II cravings). Without the craving before the first drink, there would be no "phenomenon" to discuss. But that said, if the alcoholic didn't experience the Type III Silent Craving after the first drink, *none* of the craving types would be an issue for discussion.

Obsession, Craving, or Withdrawal?

WHAT DOES IT matter, whether it's called obsession, craving, or withdrawal? Because the obsession is thinking about nothing other than alcohol. It overshadows all other thoughts. Most see giving in to the obsession by drinking as weak-willed, lacking self-control, a character flaw. But the obsession is *not* the alcoholic-craving—it is only a part of it.

Obsession or Craving?

In addition to the obsession with alcohol, the alcoholic-craving includes a compulsion—an irresistible impulse to drink that ignores consequences and sound reasoning. A dysfunctional brain causes this compulsion, replacing the choice to drink with the need to drink.

With *Type II Sober Craving*, this impaired brain uses stress, anger, remorse, sadness, fear, fatigue, and suicidal thoughts to compel drinking. Elaborate rationalizations that destroy impulse control soon follow. Then, the inability to sleep causes one to lie in misery, wishing for the end but knowing a couple of drinks would, at least temporarily, transform suffering into joy.

Moreover, if that recipe isn't enough to compel drinking, a hangover with a splitting headache, nausea, sweating, and trembling will assist.

Who could decline a liquid that changes one from feeling hopelessly lifeless and suicidal to loving life within minutes? Sober alcoholics have. They have changed in a way that has smothered the craving.

It's much easier for the alcoholic-craving to cause a relapse than a constant thought about alcohol alone. An alcohol obsession doesn't always induce a need to drink. For example, writing this book flowed from an obsession with alcohol without any compulsion to drink.

Is it Withdrawal or the Type II Sober Craving?

Differences abound whether the alcoholic's condition, when briefly sober, is *alcohol withdrawal* or the alcoholic-craving. Although the symptoms slightly overlap, they're different. For example, *physical* withdrawal symptoms may include anxiety, tremors, headache, vomiting, sleeplessness, sweating, hallucinations, and seizures, sometimes causing death. Other than anxiety, these aren't symptoms of the alcoholic-craving.

The alcoholic-craving has only emotional symptoms—anxiety, self-contempt, remorse, irritability, despair, sadness, fatigue, and suicidal thoughts.

Discovering where these feelings and symptoms come from may help the researcher and diagnostician, yet it doesn't help alcoholics in a panic trying to escape their misery.

For example, the alcoholic-craving, withdrawal, or an independent disorder could cause anxiety.* The alcoholic trusts a drink will reduce it no matter the cause.

So, withdrawal may intensify the alcoholic-craving, but withdrawal need not be present for any of the alcoholic-craving types to exist.

Submission to The Type II Sober Craving: A Decision?

"A cocktail sounds good. I wonder if I should have one?" The nonalcoholic thinks about it before answering. She may consider the time, the possible outcomes, whether she must drive,

---

*The DSM-5 defines anxiety as "anticipation of future threat." The word "anxiety" appears 1,294 times in the DSM-5. It lists 11 anxiety disorders. Anxiety appears as a diagnostic criterion for most disorders. It is listed as the seventh diagnostic criterion under "Alcohol Withdrawal." According to the DSM-5, anxiety can precede drinking (craving) and be present during alcohol intoxication.

how drinking now may affect her and others later, and other rational thoughts.

But when the alcoholic wonders if she should drink, she has already 'decided' she will. What follows isn't a decision but a justification. She'll tell herself she won't have over two drinks; what will it hurt? She can drive better after a couple, and no one will know. Finally, her mind erases thoughts of past consequences.

Rarely does the alcoholic ponder whether to drink and decide not to. Deciding weighs the pros and cons. The surrender to the Type II alcoholic-craving is now involuntary and unconscious. It's not a *decision* to drink and to continue drinking.

But she *will* reconsider in the morning when she remorsefully wonders why she drank the first one, which led to drinking too much and missing an important job interview. She's more disappointed in herself than anyone else is. (This is a good time for an intervention.)

When alcoholics need to justify their drinking, they often focus on people and events that provoke anger and resentment. These feelings fuel the alcoholic-craving and dilute feelings of guilt and remorse. This *Type II Sober Craving* causes alcoholics to falsely believe it will be different *this time*, and they can avoid the difficulties drinking causes most every other time. It quashes thoughts of drinking-related problems or any logical reason not to drink with a robust energy that motivates drinking.

This *Type II Sober Craving* is more like an emptiness confiscating thoughts and feelings—an emotional flatness—an infinite sadness. It intensifies as alcoholism progresses.

Many "maintenance" alcoholics, aware or not, maintain a blood/alcohol level to where this *Type II Sober Craving* never appears. These drinkers don't realize they're giving in to the alcoholic-craving. Still, as their condition worsens, no amount of alcohol will hide the craving's presence.

Characteristics of Type II Sober Craving

The following describes the alcoholics' thinking and behavior caused by *Type II Sober Craving*.

- Rationalizing and justifying it's okay to drink.
- Creating excuses and resentments that reduce their guilt about drinking.
- Ignoring good reasons not to drink.
- Thinking this time will be different and ignoring past consequences before drinking.
- Resenting anyone interfering with their plans to drink.
- Setting a limit on how much they will drink.
- Not eating before drinking.
- Needing to drink during and after disputes.
- Deciding to quit drinking—someday.
- Knowing the hours of every nearby liquor store.
- Feeling defensive when asked about drinking.
- Convinced others have unreasonably concerns about their drinking.
- Comparing their drinking to more 'severe' drinkers.
- Hiding most everything about drinking.
- Feeling impatient when waiting for the first drink.
- Breaking promises not to drink.
- Carrying a flask when alcohol won't be available.
- Focusing on the time left before they can drink.
- Creating good reasons to drink.
- Feeling relief after getting a bottle.
- Feeling stress and anxiety when running out of alcohol.
- Worrying about the liquor store closing.
- Questioning if alcohol will be served.
- Leaving an event early to drink.

- Creating a situation that promotes drinking.
- Convincing themselves and others that drinking is their choice, not a requirement.
- Feeling relief after planning or expecting to drink.
- Expecting to change feelings by drinking.

Type III Silent Craving

> This craving is a loss of control driven by an unconscious, *insatiable*, pervasive, and compulsive *need* to continue drinking after the first drink.

Although alcoholics don't notice this *Type III Silent Craving*, everyone else does. It's also the most popular and talked about. This *Type III Silent Craving* propels the compulsion to drink one after another. Drinkers are unaware of any force driving their continuous drinking. Yet, any break in drinking must come from an intervening source. If that occurs, they won't realize the alcoholic-craving prompted their displeasure and resentment toward those interrupting their drinking.

This craving prevents alcoholics from limiting the number of drinks once they start.

This craving causes the brain to think drinking is critical because of the higher amounts of pleasure (dopamine) rapidly released. This craving increasingly overpowers the need for food, water, and sex. The drinker knows eating will cause dopamine levels to plunge, reducing pleasure ("Eating will ruin my buzz"). The typical malnourished and dehydrated condition of the *severe* chronic alcoholic, usually with a nearly absent libido, supports this notion. So when dinner is ready, the alcoholic isn't.

THE DINNER SCENARIO

"**DINNER WILL BE** ready in 20 minutes," echoes down the hall.

"Okay. Thanks." *I have time for a quick one.*

"It'll be ready in 10 minutes."

"Thanks." *I have time for one more.*

"Dinner's ready." *Here it goes again.*

"What? That wasn't 10 minutes—it was more like six or seven. I wish you'd be more precise. Those few minutes put me in a tailspin. I'll be there in a minute." *So I have time for one more if I drink it fast.*

"It was 12 minutes. Dinner's getting cold, and we're waiting on you." *I can already hear it: "Okay. Get started."*

"Okay. Get started. I'm not feeling very good, but I'll try to join you in a minute." *So I have time to chug this last one.*

"I've covered your dinner. You can heat it when you want."

"Thanks. That was fast. Sorry." *It's this timing issue. Oh well, now I can relax and enjoy one more without feeling rushed.*

"I've got an appointment to see a lawyer tomorrow."

"Over five minutes? Whatever." *Always on my back. Well, that calls for one more.*

—

Sadly, what once brought pleasure no longer does. The compulsion to continue drinking also damages sexual relationships. For most, sex is more pleasurable than drunkenness. But the brain only knows what it knows, even when tricked into believing it. And that belief is that the alcoholic needs alcohol to survive. So, while the alcoholic's partner expects sex, the Type III Silent Craving compels continuous drinking until the drinker can't participate—not relationship-enhancing behavior. (See Chapter 8, "The Affected.")

Spending time with family, friends, and hobbies feels bland, almost depressing, so the alcoholic avoids these times. Drinking replaces hobbies. A new set of 'friends' who understand the importance of drinking replaces family and old friends. So, we hear, "All he does anymore is hang out and drink with his new friends, if you can call them that."

Many alcoholics report that one moment, they have an

almost empty drink, and then they're holding a full one, wondering how they got it. So, with this *Type III Continuous Craving*, it's as if temporary amnesia occurs during compulsive and continuous drinking.

It is well-settled science that alcohol abuse disturbs alcohol-related decisions (*prefrontal cortex*). Unconscious activity interferes with and tries to control the conscious judgment center when 'deciding' if to drink more. Drinking is now autonomic, like breathing. And if alcoholics ask themselves, "Should I have another one?" the answer will be "Yes." It's not a reasoned decision but predetermined by an irresistible impulse—a compulsive need.

And that makes sense when we consider drinking dilutes inhibitions, prompting, "Why not; what will it hurt; just one more, and that's it." Still, drinking reduces inhibitions and impulse control when anyone drinks. So why is the normal drinker able to stop?

The Type III Silent Craving and the Alcoholic and Nonalcoholic Brain: A Comparison

Alcohol produces more and a different kind of pleasure in the alcoholic brain than in the nonalcoholic brain. Both brains record the actions we take to preserve life. When the alcoholic brain needs more drinking, it orders the judgment center to focus more on drinking. This is the alcoholic-craving, which the nonalcoholic will never experience.

Alcohol has changed the alcoholic's reward network, so it doesn't work as it should, compelling the alcoholic to drink more.[57] When drinking, the silent message circulated is: "I need this to survive. Remember everything about it, and get more alcohol—now!" This command is as compelling as hunger. The brain acts the same when this Type III Silent Craving compels drinking, like hunger compels eating. Just as our misery intensifies the longer we don't eat, the more the alcoholics' misery intensifies, the longer they don't drink. So, when the brain demands drinking, the only relief for the alcoholic is to focus on drinking with no distractions.

As discussed, the satiation system related to drinking signaling satisfaction is missing in the alcoholic brain. So, the alcoholic-craving intensifies this constant command to drink more, even when the amount consumed reaches dangerous levels. This command is so compelling that it causes some to drink themselves to death—the alcohol overdose.

Conversely, the nonalcoholic brain sends this message: "This was enjoyable, so remember how to do it again if I ever want to. But my life doesn't depend on it, and I'm busy living—so don't give it too much importance." Nonalcoholics put drinking near the bottom of the "Things To Do" list. Alcohol hasn't altered the nonalcoholic brain, so the normal drinker will never *need* alcohol.

The Loss of Control

Over time, excessive drinking changes the chemistry of the alcoholic's brain. It also changes the pathways that send and receive messages between the pleasure and judgment centers. These changes cause the judgment center to become less independent. Although the judgment center is designed to control our impulses and allow us to focus and reason, the pleasure center is now in charge and orders alcoholics to focus only on drinking. These changes produce the Type III Silent Craving, which forces the judgment center to rationalize drinking as reasonable. Moreover, this dysfunction causes one to manipulate, make excuses, deceive, evade, and use other techniques that have placed the alcoholic's character in question throughout time.

Yet, problem drinkers are unaware of the craving fueling their drinking; they just drink one after another. Only when drinking is interrupted will the drinker feel this craving, just like only when our breathing is interrupted will we feel the need and craving to breathe.

The Type III Silent Craving doesn't have the features of the Type I, II, and IV alcoholic-cravings because alcohol numbs them.

But this ignored Type III Silent Craving is obvious when the drinker *repeatedly* says, "I'll have just one more. I mean it *this time.*" Or she protests when her friend calls it a night, and she's just getting started.

During this brief time, the alcoholic lives a glorious life—living in the moment.

Unless she understands alcoholism, is aware that alcoholics experience this, and accepts she's an alcoholic, she may think her loss of control is unique. Yet, she doesn't see herself as an alcoholic. She doesn't have to drink every day but doesn't stop once she starts. She knows she must change what or how she drinks or do something different other than *not drinking*.

When she experiences the prolonged Type III craving, she insists that with more practice, she can control her drinking and get it right—but she can't. She feels more isolated, constantly trying to hide her drinking. She can't discuss her problem with anyone. Alcoholics rarely discuss their lack of control unless they've been sober for a while and intend to remain sober. Admitting loss of control is admitting an alcohol problem that provokes terrorizing thoughts of abstinence.

Abnormal drinkers usually obsess about controlling their drinking for the rest of their lives unless sobriety intervenes and frees them.

Many who are sober go to support meetings often to keep the judgment center working right. It takes time for the brain to change enough until it knows it doesn't 'need' alcohol.

That's one reason many who are newly sober do better with inpatient treatment. This controlled setting makes most decisions until the judgment center improves enough to process reasonably. Still, after being released from treatment, counseling or support meetings remind alcoholics of what they learned. It's also encouraging to hear sober alcoholics tell how they solve problems and cope with sobriety, which is essential for many wishing to *enjoy* continuous sobriety.

Of course, not everyone who occasionally drinks too much is an alcoholic. Most normal drinkers have consumed more than they intended at a time or two. But, this *Type III Silent Craving* isn't an occasional overindulging. Instead, it's a *continuous* pattern of drinking more than intended.

Characteristics of the Type III Silent Craving

The following describes *Type III Silent Craving*.

- Unable to control drinking.
- Saying, "I'll just have one more," repeatedly.
- Feeling panic when hearing "last call."
- Rushing to order another drink after hearing "last call."
- Arguing about the correct time at closing, hoping to squeeze in one more drink.
- Feeling dread when finishing a bottle and unable to get more.
- Resisting food, water, or sleep when drinking.
- Late to or missing important events when drinking.
- Running to the liquor store in a panic before it closes.
- Drinking at the worst times.
- Resisting leaving an unfinished drink.
- Drinking when planning to drive.
- Feeling irritated and angry if drinking is interrupted.
- Drinking more than planned.

William D. Silkworth, MD and the Type III Silent Craving

As discussed, the "phenomenon of craving" Dr. Silkworth coined and talked about only relates to this *Type III Silent Craving*.

Dr. Silkworth believed a physical "allergy" causes this craving, which compels the alcoholic to continue drinking. However, the word allergy is confusing to some. We read words to mean their primary meaning unless an alternative definition is contextually summoned. When considering allergies, we imagine sneezing, watery red eyes, a stuffy nose, and itching. We think of it as an abnormal sensitivity to a substance, resulting in a physical reaction. The allergy is typically a brief reaction, and antihistamines treat it.

The published AA position now is, "Technically, in strictly scientific terms, alcoholism is not a true allergy, the experts now inform us. However, an allergy is a pretty good *figure of speech* to describe our condition."[58] [Italics added]

Maybe a good substitute for the word *allergy* is "sensitivity," which is the official term AA now uses when discussing the alcoholic's reaction to drinking.[59]

In light of recent scientific discoveries, Dr. Silkworth's position that a physical reaction causes nonstop drinking is more accurate than all the descriptions since. The evidence of brain damage supports his theory that stopping at one or two is "beyond [the alcoholic's] ... control."[60]

Silkworth claimed the "phenomenon of craving" only occurs with the alcoholic and never with the nonalcoholic.[61] Research now supports this. It also supports the statement of AA's co-founder, Bill Wilson: "But we are sure that our bodies were sickened as well. In our belief, any picture of the alcoholic which leaves out this physical factor is incomplete."[62]

The effects of this *Type III Silent Craving* are not silent the next morning when alcoholics regret the excesses of the night before. While enduring misery with a throbbing headache and nausea, they wonder why they drank so much, especially since they promised themselves and others that this time would be different.

Type IV Dysphoric Craving

This craving type, present after a drinking episode, seeks to avoid suicidal dysphoria (intense guilt, remorse, and self-contempt) by drinking alcohol or other self-destructive actions, including suicide.

The feelings alcoholics try to avoid surface with the *Type IV Dysphoric Craving*. This misery arrives after a drinking session. The guilt, remorse, and self-hatred are agonizing, worsening the hangover. It's so intense that suicide often seems attractive. (This is the best time for an intervention.)

This is also the time when any remaining self-respect vanishes. The alcoholic doesn't dare to look in a mirror. Their reflection repulses them. Still, they have an unyielding faith that a drink or two will provide them with enough relief, at the moment, to endure life and survive. Then, after a few drinks, they will look in every mirror they pass with increasing self-admiration. Yet, they must continue drinking to avoid feelings of hopelessness and self-contempt.

Yes, a few drinks will provide confidence and contentment. It's difficult to resist such a fast and easy escape from misery that a few ounces of the magic potion will provide. That is, if alcohol is still working. And if it isn't, the emotional pain can cause some, as Silkworth put it, "to make the supreme sacrifice rather than continue to fight."

When sober, the uncomfortable emotions of this *Type IV Disphoric Craving* may stick around for a while, longer without assistance, but eventually, they fade.

THE TEMPER TANTRUM: WITHDRAWAL

WHEN REDUCING OR stopping drinking, the alcoholic brain no longer receives what it believes it needs. So, it panics as it becomes more determined to survive. This results in the alcoholic-craving intensifying and, eventually, withdrawal.

Those who *physically* need alcohol and ignore the brain's demands by refusing to drink will cause the brain to throw a 'temper tantrum.' This tantrum includes dreadful feelings and physical discomfort—the alcoholic-craving and withdrawal symptoms. The brain has adapted to alcohol sedating it and reacts violently without it.

This 'temper tantrum' can cause sweating, increased pulse rate, hand tremors, insomnia, nausea, vomiting, hallucinations, agitation, anxiety, hostility, and seizures.[63] In many, it can be fatal if not medically managed.

These symptoms usually disappear within a few days.* Still, the *Type II Sober Craving* causing fear, uneasiness, sleep problems, and sadness may continue for days, weeks, months, or sometimes years, but they weaken.[64] To lessen these symptoms and the chance of relapsing, many sober alcoholics attend support meetings and counseling.

TOLERANCE AND CRAVING:
SURPRISE, IT STOPPED WORKING!

OUR ADAPTABLE BRAINS aren't designed to cope with large amounts of alcohol. Instead, it's always trying to maintain a chemical balance. When it senses too much pleasure (*dopamine*) caused by too much drinking, the brain corrects this by restricting the pleasure it receives.

Neuroimaging shows that the alcoholic brain restricts pleasure by reducing the 'pleasure receivers' (*dopamine receptors*). This loss of pleasure causes the alcoholic to drink more, trying to feel the effect once enjoyed when drinking less. As alcoholism progresses, the pleasure received with each drink decreases, so the alcoholic drinks more and more, looking more to the bottle as their source of happiness, satisfaction, and fun. Yet, eventually, the bottle quits producing these pleasures.

Sadly, this decrease in the brain's pleasure receivers flattens the ordinary pleasures of life.

Still, the memory of the effect and the motivation to recreate the 'good times' thrives and intensifies. While the dysfunctional brain is blocking dopamine, it's demanding more of it. If the brain doesn't quickly receive what it demands, it obsessively, compulsively, and progressively nags the alcoholic to drink more. This is the alcoholic-craving.

Suppose the brain still doesn't get what it demands. Then,

---

*For those requiring medical management during detox, 20% will die if untreated. Even with medical treatment, up to 4% will die.

it will intensify its command to drink even more by increasing stress, anxiety, irritability, sadness, and other unpleasant feelings. This is the alcoholic-craving strengthening.

The alcoholic obliges by drinking more and enjoying it less. These attempts to satisfy a dysfunctional brain can result in an alcohol overdose, which kills six people daily in the United States.[65]

Meanwhile, the massive amounts of alcohol consumed are damaging other body organs, especially the liver. As the liver becomes more impaired, it increases alcohol metabolization. This results in less alcohol reaching the brain, causing the alcoholic-craving to intensify its demand for even more drinking.

This vicious cycle of the dysfunctional alcoholic brain and liver creates the alcoholic's tolerance. This tolerance also causes more drinking without receiving the expected results while compulsively searching for the obscure euphoria once so easily found.

In time, the alcoholic must drink to feel normal and avoid the discomfort of craving and withdrawal. But normal has become as elusive as euphoria became. It's gone forever if drinking continues.

So, when one boasts they can hold their liquor better than another, they're claiming, "My brain and liver are more damaged than yours."

However, the severely damaged liver can't metabolize alcohol as it once did. This is *reverse tolerance*—the severe alcoholic now becomes drunker without drinking as much— a serious condition.

This reverse tolerance is unending unless treated by depriving the brain of what it demands—alcohol. Ironically, the decision to disobey the brain's demands must come from the same brain making the demands. And that poses a problem considering the judgment center (*prefrontal cortex*) is malfunctioning and using denial to 'protect' and 'defend' it. Most don't overcome this for long without outside help. And many who think they have don't know they haven't.

The majority who never seek sobriety will feel an expanding and impending doom. They feel deserted and stumble helplessly and hopelessly alone, with the cold winds of despair blowing through their spirits. Some will reach out and find what they've been searching for, but most will not. While deep in denial, fueled by their alcoholic-cravings, they insist they don't have a drinking problem or believe no solution exists for their 'unique' condition.

Seeking Sobriety

WHY DO ONLY 10 percent of all alcoholics ever seek recovery, and only half of those stay sober for over a year?[66] That's one out of 20 alcoholics worldwide who will ever have more than a year sober. No other fatal malady with a similar prevalence has such a low recovery rate.

As with those who began drinking alcoholically, achieving sobriety seems mostly situational, depending more on the circumstances the drinker was born into, such as genetics, environment, and, of course, good fortune.

For example, an alcoholic living now rather than 150 years ago has obvious benefits that increase the chances of sobriety. Also, the good fortune of exposure to the right people at the right time can influence the alcoholic's path.

Alcoholics Anonymous believes that becoming and staying sober hinges on the alcoholic's capacity for self-honesty. But some seem incapable of being honest with themselves. AA contends many were born with this inability. While that may be true, I think it goes beyond that. Self-honesty is often proportional to the suffering endured: *Those who have suffered the most are more motivated toward self-honesty*. Still, many motivated alcoholics seem incapable of being honest enough with themselves to escape denial.

Those who aren't as self-honest are usually fearful. Many have endured various experiences that contributed to their fear. Their guardedness prevents them from seeing or showing their true self. If confronted with this, they will quickly dismiss it as nonsense. Whether it's the highly functional professional committed to preserving their persona as 'having it all together' or one raised to hide their feelings, their armor seems impenetrable.

Just as some are more predisposed to alcoholism, others seem more susceptible to recovery. Perhaps various brain structures of those becoming and staying sober are more dominant or less impaired than those who don't. Or the pathways and neurons are different, or the neurotransmitters are balanced differently. Research is studying this.

Also, as discussed later, several drugs have proven effective in decreasing cravings. These drugs might allow one to invite sobriety with more hope and sincerity.

The Winning Ticket

The chances of recovery may be like winning the lottery but with better odds. Suppose the drinker is fortunate enough to have a chance of becoming sober. Like the lottery winner, they must still take action—good fortune alone is not enough.

Chasing the jackpot of sobriety requires effort before realizing good luck or good fortune. One must make a few right decisions and take specific action. For example, a lottery winner must:

- act to have the income to buy the lottery ticket,
- decide to invest with considerable risk of no return,
- choose the amount to invest,
- select where to buy the ticket,
- travel to buy the ticket,
- determine the number and type of tickets to buy,
- preserve the ticket in its original condition,
- get the winning ticket information,
- decide they hold the winning ticket, and finally,
- claim the prize within the claim period or forfeit it.

Congratulations! All alcoholics have the winning ticket. However, the claim periods differ for each and are unknown to all. Many have miscalculated this period, which led to their demise. So, to avoid forfeiture, one must claim their prize of sobriety... *quickly*.

SECTION FOUR

THE RESEARCH

THE NATIONAL INSTITUTE ON ALCOHOL ABUSE AND ALCOHOLISM (NIAAA) is a US government agency that provides the most global funding for alcoholism research.

The Focus of the NIAAA

The *NIAAA Strategic Plan for 2017-2021* and the NIAAA Strategic Plan for 2024-2028 is encouraging. This institute has been increasingly supporting research related to neurobiology. This research reveals Alcohol Use Disorder (AUD) is more a lifelong brain disease than a behavioral disorder. The Executive Summary put it this way:[67]

> [The] NIAAA has supported cutting-edge research [which has] significantly broadened our understanding of the factors that contribute to alcohol-related problems and ... [how] they develop. *Once viewed as a moral failing or character flaw, AUD is now widely regarded as a chronic disease of the brain with potential for recovery and recurrence.* This shift in perspective, supported by advances in neurobiological research, has helped reduce the stigma associated with AUD, led to more effective interventions, and provided support for integrating prevention and treatment services into mainstream health care. [Emphasis added]

Much of this acknowledged and published research reduces the harm alcoholism causes the alcoholic, those affected by the alcoholic, and society.

Research has Ignored the Alcoholic-craving

Until the last 10 years, researchers have mostly ignored the alcoholic-craving. They have decided the "concept of craving is much more complex" than they first thought.[68] One problem is the researchers' inability to agree on the meaning of craving.[69]

Although no agreement defining craving exists, an agreement that craving hasn't been researched enough prevails. In a paper entitled, *Assessing Craving For Alcohol*, which discusses methods of objectively measuring craving, published by the NIAAA,[70] the researchers commented:

> Despite increasing interest in this topic, little agreement exists on how best to conceptualize or measure craving.... Clinical and experimental research has [sic] confirmed the validity of the craving concept.... However, craving presents a descriptive notion, which is still impossible to measure with reliability and validity... The concept of craving has been ignored for over 30 years, only to experience its true "renaissance" in interest, research, debate, and discussion. Although many alcoholics experience craving, researchers have not yet developed a common, valid definition of the phenomenon.

Although the above quote is littered with 'reasons' why and admissions that researchers haven't adequately studied craving, it is difficult to trudge through because it provides no helpful knowledge other than confirming (a) craving exists and (b) researchers have ignored it because they can't adequately define it.

Moreover, the error in the last quoted paragraph stating "*many* alcoholics experience craving" reveals a misunderstanding of alcoholism and the alcoholic-craving. *All* drinking alcoholics experience the alcoholic-craving, not just "many," even if they're unaware they do. Without the alcoholic needing (or craving) a drink, alcoholism wouldn't exist.

Remarkably, most published information about alcoholism has been silent about craving. For example, the NIAAA published a 16-page booklet entitled *Rethinking Drinking*—the word *craving* never appears (rev. 2016).[71]

Still, the research focuses on the *craving for alcohol* rather than the alcoholic-craving. Researchers don't have the information to propose a relevant hypothesis about craving because they haven't gained this information from those with it—the alcoholic layperson. So, their conclusions aren't as helpful.

Another problem is the poor framing of research questions. To yield correct findings, these questions depend on alcoholics to self-report by essentially admitting their alcoholism. Although reliable research needs to interview a target population, the alcoholic population mainly includes those striving to hide their drinking from everyone, including themselves and researchers. The following illustrates this.

The Craving Test

Researchers have been trying to design tests to identify the existence and severity of cravings.[72]

These tests include monitoring objective vital signs such as temperature, heart rate, blood pressure, and salivation. They also include seeing how these vital signs respond to alcohol-related triggers, such as a picture of a liquor bottle or a cold, frothy beer. Neuroimaging has revealed that these triggers excite parts of the alcoholic brain.[73] Some suggest that the intensity of this excitement reveals the extent of the craving.[74]

The subjective parts of these tests claim to evaluate one's "*desire*" for alcohol by asking:

- How many times in the past year have you desired a drink?
- How much do you crave an alcoholic beverage when you've gone without a drink for 1 to 2 days?[75]
- How strong is your desire or urge to drink?

It also factors in the frequency of these desires and urges.

In a 2013 paper (modified 2021) called *Measurement of Alcohol Craving*,[76] the authors reviewed typical craving tests, identifying their strengths and weaknesses.[77] It stated, "Despite considerable research activity and application in treatment, the construct of craving remains poorly understood." Interestingly and regrettably, even this extensive review of craving tests references craving as a *desire* for alcohol instead of a *need*.

I suggest the questions must be less transparent, more effective, and the prompted answers measurable, such as:

- How many times in the past year have you debated whether to drink, resulting in your drinking? (*Drinking when not wanting to reveals the need to drink—the Type II Sober Craving.*)

- How often in the past year have you drunk more than you intended? (*This is loss of control—the Type III Silent Craving.*)

While trying to derail a diagnosis, alcoholics may not disclose every instance they were asked about but are likely to admit it occurred a few times, indicating many.

Predicting Recovery and Relapse

Many researchers believe the severity of cravings predicts the chances of recovery and relapse. They also think this prediction would help design an effective treatment plan.[78]

But predetermining any alcoholic's chances of recovery is dangerous. For example, if she knows her prognosis for recovery is 20%, she'll decide, "Why bother?" And if he learns the chance of his recovery is 80%, he'll think, "Why bother now?" Attempting to predict recovery and relapse is as likely and relevant as forecasting rainfall precisely 500 years from this moment.

These and other research dollars should be spent on

educating healthcare professionals and discovering ways to rescue 90% of all alcoholics who remain untreated and trapped in denial. These funds could treat millions afflicted, help millions more affected (including innocent bystanders), and save $249 billion yearly.*[79]

It's astonishing to see alcoholics who seem doomed recover while others who seem like perfect candidates never do. Many have seen homeless alcoholics, viewed as hopeless, recover and live productive and content lives. Then, we've watched high-functioning professionals, supported by friends and family, struggle and never stay sober.

I suspect the chances of recovery pivot more on the severity of denial, the capacity for self-honesty, and the alcoholics' motivation to quit drinking than on the severity of the craving, which is difficult to measure.

CHEMISTRY OR CHARACTER:
TREATING THE ALCOHOLIC-CRAVING WITH DRUGS

SEVERAL DRUGS HAVE received FDA approval for reducing cravings.°

Over 1,123 studies related to alcoholism are in progress.[80] Many clinical trials to discover the effectiveness of medicines in reducing the alcoholic-craving are pending.[81]

One study testing if psychedelics can reduce craving has shown encouraging results. Johns Hopkins University published a paper in the *Journal of Psychopharmacology* (May 14, 2019), finding "psychedelic use may lead to cessation or reduction in problematic alcohol use..." suggesting further studies.[82]

Also, clinical trials of the drugs Psilocybin and Ketamine

---

*According to the CDC, the yearly economic impact of alcohol misuse in the U.S. was estimated at $249 billion ($2.05 per drink) in 2010.
°According to the Surgeon General's report (11/2016), three medications help reduce cravings: Acamprosate, Naltrexone, and Disulfiram. Also, Gabapentin and Baclofen have decreased cravings.

are in progress.*

So, is it chemistry or character? The research showing that several drugs effectively reduce the alcoholic-craving suggests it is brain chemistry, rather than a moral deficiency, that fuels alcoholic drinking.

Recently, researchers at the University of Virginia have been studying low-intensity focused ultrasound, which is noninvasive and targets the part of the brain associated with craving. Early findings have been promising in reducing cravings.

CRAVING PERFORMS A DISAPPEARING ACT
(The Instant Neurobiological Change)

OCCASIONALLY, THE ALCOHOLIC has an instant psychic change and doesn't need or even want to drink. The alcoholic-craving vanishes, and the reward network doesn't need alcohol to produce pleasure. Although those experiencing this *may* need brief medical help to withdraw physically, they don't have psychological withdrawal symptoms such as anxiety, irritability, depression, fear, fatigue, and suicidal thoughts. On the contrary, these people abruptly feel wonderful.

These documented extraordinary events seem to occur when specific emotions meet *complete* emotional surrender.

Some suggest this results from an alcohol-induced psychosis or an independent mental disorder. Even if it did, many would invite this temporary condition. Those struck by this incredible change typically have no psychiatric diagnosis other than alcoholism, and many stay sober for life.°

But the alcoholic-craving may return unless the alcoholic attends a recovery program that programs the brain to remember alcohol is harmful to it and doesn't need it to cope or to feel life's pleasures.

---

*A Double-Blind Trial of Psilocybin-Assisted Treatment of Alcohol Dependence was started in June 2014 and was scheduled to be completed in December 2020 in Phase 2. Ketamine is also in clinical trials.

°Some reference this as a "spiritual experience," discussed in Chapter 11.

SO, THE DIFFERENCE between the alcoholic and nonalcoholic is mainly within the brain's reward network.

The alcoholic-craving can ebb and flow as it weaves through the alcoholic's mind. If not adequately prepared, it can quickly attack, resulting in a relapse. If the nonalcoholic had the alcoholic's brain, a similar inability to resist would exist. Of course, the nonalcoholic would then be alcoholic.

Not that neurobiology alone decides fate. Various other influences, including environmental and life experiences, play a significant role. So, the alcoholic has a say in seeking sobriety—some apparently more than others.

Although no one experiences the alcoholic-craving the same, this look inside the alcoholic's mind vitalizes a much-needed comprehensive view of the ignored alcoholic-craving.

QUESTIONS FOR DISCUSSION

1. Has this chapter affected you? How?
2. Has this chapter altered your understanding of the alcoholic-craving?
3. If you're an alcoholic, have you ever experienced any of the four craving types discussed in this chapter?
4. Do you identify with any of the listed characteristics of the craving types? If so, which ones?
5. Did the neuroscience discussion increase your understanding of alcoholism (particularly craving)? Explain.
6. After the neuroscience discussion, did you believe alcoholism is more physiological than behavioral? More disease than misbehavior?
7. Do you believe the neuroscience discussion was helpful? If so, in what way? Discuss.
8. Before reading this chapter, did you believe there was a difference between alcohol obsession, alcohol craving, and alcohol withdrawal?
9. How has this chapter helped you?
10. Do you strongly agree or disagree with anything in this chapter? If so, what? Why?
11. Have you learned anything from this chapter? If yes, please discuss.

THE ALCOHOLIC STIGMA
A Blessing in Disguise?

CHAPTER 4

*You're probably an alcoholic if
you've ever alternated liquor stores, so the
clerks don't think you have a drinking problem.*

—

WHAT DO THE *drinking* alcoholic and the leper have in common? The public views them with the same scorn and repulsion, according to sociologists.*[1]

When I mentioned this to an alcoholic 35 years sober, he insisted, "No way! I don't believe it! They won't even let lepers around the rest of us; they're so contagious!" Although he's intelligent, knowledgeable, and a successful professional, he mistakenly believes what most of us do—that leprosy remains a severe threat.

Most are unaware that a cure for leprosy was discovered in the 1940s and that a vaccine is still available.[2] Today, it's one of the least contagious diseases.[3] Still, knowing that will not encourage many of us to book a weekend island getaway to the nearest leper colony.° It exemplifies the stigma's power, causing many to believe something undeniably false.

This chapter explores whether the alcoholic stigma can

---

*Erving Goffman, a renowned sociologist, defined the "leper stigma" as associated with physical deformities and "blemishes of character, *such as are associated with alcoholism.*"

°I'm not disparaging the person with leprosy. My intent is to show the power of stigmas. Indeed, many areas with leper colonies globally are luxurious vacation destinations.

change, and if it can change, should it change? It also discusses methods of rendering the stigma powerless for 90% of all alcoholics who are untreated because, in part, they are shackled by the stigma.

The Meaning of Stigma

The term stigma is derived from Latin and Greek, meaning to mark, brand, or tattoo someone to disgrace them publicly. A social stigma is a set of negative and *often* unfair beliefs that a society or group has about another group. It's the disapproval of those who are different.[4] The stigmatized are shamed, disgraced, dishonored, and humiliated.[5] Stigmas manifest by name-calling (labeling), ostracizing, prejudicing, and discriminating.[6]

The most stigmatized disorders are those society views as self-inflicted or caused by poor moral character.[7] Alcoholics are one of the most harshly stigmatized groups.[8]

Missing the Mark

All prominent organizations insist that ending the alcoholic stigma is critical in combating alcoholism.[*] Yet they don't see that the alcoholic stigma often benefits both sober *and* drinking alcoholics. It can encourage recovery, reduce relapses, and promote companionship through community, thus improving lives.

These organizations contend that the public's opinion of alcoholics would shift if it understood alcoholism is a disease, not a moral issue. This understanding would dissolve the stigma, causing many who no longer feared the label of "alcoholic" to seek sobriety. Although that may be true, what do we do until this lofty dream becomes a reality, if ever?

The World Health Organization (WHO) released a 62-page publication, *Stigma: A Guidebook for Action*, available as

---

[*]These organizations include the NIAAA, NCADD, CDC, WHO, SAMSHA, NOFAS, AMA, Surgeon General's Office, American Psychiatric Association, American Psychological Association, American Council on Alcoholism, etc.

a download.[9] However, even this guide recognizes the questionable chances of success and, to diminish the likely frustration from failure, cautions against optimism by stating:

> Discrimination and stigma is [sic] so widespread throughout every level of society, that tackling it [sic] can seem an impossible task. (p29)

It further gives the following insightful fatalistic forecast:

> It is important to learn from the things that do not work—things *often* do not turn out as planned! (p32) [Italics added]

Although this guidebook is a noble effort, the above quotes inherently recognize that removing the stigma is unlikely.

The message that alcoholism is a disease and not a moral issue from well-respected organizations is aimed at everyone *except* the drinking alcoholic. This message misses the mark because it's the *self*-stigma, not the social stigma, that creates a daunting barrier for the drinker who is considering sobriety.

The Alcoholic Stigma

EVIDENCE OF THE alcoholic stigma is abundant. For instance, through leading health associations, insurance carriers, government agencies, and the law, society *says* alcoholism is a deadly disease. Yet, society doesn't treat it like any other fatal illness, such as cancer and heart disease. Doesn't society treat it as a shameful condition voluntarily brought on by the alcoholic's moral depravity?

For example, when was the last time a school had a charitable run or fundraiser to help fight the disease of alcoholism?

Over 80 unique awareness ribbon colors and designs

exist.[10] But the fight against alcoholism doesn't have one.* No little flags in front yards exclaiming:

**CRUSADE AGAINST ALCOHOLISM
EARLY DIAGNOSIS SAVES LIVES!**

No buttons inscribed with:

JOIN US IN THE FIGHT AGAINST ALCOHOLISM!

No bumper stickers imprinted with:

**I'M PROUD TO HAVE SURVIVED
MANY ALCOHOLIC RELAPSES!**

No balloons that say:

WALK THE WALK—UNITED AGAINST ALCOHOLISM!

No t-shirts that read:

I'M AN ALCOHOL SURVIVOR!

IN 1981, THE USPS issued this commemorative postage stamp stating, "Alcoholism—You can beat it!" According to the USPS, this controversial stamp prompted more complaints than any other. Many who received mail with this stamp were offended, even if they didn't drink. Only 90 million were printed.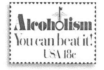

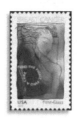 In contrast, the post office issued this breast cancer research stamp in 1998. According to the USPS, over one billion stamps have been sold, generating over $92.6 million to support breast cancer research.°

The alcoholism stamp wasn't a fundraiser

---

*Recently, the red ribbon has been associated with substance abuse awareness, which includes all substances, not just alcohol abuse, which is more widespread than every other substance. In 2011, President Obama issued the first-ever Presidential Proclamation designating October as National Substance Abuse Prevention Month.

°This type of stamp is a fundraising stamp. The price of the stamp includes the first-class postage rate plus an amount to fund a specific cause.

stamp, so it raised nothing. No one receiving the cancer stamp complained. Yet there are 42,000 breast cancer deaths and 178,000 alcohol-related deaths yearly. And there are 40 times more alcoholics than those with breast cancer; still, the cancer stamp sold over 12 times more.

Undoubtedly, society doesn't view alcoholism as it does other deadly diseases, which further shows that the alcoholic stigma remains one of the strongest stigmas.

FIVE ALCOHOLIC STIGMAS

I'VE OBSERVED WHAT appears to be five types of alcoholic stigmas: 1) the stigma of sober alcoholics, 2) the *self*-stigma of drinking alcoholics, 3) the stigma of drinking alcoholics, 4) the stigma of dry alcoholics, and 5) the stigma of women alcoholics.

1) The Stigma of Sober Alcoholics

I've never spoken with a sober alcoholic who feels *significantly* stigmatized. Those sober for years often receive praise for their strong 'willpower.'* This confirms the prevalence of the common misconception that it takes willpower for the alcoholic not to drink, which supports the stigma. Although the sober alcoholic stigma is much less noticed than the drinking alcoholic stigma, *both exist.*

Also, one's status seems to affect the impact of the stigma relating to whether they admit their alcoholism. For example, a sober political candidate is more reluctant to disclose their alcoholism than one sober applying for work on a painting crew comprised of other sober alcoholics.

Still, I've often noticed sober alcoholics lower their voices when discussing alcoholism publicly. At some level, they know the sober alcoholic stigma exists. Yet, they have ignored it enough, so it barely affects them.

---

*It doesn't involve a strong will when one doesn't want or need to drink, nor is strong will enough to refuse a drink when *needing* one.

I recently talked with an intelligent and successful professional woman who is a three-year sober alcoholic about the alcoholic stigma. She insisted it doesn't exist. I tried convincing her that it did. She remained unconvinced.

After considering it, I decided she was right. A stigma can only exist if the ones targeted fuel it by self-stigmatizing. She doesn't think it exists, so for her, it doesn't.*

But it's not the stigma of sober alcoholics that interferes with one seeking sobriety. Instead, it's the self-stigma of drinking alcoholics coupled with the social stigma that creates the barrier.

2) The Self-Stigma of Drinking Alcoholics

For a stigma to harm, the targeted group must feel stigmatized. It's common for those stigmatized to act in ways the stigmatizer expects.[11] Drinking alcoholics self-stigmatize by adopting the public's shaming of them.[12] Their negative self-talk results in persistent embarrassment, humiliation, guilt, shame, remorse, and self-loathing. It's worse after a drinking episode; then, it declines until revived by the next hangover. This self-stigma feeds the social stigma, worsening the alcoholic's condition.

Drinking alcoholics feel inferior—feeling like they're a disappointment to everyone, including themselves. They're convinced that someday they will get it together, quit drinking, and maturely cope with life. But that goal remains elusive. While blaming themselves for their affliction, they're too embarrassed to seek help as they slip further into their progressing disease.

This self-stigma intensifies as alcoholism progresses. At some point, these drinkers will stigmatize themselves more than others do. The public stigma becomes irrelevant when alcoholics think less of themselves than others think of them, and misery entombs them. When the will to survive eclipses

---

*Still, she glanced around and lowered her voice when she whispered, "Alcoholism." Nor has she revealed her alcoholism to her employer.

the opinions of others, self-stigmatization will not interfere with sobriety. And, as we'll see, drinking alcoholics who are *desperate* enough will seek sobriety despite their self-stigmatization.

3) The Stigma of Drinking Alcoholics

A 2010 Oxford University study reveals that most people prefer distancing from drinking alcoholics much more than they do from those with other mental disorders.[13]

According to this study, despite respected organizations officially supporting the disease concept, most people don't, including most members of these organizations. Instead, they believe alcoholics can control their drinking.

Not surprisingly, this study found that drunks excite more irritation, anger, and repulsion than anyone else with any other mental disorder. It also reported that many oppose spending money on alcoholism research.[14]

Moreover, this study found that people view drunks as unpredictable, untrustworthy, dangerous, obnoxious, repulsive, dishonest, and self-absorbed.[15] These traits aren't present with intoxication from other substances such as opioids, cannabis, hallucinogens, amphetamines, cocaine, and sedatives.

We've heard or said, "Drinking is a choice. Millions of alcoholics have stopped, so those who keep drinking must be weak-willed and character-flawed." Although that thinking creates what it condemns, it prevails. That is, the drinker in denial thinks their drinking is a secret, which it rarely is. So, they 'avoid' the label of "weak-willed and character-flawed" by remaining silent, fearing treatment will reveal their secret and invite this labeling. Consequently, their silence feeds their belief in this stigma, which fuels it more.

4) The Stigma of Dry Alcoholics

Few realize, including many sober *and* drinking alcoholics, that drinking is merely a symptom of alcoholism.[16] That means the underlying disorder—the maladjustment and inability to cope with life on life's terms—remains when drinking stops.

Since alcoholism is treatable but incurable, other symptoms become more noticeable when the alcoholic stops drinking.

Recovery treats the underlying cause of this dry condition. Still, many alcoholics claim they don't need help to quit. Unfortunately, they mistakenly believe that the only purpose of continuous treatment is not drinking.

The untreated, dry alcoholic, commonly referred to as a "dry drunk," causes some to silently scream: "He was easier to deal with when he was drinking. I almost wish he never quit!" As a result, dry drunks often contribute to the alcoholic stigma.

5) The Stigma of Women Alcoholics

Society stigmatizes women alcoholics more than it does men.[17] Only 5.4% of alcoholic women, compared with 7.4% of alcoholic men, seek treatment.[18] One reason is the traditional role society has assigned to women as family caregivers. The responsibilities associated with caring for others leave little time for themselves or their ambitions, which makes it more challenging to receive inpatient or outpatient care. And the financial barriers that are often unique to women increase this challenge. Still, society criticizes women for not getting help.

When alcoholic women need a break, they drink to cope. They hide their drinking more than men, fearing the label of "bad mother."

Women are diagnosed with eating, anxiety, depression, and trauma-related disorders at double the rate of men.[19] Dual-disordered women—those with one of these disorders, plus alcoholism—boost society's disapproval of them and them of themselves.

Women react biologically differently to alcohol.[20] They metabolize it slower, becoming drunk sooner while drinking less.[21] Additionally, they develop more alcohol-related medical issues much earlier.[22] Also, neuroimaging reflects that women's brains are more susceptible to damage from drinking.[23]

Hormonal issues further complicate their alcoholism.[24] Premenstrual syndrome (also known as premenstrual dysphoric disorder) in some women causes severe depression, anxiety, insomnia, fatigue, and physical pain. This syndrome intensifies the alcoholic-craving, making it more difficult to abstain. Menopause also causes other complex issues affecting sobriety. Women also incur more alcohol-related consequences.* All of this increases the disparate stigma of women alcoholics.

Potential pregnancy presents another issue. If fetal alcohol syndrome results,° the shame and guilt are devastating, usually lasting a lifetime. The stigma toward these mothers exceeds most stigmas.[25]

So, while society sees alcoholic men as weak-willed, it views alcoholic women as reckless, lazy, and selfish.

CAN AND SHOULD THE ALCOHOLIC STIGMA CHANGE?

WHETHER THE ALCOHOLIC stigma can change depends on whether it's rational, irrational, or both, the strength of the fear that powers it, and whether this fear is reasonable, unreasonable, or both.

Fear and Stigmas

Fear is the power plant of the stigma. Fear breeds stigmas: the stigmatizer and the stigmatized fear one another.

Although we typically think of fear as a negative emotion, we know the human race would have perished long ago had

---

*Alcohol-related emergency department visits for women are 55.5% and 43.4% for men.
°Fetal Alcohol Spectrum Disorders, also known as FAS, includes fetal alcohol syndrome. Women who consume alcohol while pregnant risk their babies having learning, physical, and/or behavioral problems.

we never feared. Fear energizes us to protect ourselves from life-threatening danger. If we ignore fear, it will intensify until we recognize it and act to protect ourselves.

Fear is often contagious. When facing a threat, we invite others to unite, fostering strength and protection for us and those who join us—division maintains weakness. This instinctive need to unify and protect us from those we fear incites the stigma.

We're designed to overfear a threat and survive than to underfear it and perish. Yet occasionally, our fears far exceed this design, resulting in unreasonable fear. Reasonable fear creates rational stigmas, unreasonable fear drives irrational stigmas, and a mix of reasonable and unreasonable fear fuels other hybrid stigmas.

The Rational, Irrational, and Hybrid Stigmas

Although most consider stigmas harmful, some can be helpful. Whether the alcoholic stigma is harmful or helpful and subject to change depends on whether it fits within one of these three categories: 1) *The Rational Stigma*, 2) *The Irrational Stigma*, or 3) *The Hybrid Stigma: Rational and Irrational.*

1) The Rational Stigma

Rational stigmas are reasonably related to fear, have beneficial qualities, and can be logically explained.

For instance, the stigma of the convicted criminal is rationally based. The more violent and abhorrent the crime is, the more we fear and ostracize the offender. And the more we fear, the more the stigma intensifies and the longer it lives.

Society isolates those with infectious diseases during epidemics to protect the healthy ones. For example, a recent COVID-19 pandemic caused a reasonable fear, requiring those infected, including those exposed to infection, to quarantine. While isolated, others whispered about their condition, which resulted in a rational stigma.

So, the benefit of rational stigmas is protection and survival. A rational stigma rarely, if ever, disappears. But at times, we go too far and fear irrationally.

2) The Irrational Stigma

The irrational stigma includes negative feelings toward a group merely because they look, believe, or act differently. This stigma is harmful.

When a group ostracizes and stigmatizes others because of their religious beliefs, sexual orientation, spoken language, gender, or race, with no rational basis, it is an irrational stigma powered by fearing a threat that doesn't exist. Changing *pervasive* stigmas without logical roots can be challenging, but they have changed.

Affirmative action and other legislation have partially equalized the playing field and mitigated the effects of many irrational stigmas.

3) The Hybrid Stigma: Rational and Irrational

The Hybrid Stigma is both rational and irrational. This stigma resists change more than an irrational stigma because it includes rational fear.

For example, the terrorist's primary weapon *is* fear. They program their victim to fear a danger that doesn't exist by occasionally doing what they constantly threaten. Terrorism creates an irrational fear, often resulting in post-traumatic stress disorder (PTSD).[26] These irrational fears cause an excessive and costly overreaction, including using security measures that outweigh the risk.

We see the effects of irrational fear globally at airports, triggered by one terrorist act nearly 25 years ago, known as the 9/11 attack. It has cost billions and caused great inconvenience to reduce the chances of not only a potential attack but also the *fear* of such an attack. The irrational part of the stigma is so tangled up with the rational part that it isn't prone to untangling. Therefore, even the irrational or unreasonable portion of the stigma doesn't lend itself to weakening.

KNOWING IF THE stigmas that have changed are rational or irrational will help us decide if the alcoholic stigma is a candidate for alteration.

A Brief Review of Evaporating Stigmas

HISTORY IS RIDDLED with stigmas. We've stigmatized mental disorders, physical disabilities, infectious diseases (e.g., leprosy, smallpox, AIDS, COVID-19), illegitimacy, sexual orientation, gender identity, skin color, nationality, paupers, welfare recipients, ethnicity, religion, occupations, criminality, and much more.

This historical glance at stigmas that have drastically *weakened* will help answer whether the alcoholic stigma is subject to shrinking.

The Sexual Orientation Stigma

Same-sex attraction was heavily stigmatized 50 years ago. Although the stigma has softened, we know it exists. The related slang terms further evidence its presence.

We reacted fearfully as closet doors increasingly opened. Could same-sex orientation ever threaten the extinction of humans and, therefore, be a rational stigma? Theoretically, yes, if everyone were same-sex-oriented, we would no longer reproduce, and humanity would end. But everyone isn't.

We become more open-minded and receptive to truth once we allow logical reasoning to prevail over our emotions. Unjustified and unproductive fear then dissolves, allowing the stigma to evaporate. For example, the laws providing for same-sex marriages show that the stigma is fading.

Occasionally, the actions of those condemning others become so offensive that it triggers a 'rebound compassion' for the stigmatized group and weakens the stigma by branding the

The Gender Stigma

Although stigmatizing women in the United States and elsewhere has been slowly changing, it remains.

Women's status in the workplace is still disproportionately lower.* On average, women receive lower pay for equal work unsupported by any rational basis.[27]

Historically, this stigma was partly rational. Women delivered and nurtured newborns, a biological impossibility for men. Society believed mothers could raise children better than fathers. Women were homemakers and expected not to work outside the home.

But WWII changed that. Women filled positions left by men who enlisted. Before the war, women were fewer than 25% of the workforce. Today, 47% of all employees are women. More women than men have bachelor's degrees by age 29.[28] During this change, women became more vocal, insisting on parity.

One hundred years ago, women couldn't vote.° The first woman to sit on the U.S. Supreme Court was in 1981. Today, 43 years later, four of the nine justices are women. In 2016, this country nominated a woman for president for the first time, winning 2.1% more of the popular vote than the elected president. In 2020, a woman became the first U.S. vice president, and in 2024, she ran for president.

All the evidence shows that this prejudice is irrational. As time passes, gender-based economic, political, and social disparities have improved, reducing the stigma.

---

*Women occupy less than 20% of political offices, although they make up 50.8% of the U.S. population. They account for 78.4% of the labor force in healthcare and social aid, but only 14.6% of executive officers and 12.4% of board directors of healthcare companies are women. None of the CEOs of these businesses are women. There are many other instances of similar disparities.

°In 1920, the 19th Amendment allowed women to vote.

The Racial Stigma

The stigma attached to African Americans is unique in that, unlike the other irrational stigmas, it was never conceivably rational.

Wide racial gaps still exist despite slavery ending nearly 160 years ago, the Civil Rights Act of 1968, and desegregation. Although the earning disparity between Blacks and whites has narrowed, it remains vast, with Blacks earning about a third less than whites.

Black physicians have doubled since 1940, yet despite a Black population of over 13%, they still only make up 5.4% of all physicians. Further, only 5% of lawyers are Black. Additionally, while Black teachers increased by 25% in the past 25 years, only 6.1% of public school teachers are Black. And only 34% of Black people have associate degrees or higher compared with 50% of whites. The disparities continue.

It wasn't until 1965 that the first Black man became a Supreme Court Justice. In 2008, 43 years later, the first Black President of the United States was finally elected. In 2020, a woman of African American descent became the first vice president, and in 2024, she ran for president.

The slow shrinking of this stigma shows that even a pervasive and severe irrational stigma can and will *eventually* diminish.

The Mental Illness Stigma

It's undisputed that the mental illness stigma exists. Historically, the brutal and cruel treatment of the mentally ill was standard.[29]

Until a couple of hundred years ago, people believed evil caused mental illness.[30]

Many, embarrassed and ashamed of their mentally ill children, hid them from the public, forcing them to live in cellars and basements. Eventually, insane asylums multiplied and caged the "insane" in small rooms that were never cleaned. These people were chained, preventing them from lying down to sleep, and forced to sit in their waste. And it was often much worse than that.*[31]

Society stigmatizes psychological more than physical suffering.[32] It's widely accepted that many afflicted with bipolar, depression, schizophrenia, and other mental disorders have a tough time getting well solely because of the stigma.

Although the mental illness stigma is part rational and part irrational, the discovery of effective treatments has been reducing the irrational portions of the stigma.

Until recently, the law has unreasonably restricted the rights of those with mental disorders.° However, new laws are protecting their rights, which reveals the irrational portions of the mental illness stigma are fading.

The Japanese-American Stigma

It was purportedly the *fear* of Japanese disloyalty that propelled the internment of Japanese Americans during WWII. Many were natural-born U.S. citizens, including 60,000 mothers and their young children who were forcibly relocated to camps.[33]

However, according to the Commission on Wartime Relocation and Internment of Civilians (CWRIC), no evidence existed to support the prevalent and pervasive fear of disloyalty and found that "race prejudice, war hysteria, and a failure of political leadership" fueled the stigma which resulted in the acts of internment.[34] Although conceivably rationally based initially, as the irrationality soon surfaced, the stigma quickly weakened, and it is now mostly abated.

ALTHOUGH THIS IS a partial list, it shows the softening of

---

*'Treatment' included drilling holes in scalps, bloodletting (phlebotomy), laxatives, removing or mutilating brain sections (lobotomy), shock treatment causing bone fractures, the "gyrating chair" (shook the patient unconscious), beatings, torture, punishment, confinement, restraints, padded cells.

°For example, laws restricting owning handguns and disparate treatment of mentally ill intruders in one's home are abundant.

irrational stigmas in the past century. Therefore, we can initially conclude that an irrational stigma can and will eventually fade.

IDENTIFYING THE ALCOHOLIC STIGMA: IRRATIONAL, RATIONAL, OR BOTH?

DECIDING WHETHER THE alcoholic stigma is rational, irrational, or both will tell us if it's even a candidate for modification. Doing this requires identifying the stigma. It's also necessary to trace the source of the stigma and determine if any part is valid.

We have seen that the alcoholic stigma is real and pervasive—playing a leading role in the denial of alcoholism. It has been an obstacle for many in deciding whether to seek sobriety.

However, the alcoholic stigma did not arise from a vacuum—it had a beginning. According to archaeological discoveries, the first fermented drink made and drunk was 7000-6600 BC during the Neolithic period (10,000-5,000 BC).[35] The consensus is that drunkenness existed as far back as recorded history. The birth of the stigma likely occurred the first time a drunk acted offensively.

So, let's travel back to the place and time where the alcoholic stigma began.[*]

THE STORY OF
THE ALCOHOLIC WHO STARTED THE STIGMA

THIS SETTING IS the small village of Jiahu in the Henan province of Northern China. The landscape is beautiful, with rolling green hills framed by massive, deep chestnut brown rock formations and hundreds of cliffs. A large cobalt blue lake centers the village, creating a mirrored reflection.

Seven thousand years ago, a villager wanders the countryside on a gorgeous morning and stumbles on some

---

[*]Although fictional, it's loosely based on anthropological archaeology.

fallen fruit. It's not fresh fruit. He kicks some out of the way and tramples a few, which squirts juice. He pauses, looks around, and walks off his beaten path to tour the area. He avoids stepping on the undamaged fruit. He sees that some look better than others, but none has freshly fallen. He bends over, picks one up, and inspects it.

He blows off some dirt and gently squeezes it—it's soft. He smells it—smells okay. With his sharpbone, he makes a small cut on the cleaner side. Some juice oozes. He touches the droplet and rubs it between the tips of his forefinger and thumb until it disappears. He then touches the end of his nose. Looking puzzled, he flicks his tongue across his fingertips with a curious facial expression. He cuts the fruit deeper and squeezes a few drops on his tongue. After a few minutes, he squeezes more on his tongue. His eyes squint, and his mouth puckers.

After 15 minutes, he leans his head back, opens his mouth, and squeezes out the remaining juice.

Minutes later, he's smiling from ear to ear, bursting out in laughter and humming a melody. He makes his way to the village with a skip in his walk to find Barney.

"Hey, Barney, come see what I found!"

Barney is busy and resists, but Fred insists. "Okay, Fred, give me a minute. I'm coming."

"Hurry up, Barney. The good ones might disappear unless we hurry!"

"What is it, Fred? Tell me, tell me!"

"Oh, my little buddy, this is beyond telling. This needs showing."

They arrive.

"What, Fred?" Barney looks around and shakes his head. "All I see, Fred, is a bare tree." He squints his face, covers his mouth and nose with his hand, then steps back and moans, "And all this rotten fruit on the ground."

"That's it, Barney! Taste one!"

"Fred, you're acting weird. I'm not eating one of those

rotten things. They look and smell nasty."

"Barney! You don't have to *eat* it. Just squeeze the juice into your mouth like this." So, Fred cuts one and empties the juice into his mouth. He pierces another one and hands it to Barney. "Now squeeze it in your mouth ... I won't tell you again." Fred is more aggressive than usual.

"Okay, Fred, if it'll make you happy."

"Barney, it's going to make *you* happy, very happy!"

So, Barney squeezes and swallows the juice—slowly. Then, a few minutes later, he squeezes another one—less slowly. And then, he squeezes the third one, and after a few minutes, he turns to Fred and yells, "Yabba Dabba Doo! I just discovered the meaning of life!" Both squeeze one after another.

OVER THE NEXT few days, Barney spends all his time squeezing the fruit into pottery jugs. He ferments the drink with rice, honey, and hawthorn fruit, sometimes adding grapes.

He offers it to the villagers. Some try and like it, but no one wants more than a few swigs. They feel good, but more than half a mug causes them to feel uncomfortable and disoriented.

The more Barney drinks, the faster he drinks. He's now drinking nonstop and acting like a different person. The villagers don't know what to think.

Everyone loved Barney, the top producer in the village ... before he started drinking. Now, he's slurring his words, staggering, and bumping into others.

He's no longer working—he spends all his time making the fermented drinks and drinking. He drinks from sunrise until he collapses. He misses important meetings and gets nowhere on time. He's dangerous, risking his life and the lives of others.

He's unprovocatively aggressive. He talks nonstop about bizarre ideas—even when no one is around to hear him. When anything goes wrong, he blames someone else.

He becomes enraged when anyone mentions his drinking.

He used to be respectful of the women, but now he shouts inappropriate comments, so they avoid him. As he's casting provocations at the men, he postures into a fighting stance. A moment later, he insists they hug it out.

Lately, he's been careless while trying to spear the moon. When his spear lands, it often barely misses strolling villagers.

He becomes loud and angry, and then, seconds later, he sobs. His sobbing is loud and is lasting longer. He calls a village meeting, apologizing for his actions and promising to change. But despite his apologies and promises, he continues drinking and remains dangerous and offensive.

Fred decides to end this nonsense and meets Barney to discuss his drinking, but it's not as easy as he thought. "Barney, I want to talk to you about your drinking, but it looks like you've already had a few."

"I've only had a couple, Fred."

But Fred marked the jugs and knows he's had more. "Barney, if you don't stop drinking this stuff, we're going to have some real problems."

"Fred, don't make me kill you."

"What'd you just say?"

While Barney reaches for his spear, he asks, "Hey Fred, is that a fish on your face?"

"Why would you ask me that? Of course, there's no fish on my face."

"Well, I see one, and I'm getting ready to spearfish!"

Barney gives Fred a chilling glare, pulls back his spear, and aims it at him. Fred runs for his life.

Barney yells a threat that echoes off Stone Mountain, "Fred, you'll have to sleep sometime ... time ... time ... time ... time!"

EVERYONE QUICKLY LEARNS that confronting Barney about his drinking is a bad idea, so things are a bit tense.

Barney tries to control his drinking by using more rice or less honey when making the beverage. He tries other methods, but nothing works. Then, in a moment of intense remorse over a villager he injured with his reckless spearing, he promises never to drink again.

Fred and the villagers celebrate. But the next day, he's drunk. The villagers meet to decide what to do with Barney, who has become the village's nuisance and a menace. While deciding Barney's fate, they scratch their heads, run their fingers through their long, tangled beards, and mumble a few words. Then the village leader stands and, in a deep, monotone voice, slowly and loudly announces: "We will shackle him to Shackle Rock in the center of the village until we know he will never drink again."

So, the shacklers search for Barney, but they can't find him because he's with the leader, talking his way out of shackles with a flood of promises. The village leader gives him one more chance.

During that same moonlit night, while standing on the edge of Starview Cliff trying to spear the moon, Barney slips and falls to his death.

From then on, every seventh sunset, while sitting around the fire, the villagers tell stories about Barney, the village drunk, hoping to dissuade others from following his path. And these fireside chats were the origin of the alcoholic stigma—or something like that.

SINCE THE STIGMA began, it has been twisted by the drunk alcoholic's behavior, bent by the opinion of nonalcoholics, warped by hundreds of years of rhetoric trying to classify alcoholism, and squeezed by plenty of studies. But thousands of years later, the alcoholic stigma shows few signs of damage. It's almost as robust as ever. So why hasn't much change occurred like we saw with irrational stigmas? Could it be that the alcoholic stigma is at least partly rational?

Assume everyone understands that the drunk alcoholic who is loud, aggressive, offensive, repetitive, emotive, invasive, repulsive, disruptive, and insensitive is a sick and blameless person. Will people change their feelings about the drunk? Undoubtedly, no policy changes, declarations, legislation, or reliable scientific studies will change our reflexive attitude toward the excessively drunk alcoholic, convinced he's enlightening us with slurred words treated with spit mists.

THEY CAN RUN, BUT THEY CAN'T HIDE

THE LEPROSY STIGMA was once rationally based. People feared the disease because it caused disfigurement and was highly contagious. Society ostracized lepers by banishing them to remote islands and isolated places with others who were infected.[36] Although leper colonies still exist, they're occupied voluntarily, and many are tourist spots with museums.*[37]

Groups have worked hard toward removing the leprosy stigma, with little success—the stigma remains.[38]

Those interested in minimizing the leprosy and alcoholic stigmas have promoted name changes.[39] They believe the terms leper and alcoholic are stigmatizing.[40]

The Leprosy Mission thinks the word "leper" is "derogatory, ostracizing, and outdated." Rather than the term leper, they now suggest "People/Person with Leprosy."°[41]

Similarly, the American Psychiatric Association (APA) now replaces the terms alcoholism and addiction with "mild, moderate, or severe alcohol use disorder (AUD)," preferring this "more neutral term" to alcoholism with its "uncertain definition and potentially negative connotation."[42] What about using the acronym PWL for the leper? Wouldn't that camouflage the leper as well as AUD hides the alcoholic?**

Undoubtedly, the pure motives and good intentions be-

---

*Over the years, communities of Lepers have developed, and many are undisturbed because that is where they feel a sense of community and can escape stigmatization. Many of these communities have become tourist spots. I wonder whether tourists would visit a community of drunk alcoholics.

°In 1931, a group of lepers advocated changing the name leprosy to Hansen's disease to mitigate stigma. It is now known and referred to as Leprosy/Hansen's disease.

**Why hasn't the National Institute on Alcohol Abuse and Alcoholism changed its name to the National Institute on Alcohol Use Disorder?

hind these name changes are to label the disease rather than the person, allowing people to distance themselves from the condition since it's not who they are but what they have. It's no longer name-calling. Still, whether name-calling is insulting depends on the name. For example, calling someone a saint doesn't offend. So, none of this would be an issue if health care didn't hold the stereotypical view of the alcoholic (person with AUD) as a pathetically self-absorbed, undisciplined waste of time.

These name changes suggest that the alcoholic and the leper must hide *more* from the stigma. But if one has nothing to hide, why hide? Moreover, hiding a condition implies that it's shameful and needs hiding, which further feeds the stigma and bolsters shame. It's like an infamous person legally changing their name, trying to hide their identity and reputation. Eventually, the new name will identify the condition of the group it's trying to conceal.

Another problem with this terminology change is its potential effect on the denial of drinking alcoholics. For example, one branded with only *mild* AUD will likely decide there's plenty of time left to drink before seeking sobriety. It's the perfect excuse and solidifies denial. When their AUD is *moderate*, they will consider doing something about it, and if it becomes *severe*, they will take prompt action, but certainly not now.

Changing the name of the targeted group is ineffective, offensive, and will likely have an unintended outcome.

A Comparison of the Alcoholic and Leper Stigmas

Comparing the leper and alcoholic stigmas will further identify and discover whether the alcoholic stigma can change.

Similarities

- Both stigmas originated thousands of years ago.
- Both conditions cause embarrassment and shame.

- Both refrain from admitting their condition and receiving treatment, fearing further stigmatization.
- Both have advocates unsuccessfully trying to end or, at least, reduce the stigma (e.g., name changes).
- The stigmatizing group considers both second-class people.
- Society has shunned and ostracized the leper and the alcoholic.
- The families of both also suffer from stigma.
- Both stigmas are mainly based on misinformation. People think the leper is still highly contagious, and the drinking alcoholic has a flawed character.
- Both are stereotyped as impoverished (e.g., the skid row homeless drunk and the leper colony resident on a deserted island).
- Both have derogatory references to them in the Bible (according to many theological interpretations, drunkenness and leprosy are punishments for past sins).
- Both have been confined to sanitariums.
- People insist on 'safe' distancing from both.
- Lepers were physically cast away and forced to colonize deserted islands—alcoholics were emotionally banished and forced to colonize emotionally deserted islands (isolation).

Dissimilarities

- Often, the active alcoholic has alienated family and friends while the leper's family remains close.
- Alcoholism is much more prevalent than leprosy.*
- The symptoms of leprosy are not aggression, improper sexual conduct, rapid mood swings, and inappropriate

---

*According to the World Health Organization, globally, there are 2-3 million people with leprosy and 380 million alcoholics.

reactions, which terrorize those present.

- Leprosy has a vaccine and has had a cure for 75 years, while alcoholism has neither.
- Alcoholics can more easily disguise their condition (when sober) while the leper can't.
- Society forced Lepers to colonize deserted islands in remote regions, but alcoholics were not.
- Leprosy is a disease—the debate about whether alcoholism is a disease continues. Most of the public believes it is not.
- Most believe the alcoholic's condition results from willful misconduct, while leprosy results from misfortune.

Alcohol Intoxication is Unique and Supports the Stigma

ALTHOUGH ALCOHOL IS clumped with other substances, in the *Substance Abuse* section of the DSM-5, it is different.*[43] Though it directly affects the brain's reward network, like other substances, the alcoholic brain processes it differently.[44]

Alcohol is legal and socially acceptable, and the conviviality with others encourages its open consumption. In small doses, it *may* be healthy.° In moderate amounts, it acts as a social lubricant, inspiring a festive time. But alcoholics don't drink small doses or moderately. When alcoholics drink, it's usually excessive and often offensive. And this offensive conduct supports the rational portion of the alcoholic stigma.

Symptoms of Alcohol Intoxication are Unique

The symptoms of alcohol intoxication *include* 1) inappropriate sexual behavior, 2) aggression, 3) mood lability (rapid mood changes), 4) impaired judgment, 5) reduced memory

---

*The other substances in this section are amphetamines, cocaine, cannabis, hallucinogens, inhalants, hypnotics and anxiolytics, sedatives, and other unknown substances.

°Recent studies now suggest that any alcohol consumption may be unhealthy.

and attention, 6) unsteady gait (staggering), 7) slurred speech, 8) incoordination, 9) stupor or coma, and 10) nystagmus (involuntary eye movement).[45]

Seven of these 10 symptoms are also present when under the influence of other substances. The three symptoms collectively present and unique to excessive drinking are 1) sexual impropriety, 2) labile mood, and 3) aggression.[46]

Labile mood is intense mood swings occurring quickly (usually within seconds or minutes) with emotional reactions outside an expected response. These reactions may include outbursts, throwing items, threats of homicide or suicide, aggression toward oneself or others, and terrorizing behavior.

When drinkers are aggressive, they emotionally and physically harm the target of their aggression. Aggression, combined with sexually inappropriate conduct, gestures, or comments, increases this harm.

This behavior explains why drunkenness is more offensive and dangerous than intoxication from all other substances, causing others to protect themselves by distancing from the offender, which increases stigmatization.

To illustrate, imagine a drunk making offensive comments to a woman while inappropriately touching her. She resists his aggression by walking away. The drunk's reaction to the rejection includes slurring obscene and threatening words, throwing an item in her direction, bumping into and damaging property, ignoring pleas not to drink another one, and loudly repeating slurred words until passing out with little or no recall the following day.

Her thoughts and feelings about the 'obnoxious drunk' will not likely change, even if she's convinced his conduct is symptomatic of a disease. *It is not stigma-reducing conduct.* Who wouldn't ostracize and stigmatize a person acting this way?

Drinking Appears Voluntary

We also condemn drunken behavior because it *appears* voluntary (e.g., "Why did he drink so much?"). The non-alcoholic sees a sober person pour alcohol into a glass, bring it to their mouth, drink, and swallow. They know this action results in drunkenness and consequences (e.g., "They brought it on themselves."). It looks like a choice—a lack of willpower. Because they have never experienced the alcoholic-craving, as discussed in Chapter 3, they will have no empathic source of understanding.

Stigma and Empathy

We can't truly empathize with one having feelings we've never felt. It's like someone childless understanding the flood of new feelings saturating parents the moment their child is born—feelings incapable of imagining before feeling them.

A stigma vulnerable to empathy will improve. We feel uneasy condemning those with whom we can relate. Most can't empathize with a leper. So, fear, rational or not, will lessen any concern for the leper's inhumane treatment. It's the same with alcoholics.

Those who can't empathize with alcoholics are less concerned about their suffering. Yet those who can empathize know that the drinker's distress is necessary to motivate change. Still, they also find the drunk's actions repulsive. They eventually walk away from compassion unless the alcoholic is ready and willing to change.

The Benefits of the Alcoholic Stigma

SINCE THE ALCOHOLIC stigma is real, extensive, and partly rational, it will not change significantly soon, if ever.

Despite this, the alcoholic stigma offers at least four benefits for the sober and the drinking alcoholic—it promotes recovery, reduces relapses, promotes fellowship and community, enhancing many lives.

1) Promotes Recovery

Although the alcoholic stigma plays a role in whether one quits drinking, it's absurd for the stigma to prevent one from escaping the group it stigmatizes. Ironically, most alcoholics will not leave the group, fearing more exposure and stigmatization.

Yet, for some, the remorse, discouragement, guilt, shame, and self-loathing created by the stigma become so unbearable that these feelings propel many alcoholics from denial into recovery. The consensus is that the best time to approach the alcoholic about recovery is during periods of genuine remorse, usually the morning after a night of heavy drinking.

2) Reduces Relapses

Sober alcoholics stigmatizing drinking alcoholics prevents many relapses. Sober alcoholics don't want to rejoin a group they now stigmatize—especially a group from which they narrowly escaped.

One symptom of alcoholism is glamorizing drinking while ignoring its consequences. The thoughts that sober alcoholics have about active alcoholics fortify the stigma and motivate memories of these consequences, which supports their sobriety. This thinking often provokes drinking alcoholics to seek sobriety.

3) Promotes Fellowship and Community

People bond during a crisis. We see this often with natural disasters. For example, people connect uniquely to help their neighbors and even those in distant lands after a tsunami, earthquake, tornado, hurricane, or other disaster. Their innate need to survive and desire to share in this humanitarian action continues for weeks, months, and sometimes years. Many remember this as one of their most fulfilling experiences.

M. Scott Peck, MD, a psychiatrist and best-selling author, discusses this in his book *Further Along the Road Less*

Traveled.[47] Peck credits this phenomenon with AA's success.* He suggests alcoholism is a lifelong crisis producing the same longing to band together and survive the peril as those enduring a natural disaster. And those who belong to the stigmatized group also seek solace and fellowship with each other.

This fellowship is a significant part of Alcoholics Anonymous and other support groups. It promotes lasting friendships, which would have never formed without the lifelong common peril of alcoholism. Most members of that society appear happier and more content than many without this membership.

It promotes community, belonging, and connection to something more significant, which is essential for healthy living. It provides an opportunity for other-centeredness, producing a sensation of well-being and genuine happiness.

Although it's puzzling that some are so open about their recovery from alcoholism, a 2013 study showed that sober alcoholics in a recovery program (the researchers used AA members) who embrace and express that they are recovering alcoholics have longer and more satisfying sobriety than those on the sidelines guarding their anonymity.[48] Nor does it matter how people react to them. It invites embracing a new social identity associated with healing.[49]

The researchers hypothesized that the more involved someone is in their recovery, the less they experience the alcoholic-craving, so this social connection lessens the chances of relapsing. The preliminary findings support their theory. Without the stigma, this social connection that reduces relapses would not exist.

4) Improves Life

As shown, the alcoholic stigma improves lives. It provides

---

*Estimates are that Alcoholics Anonymous currently has two million sober members worldwide, *excluding* the millions who have become sober but no longer attend regular meetings and those who died sober.

many with a new meaning—a higher purpose. It reduces relapses and encourages connecting with a higher power. It significantly decreases dysphoria and increases self-esteem, self-confidence, and self-respect. These alcoholics no longer feel useless nor wallow in self-pity. Instead, they are grateful and happy to be responsible members of society.

Beyond Rational

Undoubtedly, the alcoholic stigma is not all beneficial. Portions of the stigma exceed its rational basis. Substandard health care is a noticeable consequence, flowing from the irrational part of the stigma. These practices must end when the stigma results in unfair and discriminatory practices.

However, ending these practices is not a simple task. One may intellectually disagree with the alcoholic stigma but emotionally agree with it, which is especially true for healthcare providers who routinely treat alcoholics. Their early indoctrination and experience with drinking alcoholics cause this. Healthcare's frustration and approach are unique and discussed thoroughly in Chapter 7, "Health Care, Alcoholism, and the DSM."

The Disease Concept and the Stigma

As stated in this chapter's introduction, reputable associations and organizations believe that educating society about alcoholism as a disease that innocently afflicts alcoholics would lessen the alcoholic stigma. Yet, that thinking seems naïve. The stigma has remained robust despite the widely touted and scientifically proven disease concept, which is not new.

For instance, in 1784, Dr. Benjamin Rush, surgeon general of the Continental Army and signor of the Declaration of Independence, classified alcoholism as a disease.

In 1904, this newspaper advertisement appeared. The first paragraph states:

> It is now a well-known fact to the medical fraternity and the laity, that drunkenness is a disease of the entire nervous system, and it is curable, the same as any other malady.

In 1956, the American Medical Association called it an illness, then a disease in 1965.

In 2004, the American Psychiatric Association (APA) and the World Health Organization considered alcoholism a disorder.

In 2007, the American Bar Association affirmed that it is a disease, encouraging insurance coverage equal to other illnesses.

The Americans with Disabilities Act lists alcoholism as a disease. The NIAAA and many other respected associations consider it a disease. All publicly declare that the alcoholic does not drink because of a flawed character or willful misconduct, although privately, most individual members believe otherwise.

Still, would wholesale adoption of the disease concept and total elimination of the stigma benefit society and the alcoholic?

IMAGINE OUR WORLD without the alcoholic stigma. . . . The World Health Organization, the NIAAA, and many others have met their goal of ending the alcoholic stigma. Everyone now finally knows that drinking is merely a symptom of a deadly epidemic disease—not a character flaw or a moral failing.

The laws against public intoxication have carved out an exception for alcoholics because intoxication is symptomatic.

Since alcoholics can't be held criminally liable for their *unintentional* drunkenness in public, a diagnosis of AUD has become a common legal defense. It only applies to nonalcoholics who drink voluntarily in public.*

Suddenly, the problem drinker feels no remorse about being drunk or being a drunk because they are not guilty of anything—their actions are merely symptoms of their condition.

Sure, it disappoints their family when they miss dinner and are gone for days, but they understand. So, their loved ones resist separating from them—it wouldn't feel right to desert someone because they're sick.

Alcoholics are becoming sicker as the disease progresses. Many wish they could do more for them. They can't function well physically or mentally. Perhaps they haven't bathed in days, and bodily functions occur while clothed.

As expected, the drinker is unsteady, occasionally bumping into and damaging property and people.

The alcoholic is moody and, at moments, so in love with everyone, demanding lengthy hugs from anyone within staggering distance. Moments later, they've fallen out of love, yelling empty threats at those they just hugged. No one reacts because "they're just sick." Everybody feels compassion for them having to endure this terminal disease.

With the stigma removed, alcoholics can now be themselves. Uncontrolled. Free. When late to work, they don't need an excuse. When not *too* drunk to call in, they tell their boss they had an unexpected flare-up of alcoholism, "partied too hardy," but hope to make it in tomorrow. Their employer understands and prefers they not come in—he remembers the last few times they showed up drunk.

---

*In 1968, in *Powell v Texas*, 392 U.S. 514 (1968), the U.S. Supreme Court heard a case wherein a self-proclaimed alcoholic was charged with public intoxication. The Defendant claimed constitutional violations, alleging he couldn't be prosecuted for displaying the symptoms of an illness. The Court disagreed.

And since their actions are symptomatic of their disease and not willful misconduct, they're paid sick time when missing or late to work because of excessive drinking. But soon, employment won't be an issue since they will receive permanent disability.

Next, a program called *Adopt-a-Drunk* is launched. An alcoholic is 'adopted' for a week and enabled to do whatever they want without consequences because they have suffered enough. The alcoholic shouldn't have to endure the natural results flowing from drunken behavior. This way, they won't burden themselves with trying to get sober since they have a disease.

Although fictionalized, all this illustrates flaws in trying to remove the alcoholic stigma and highlights how the stigma has some benefits.

SOLUTIONS

ALCOHOLICS EITHER KNOW, don't know, or suspect they might have a drinking problem. However, most public service announcements only focus on those who know they're alcoholics by providing a number to call for help (e.g., "If you have a drinking problem, call ..."). Those who don't know or briefly question whether they have a drinking problem are typically ignored.

It's time to candidly address the stigma and rescue the millions of professional and highly functioning alcoholics, alcoholics who don't drink daily (periodic alcoholics), and others who don't see their drinking problem by beaming the light in their direction and exposing their denial.

Unfortunately, ignoring these alcoholics who don't know they're alcoholics doesn't reduce the silent misery they and those around them suffer. These alcoholics who are in denial are the most neglected and affected by the stigma.

The following are six methods of reaching unseen and untreated alcoholics by shining the light on their denial.

1) Openly Addressing the Alcoholic Stigma

Recovery messages need to discuss the alcoholic stigma openly. Knowing the stigma exists but pretending it doesn't is disingenuous and supports it.

A 30-second announcement discussing the alcoholic stigma and its absurdity would expose the "elephant in the room." It would describe how the stigma prevents one from escaping it. It would also explain how the drinker, who 'hides' their drinking and isolates to avoid the stigma, self-imposes a life sentence of alcoholic torture.

2) Focus on the Neglected Functional and Periodic Alcoholic

An effective media spot targeting the functional and the periodic alcoholic in denial might be the following.

> **Alcoholic:** "I'm not an alcoholic. I don't *have* to drink. I enjoy drinking. I don't even drink *every* day. It's just that I don't *want* to stop once I start."
>
> **Announcer:** Did you know that:
> - Most alcoholics don't drink every day.
> - Most alcoholics are employed and functional.
> - Most alcoholics aren't homeless.
> - Many alcoholics drink less than nonalcoholics.
> - Most alcoholics have never slept on a park bench.
> - Many alcoholics are doctors, lawyers, teachers, pilots, and other professionals.
> - Most alcoholics don't drink during the day.
> - Most alcoholics don't think they're alcoholics.
> - Most alcoholics seem like everyone else.

2) Assurance of Confidentiality

To withstand the stigma, a service announcement recognizing the prospect's fears of exposure would explain that alcoholics have an absolute legal right to privacy and that ample safeguards are required and in place to ensure confidentiality. Like other health conditions, alcoholics considering treatment and the rest of the public should understand that their privacy is protected—no one can or will know of their treatment except those the drinker wants to know.

It could follow with focusing on the alcoholic resisting sobriety, fearing exposure of their alcoholism, by asking these three questions:

> - Has anyone ever mentioned your drinking?
> - Have you ever wondered if you might have a drinking problem?
> - Did either question cause you discomfort?

This message would target the estimated 90% of alcoholics who have done nothing about their drinking.[50]

3) Minimizing the Stigma's Power

The stigma's power can be destroyed at once by the actions and thinking of the alcoholic. The alcoholic stigma is powerless unless one *self*-stigmatizes.

An ignored stigma is no longer an effective stigma or a barrier to treatment, as shown earlier when discussing the man 35 years sober and the professional woman who believes the sober alcoholic stigma doesn't exist.

Why would one refuse sobriety and life and choose to remain in alcoholic bondage based on their fear of what others might think? It's done all the time because of the drinker's distorted thinking, drenched with negative self-talk. The alcoholic doesn't logically consider that it makes no sense since the social and self-stigmatization of drinking alcoholics is much harsher than that of sober alcoholics. Also, others already know much more about their drinking than they suspect. So, they're not subjecting themselves to more of a stigma by becoming sober but less of it.

Rather than seeing the stigma as some vast, dark, ominous,

judgmental mass hovering above, one can reduce self-stigmatizing and the stigma's effects using many methods. These methods include guided or unguided meditation, cognitive or dialectical behavioral therapy, motivational therapy, peer support groups, family and couples therapy, interventions, and other techniques psychology offers.

4) Knowledge is the Answer

We must inform society, including pre-alcoholics, healthcare providers, and legislators, about alcoholism, which should start in first grade and continue through 12th grade as part of the school curriculum. Initially, this would be minimal.* The goal wouldn't be to end the stigma but to teach the symptoms and signs of early alcoholism and deter self-stigmatization.

This information would enable students to recognize problem drinking in themselves and their peers as they enter adolescence. Almost half of 12th-grade students admit they were "drunk in the past year."[51] Most drinkers experienced their first intoxication at about 15 years old.[52] Research also shows that most alcoholics start drinking as teenagers,[53] and the earlier they drink, the likelier they are to develop alcoholism.[54,55,56]

It is important to teach that alcoholism is a treatable illness, and briefly introducing this early and regularly, such as one hour each year, would lessen the irrational part of the stigma, making it easier for those students in an alcoholic home and those who develop a drinking problem to ask for help. Moreover, the students who become healthcare professionals will provide better care. Also, those who become legislators will likely introduce and pass better, more evidence-based laws.

---

*For example: 1st grade: *What is alcohol?* 2nd grade: *The effects of alcohol.* 3rd grade: *The signs and symptoms of intoxication.* 4th grade: *The neurobiology of alcoholism.* 5th grade: *The disease concept of alcoholism.* 6th grade: *The signs and symptoms of alcoholism.* 7th grade: *The trauma to those affected by alcoholism.* 8th grade: *Alcoholism's effect on society* (e.g., traffic deaths, accidents, injuries, premature deaths, trauma to those living with an alcoholic, the costs, and the misery). 9th grade: *The interventions and treatments available.* Grades 10-12: A recap including new research findings about that taught in grades 1-9.

As with most diseases, early education and detection are vital.

5) Reaching the Untreated Alcoholic Majority

A practical approach to reaching those not considering sobriety (most alcoholics) is to lighten the darkness that shrouds them.

For example, imagine friends and family gathered to watch a Super Bowl broadcast. Many are drinking. By halftime, the alcoholic is identifiable—the loudest, screaming derogatory comments about the halftime show, the coach's decisions, the substandard players, and the wrong calls.

The announcement could mirror the scene of this Super Bowl party watching the halftime show. It would focus on the alcoholic's behavior, reflecting the viewer's environment. Although perhaps extreme, it would show the drinker's impact on their friends and family.

6) Providing Information at the Retail Level

The government could require wholesalers or retailers to include information with alcohol sales. An example of this could be a card attached to the bottleneck, including any three of these eight questions:

- Does your drinking worry anyone?
- Have you ever wondered if you *might* have a drinking problem?
- Within the past year, did you drink more than you planned?
- Do you ever feel the urge to apologize for your drinking?
- Have you ever thought about quitting or reducing your drinking?
- Have you ever tried to keep *anything* about your drinking a secret (e.g., buying alcohol, making a drink, drinking, the number of drinks you've had, "acting" sober, reading this, thoughts and feelings about your drinking, the time you drink, injuries and other effects of drinking, improper conduct while drinking, false responses about drinking,

> etc.)?
> • Does drinking affect your life?
> • Do you feel uneasy answering these questions?
>
> **If you answered yes to *any* of these, call 1-800-PRI-VATE for information. Your call is 100% confidential, with no obligations.**

This card is a screening, not a diagnosis. When calling the number on the card, the caller will reach a well-trained person who will explore whether a drinking problem *may* exist. If so, they could recommend further action.

SOME SPEAK OUT AGAINST THE ALCOHOLIC STIGMA

ON FEBRUARY 22, 1842, 19 years before Abraham Lincoln became president, the 33-year-old lawyer spoke to the Springfield Washingtonian Temperance Society and other curious attendees. His speech was different from what most expected. He expressed compassion for the alcoholic, suggesting the nonalcoholic was not any better but was merely fortunate to have dodged the affliction. He spoke highly of the alcoholic's character. The following is an excerpt from his 30-minute speech.

> *In my judgment, such of us as have never fallen victims [to alcoholism], have been spared more by the absence of appetite, than from any mental or moral superiority over those who have.*
>
> *Indeed, I believe, if we take habitual drunkards as a class, their heads and their hearts will bear an advantageous comparison with those of any other class. There seems ever to have been a proneness in the brilliant, and warm-blooded to fall into this vice.*
>
> *–Abraham Lincoln*

However, not all prominent people and organizations have acted to reduce the stigma.

Special Recognition of the Contributors to the Alcoholic Stigma

IT'S NOW TIME to pay special tribute to the influential and respected organizations, institutions, and people who have enlarged the alcoholic stereotype and the stigma.

Ten Contributors to the Alcoholic Stigma

Drum Roll, Please!

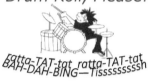

Dr. Benjamin Franklin

BENJAMIN FRANKLIN BELIEVED that a flawed character caused alcoholism. This view inspired him to write several serious essays about drinking, including the famous and less serious *The Drinkers Dictionary,* published January 13, 1736. It has over 200 slang terms describing drunkenness, which he had heard in taverns. Dr. Franklin* published it in the *Pennsylvania Gazette.* The subtitle is *Nothing More Like a Fool Than a Drunken Man.*

Well-skilled in diplomacy, Benjamin Franklin would not risk offending anyone unless their behavior was much more offensive. His advice was, "Never speak your mind." Yet the drunk behaved in a way that provoked Dr. Franklin to ignore his own advice. His widely *published* writings were observably stigmatizing.

---

*Dr. Franklin received an honorary Doctor of Laws degree on February 12, 1759, from the University of St. Andrews and again in 1762 from Oxford University. Although he never formally attended a college or university, he preferred being called Dr. Franklin.

⑨
THE UNITED STATES SUPREME COURT

IN 1988, THE U.S. Supreme Court heard a compelling case related to the alcoholic stigma.[56] It's a split-decision case (4-3) in which the Court goes into an in-depth study and analysis of alcoholism in its 36-page opinion. The issue: *Is alcoholism a disease or the result of willful misconduct?*[*]

The case is *Traynor v. Turnage*, 485 US 535 (1988), which involved two alcoholic Vietnam veterans who could not complete their education within 10 years to qualify for payment under the GI Bill. Only "a physical or mental disorder which was not the result of ... willful misconduct" could extend this limit. The veterans claimed alcoholism disabled them during much of those 10 years. The Veterans Administration (VA) disagreed, defining alcoholism as *"willful misconduct"* and didn't allow the extension.

The dissenting (minority) opinion by Justice Blackmun is undeniable. He wrote that the VA presumed "willful misconduct" caused the veterans' alcoholism, but it failed to show that *every* alcoholic knew their first drink would result in alcoholism.

The VA argued that any drinking beyond normal drinking was the willful act of *"voluntarily drinking poison."* Blackmun disagreed:

> Indeed, I wonder how one meaningfully can ascribe such intent and appreciation of long-range consequences to a 9- or 13-year-old boy who follows the lead of his adult role models in taking his first drinks.

The majority held that consuming the first drink is

---

[*]The AMA, National Council on Alcoholism, and Vietnam Veterans of America filed *amicus curiae* briefs. *Amicus curiae* is Latin for "friend of the court," and an *amicus curiae* brief is filed by an entity that is not a party in the case but has strong views on the subject matter or a strong interest in the case. They are usually filed in cases wherein the subject matter involves broad public interest.

voluntary. So, it's *willful misconduct* if alcoholism results. But Blackmun found this rule only applied to alcoholism and no other addictions such as smoking, a "causative factor in the high incidence of cancer, emphysema, and heart disease... Yet smoking has not been considered misconduct." He said it's unlawful to treat alcoholism differently.

Blackmun stressed that the majority are stereotyping alcoholics and supporting the alcoholic stigma.

The highest Court's opinions are influential and have far-reaching implications in other pending or contemplated litigation. They also affect public opinion, and this decision boosted the alcoholic stigma.*

OTIS CAMPBELL OF THE ANDY GRIFFITH SHOW

AND LET'S NOT forget Otis Campbell from the television series *The Andy Griffith Show*, which ran for eight years (1960-1968) and was one of the most popular series ever aired.[57] Reruns continue today.

Otis was the town drunk of Mayberry (a fictional dry county) who *voluntarily* staggered to the jail every weekend, locked the cell door behind him, and hung the keys within reach to release himself when sober. Not only did he have the keys to his cell, but also the courthouse.

Otis was a periodic alcoholic and would 'voluntarily' binge drink on weekends. His intoxication and everything he did appeared *voluntary*. He was the subject of many practical jokes highlighting his drunkenness in the subtle Mayberry fashion.

This series portrays alcoholism as willful misconduct and

---

*Congress disagreed with the Court's decision, and 44 days later, on June 3, 1988, introduced a new bill that abrogated the holding of the highest Court's decision by enacting the Veterans' Benefits Improvement Act of 1988, providing that alcoholism is not willful misconduct. On October 18, 1988, the bill passed the Senate, and the President signed it.

is a contributor to the alcoholic stigma.

The Expert's Definition of the Alcoholic Craving

The prevailing expert's definition of the alcoholic-craving supports the alcoholic stigma. As detailed in Chapter 3, "The Alcoholic-Craving," using the word "desire" instead of "need" to define the alcoholic's craving for alcohol implies drinking is voluntary misconduct and not an uncontrollable, compulsive need to drink. This incorrect view, contrary to reliable and convincing evidence, strengthens the alcoholic stereotype and contributes to the alcoholic stigma.

The American Psychiatric Association and Health Care Professionals

Most healthcare professionals silently believe alcoholism is immoral behavior spawned by willful misconduct and lack of willpower.

It was not until 2004 that the American Psychiatric Association announced alcoholism as a disorder. Their failure to broadcast this sooner implied drunkenness was willful misconduct, contributing to the stigma.

Other associations supported the stigma by withholding their decision to consider alcoholism a disease or a disorder until after the APA's announcement.

The Bible

The Old and New Testaments mention alcohol use often. Although room for differences exists with biblical interpretations, the theologians' consensus is that drinking alcohol (wine) in moderation was acceptable, but drinking too much was sinful—a severe moral and spiritual failing. It is no different today. There are about 70 disparaging biblical references to drunkenness. Undoubtedly, the Bible contributes to the alcoholic stigma.

Alcoholics Anonymous

ALCOHOLICS ANONYMOUS HAS been and is a significant contributor to the stigma. The name suggests that members must hide. But something hidden is usually shameful and dishonored, not cherished.

While anonymity in AA now has various purposes,[58] the name's original intent was to ensure alcoholics felt protected when becoming members of AA. The co-founders understood alcoholics were ashamed of their drinking, fearing public exposure and reprisals. Without assuring anonymity, most members would not have joined and sought sobriety.*[59]

This Book

THIS BOOK HAS contributed to the stigma by highlighting its benefits and stressing that the drunk's conduct has invited the stigma.

The Sober Alcoholic

SOBER ALCOHOLICS STIGMATIZE drinking alcoholics. Most sober alcoholics see themselves as more fortunate than wet

---

*As time passed, anonymity meant much more, evolving into a spiritual foundation and stimulating the drafting of the last two traditions: 11. "Our public relations policy is based on attraction rather than promotion; we need always maintain personal anonymity at the level of press, radio, and films," and 12. "Anonymity is the spiritual foundation of all our Traditions, ever reminding us to place principles before personalities."

alcoholics. And why shouldn't they? They have accepted a reprieve also offered to, yet rejected by, drinking alcoholics. This thinking refreshes memories about a place they never want to return to, increasing their negative perception of the drinking alcoholic.

And The Number ONE
Contributor To The Alcoholic Stigma:

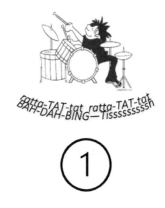

①

DRINKING AND DRY ALCOHOLICS

SIMPLY PUT, THE leading contributor to the alcoholic stigma is the offensive behavior of the drunk alcoholic and the untreated, dry alcoholic who is not in recovery.

—

TO CONCLUDE, THE alcoholic stigma is rational *and* irrational—it will not disappear soon, if ever. Still, the benefits of the stigma often outweigh the harms.

Although the stigma usually impedes those seeking sobriety, it doesn't prevent it. For desperate alcoholics who have drunk the value out of drinking, the stigma won't stop them.

In short, the alcoholic stigma *is* a blessing in disguise.

Questions for Discussion

1. Do you believe the alcoholic stigma has ever affected you? If so, how?
2. Has this chapter altered your thinking about how the alcoholic stigma may have affected you?
3. Do you agree with the author that the alcoholic stigma is helpful?
4. Are there ways the stigma is helpful other than the ways identified in the chapter?
5. Do you believe the alcoholic stigma could change? If yes, what part could change, and when will it change?
6. Do you believe alcoholism is a disease? Why or why not?
7. Has anything in this chapter affected you? Explain.
8. Has this chapter affected you? How?
9. Have you learned anything from this chapter? If yes, please discuss.

Contact Information

Suicide & Crisis Lifeline:
Call or text 988 or chat at 988lifeline.org

Suicide Prevention Lifeline:
1-800-273-TALK (8255)

For confidential information about help for alcohol dependence, contact one or more of the following:

NIAAA ALCOHOL TREATMENT NAVIGATOR
"Pointing the way to evidence-based care"

A service of the U.S. federal government providing unbiased information for finding quality alcohol treatment through mutual support groups, therapists, doctors, and outpatient & inpatient care.
www.alcoholtreatment.niaaa.nih.gov

Mutual-Support Groups

(AA) Alcoholics Anonymous
www.aa.org | 212–870–3400
(or local phone directory)

Al-Anon Family Services/Alateen
For Those Affected by Another's Drinking
www.al-anon.org | 888-425-2666 for meetings

Adult Children of Alcoholics & Dysfunctional Families
www.adultchildren.org | 310–534–1815

AA Agnostica
A space for AA agnostics, atheists and freethinkers worldwide
www.aaagnostica.org | admin@aaagnostica.org.

Celebrate Recovery
A Christ-Centered Recovery Program
www.celebraterecovery.com | 800-723-3532

LifeRing
Secular (nonreligious) Recovery
www.LifeRing.org | 800-811-4142

Moderation Management
www.moderation.org | 212–871–0974

Secular Organizations for Sobriety
www.sossobriety.org | 314-353–-3532

Secular Alcoholics Anonymous
AA meetings for agnostics, atheists and freethinkers
www.secularaa.org

SMART Recovery
An Alternative to AA, Al-Anon, and other 12-Step Programs
www.smartrecovery.org | 440-951-5357

Women for Sobriety
www.womenforsobriety.org | 215–536–8026

INFORMATION RESOURCES

The Alcohol and Drug Addiction Resource Center
(800) 390-4056

Alcohol and Drug Helpline
www.alcoholanddrughelpline.com | (800) 821-4357

Alcohol Hotline Support & Information
(800) 331-2900

American Council on Alcoholism (ACA)
www.recoverymonth.gov | (800) 527-5344

National Child Abuse Hotline
1-800-25-ABUSE

National Clearinghouse for Alcohol and Drug Information
www.ncadi.samhsa.gov | (800) 729–6686

National Council on Alcoholism & Drug Dependence, Inc.
www.ncadd.org | *HOPE LINE*: 800/NCA-CALL (24-hour)

National Domestic Abuse Hotline
1-800-799-SAFE

National Helpline
Treatment referral and information 24-7
www.samhsa.gov | 1-800-662-HELP (4357)

National Institute on Alcohol Abuse and Alcoholism
www.niaaa.nih.gov | (301) 443–3860

National Institute on Drug Abuse
www.nida.nih.gov | (301) 443–1124

National Institute of Mental Health
www.nimh.nih.gov | (866) 615–6464

THE DARKNESS AND LIGHTNESS OF DENIAL
and the Alcoholic's Entourage

CHAPTER 5

*You're probably an alcoholic
if you've ever denied being an alcoholic.*
—

DENIAL IS CONTAGIOUS. Drinking alcoholics don't have a monopoly on denial. Those in a position to help the alcoholic seldom do because they are also in denial. This includes loved ones, friends, co-workers, employers, employees, treating doctors, therapists, and the courts. I call them the *alcoholic's entourage*.

This entourage, in some way, benefits from the alcoholic's drinking. Their concern for the alcoholic, themselves, and others fuels this 'unrecognized' denial. And their kindness, lack of knowledge, fear, and reasons discussed below fuel this denial even more. Still, the alcoholic stereotype contributes the most.

And it's worse when members of the entourage are in denial about their own drinking. Recognizing alcoholism in another is more challenging when we don't see it in ourselves.

The entourage's denial isn't as problematic when the alcoholic is in the advanced stages, and it's obvious to everyone. Still, the symptoms are easily missed in the early and middle stages, often lasting years.

I say none of this to reduce the alcoholic's responsibility by deflecting 'blame.' However, it is meant to identify a lingering problem created and skillfully manipulated by the alcoholic to avoid the terrorizing thought of living sober, which the alcoholic sees as living a life of misery. And this revelation recognizes the widespread effect alcoholics have on those surrounding them. Still, not every member of the entourage is in denial—just most.

What is Denial?

"DENIAL AIN'T A river in Egypt," Mark Twain once quipped. Yet, isn't it like *The Nile* River? Both can be powerful, unyielding, and deadly. But rather than a river of water, denial acts like a dam on a river of information and controls its flow.

The Lightness of Denial

This 'dam of denial' is our mind acting as a shield—a gentle regulator—controlling and restricting the release of emotionally provoking information from flowing downstream, flooding our awareness.

When our awareness can absorb and cope with more truth, the dam releases a measured amount. It continually performs a cost-benefit analysis: Does the emotional cost of knowing exceed the benefit of not knowing? The dam of denial is designed to release information we need to know and protect us from a flood of distressful information we lack the coping skills[*] to absorb.

Living life without denial would be difficult. Denial protects us—keeping us in the dark about issues that would harm us and others if seen. At times, we're not ready to see the whole truth.

Denial protects us from knowing something that, if revealed, could threaten our self-image, health, safety, or survival.

Denial often provides a grace period, giving our minds time to adapt and prepare for disturbing information. It's like

---

[*]For the alcoholic, alcohol substitutes for this lack of coping skills.

a safety net cushioning the impact of our fall when we occasionally lose our grip after receiving troubling information.

For example, consider those who suffered childhood trauma and repressed it for years. To cope, they may ignore some reality. Another example is the sober alcoholic mother, who had emotionally abandoned her children so she could drink. To avoid paralyzing guilt, she nurtures her denial by cultivating 'reasons' why she has a strained relationship with her children.

And finally, there's the drunk driver who crossed the center median, colliding with oncoming traffic, resulting in casualties. To cope, he *temporarily* ignores some truth by rationalizing that it was probably a mechanical problem, the poorly-designed center median, or oncoming traffic was speeding—anything other than his drinking.

It could be devastating if struck with a bolt of hurtful truth during a board meeting, critical exam, job interview, family reunion, or while driving. Discovering information at the wrong time could cause us to act irrationally—saying or doing things that could harm ourselves or others.

Denial often reduces our anxiety, making us calmer and more collected—more focused and productive. Denial gives us time to respond rather than react impulsively and ineffectively.

Haven't most of us acted as the dam of denial for others, restricting the flow of information to protect them from the truth? Before we reveal anything too sensitive, we compare the likely benefit with the possible harm it could cause them or others. We distort the truth to spare feelings—the 'white lie,' or we say nothing—the 'silent lie.'

As loving parents, we protect our children from those truths we deem age-inappropriate or hurtful. We also do this with loved ones to lighten their concerns.

Still, too much denial can fail to warn us of a severe threat. So, while denial may be temporarily beneficial, it can eventually become destructive if unresolved.

The Darkness of Denial

When denial malfunctions, preventing us from seeing a threat we need to see—a threat to our survival—it's failing and destructive. The denial of alcoholism is an example of this.

One symptom of alcoholism is blocking the light of truth, allowing the alcoholic to hide in the shadows and alcoholism to flourish. As discussed in Chapter 3, "The Alcoholic-Craving," the alcoholic brain believes drinking is necessary to survive and dismisses other perspectives.

So, denial, a key symptom of alcoholism, prevents one from seeking sobriety. Denial can also narrow the dam's spillway, causing those who suspect they might have a drinking problem to minimize its severity. Denying that drinking is a *severe* problem can avoid terrorizing thoughts of not drinking and invite rationalizations that they will do something about it before it gets too bad.

Rationalization supplies us with reasons that sound good for everything we do. It strengthens denial, and alcoholics will do almost anything to nurse their denial, which includes comparing themselves to those who drink more, drink earlier in the day, or have more drinking-related problems.

We cultivate denial by blaming others. We interrupt others to avoid hearing the truth. We engage in unhealthy and harmful behaviors to smother thoughts that soften denial—many drink to block the truth about their drinking problem. The maneuvers employed to avoid the light are endless.

Yet, aren't we all in denial about some issues to an extent? Can we be in denial if we know we're in denial? We can and are. Don't we occasionally bury our heads in the sand to postpone dealing with something we've predecided is unpleasant?

And then we're *unknowingly* in denial about other issues. We know this when the truth stuns us. We then see that we ignored the clues that were obvious to others. The reason is as obvious as the clues were—we didn't want, or weren't ready, to cope with the truth.

So, denial adjusts the amount of information flowing from the darkness into the light—from our unawareness to our awareness.

Denial: Awareness and Unawareness

There is a reason why our awareness (consciousness) and our unawareness (unconsciousness) exist.[*] We were designed to be aware of some and unaware of other information. Our brains accommodate denial.

Those who strive toward higher consciousness attempt to discover their unconscious thinking. This effort, known as mindfulness, is an effort to prevent instincts and emotions from controlling our reasoning and actions.

It's challenging to manage our unconscious by issuing conscious demands. Our conscious mind may request that our unconsciousness release certain information, adjust our behavior, or allow us to think and feel differently. Although our unconscious may consider these requests, it stubbornly decides what it will do—whether we like it or not.

For example, if we demand that grief, fear, or the alcoholic-craving vanish, it likely won't. However, these may partially fade by using various methods such as psychotherapy, cognitive-behavioral therapy, peer-support meetings, prayer, meditation, self-affirmation, visualization, hypnosis, and other techniques.

An example of our dominating unconscious is when a name, phone number, or word is on the 'tip of our tongue' or we can't find something we've 'misplaced.' Still, we know the name, phone number, and where we placed an item; we're merely having difficulty retrieving the stored information. So, we didn't misplace our item; we misplaced where we stored

---

[*]Some suggest this information we have access to is in our "preconscious" also referred to as our subconscious.

the information about the item's location.

We can plead with our brains to stop our grief. Yet, since we can only slightly affect the intensity and length of grief, it must have benefits. Our brain disregards those pleas that could be harmful if granted. Although we're unaware of any benefits, our unconscious is, and it's in charge.

Despite the design of our minds to be aware and unaware of certain information, alcohol disrupts this design. An example is the alcoholic trying to support their denial by controlling their drinking. They do this by instructing their brain not to exceed a preset drinking limit. But the unconscious doesn't obey.

We might instruct our brain to stop obsessing about drinking or remove the compulsion to drink. Yet our brain ignores these instructions because it believes drinking is beneficial. So, we must replace these instructions with self-affirming messages infinitely repeated—a form of programming or 'brainwashing,' which is often successful.

The Defense Mechanism of Denial

Consider those grieving a significant loss, such as the loss of a loved one, a divorce, an ending romance, or a job loss. They typically process acceptance of the loss by walking through five stages of grief.*

The first stage is denial, during which the person may make statements like, "They must have tested the wrong specimen," "But he looks like he's feeling better," "We'll reconcile someday," or "They'll rehire me when they realize how much they need me."

It's like alcoholics accepting their condition. It starts with denying their alcoholism: "I don't have to drink every day," "I don't drink as much as he does," "I have a good job, never miss work and earn a good income," or "I'm not homeless."

---

*According to the Kübler-Ross model, the five stages of grief are denial, anger, bargaining, depression, and acceptance. But not everyone experiences all these stages, and not always in this order.

For the fortunate few who struggle through the stages of denial until acceptance, they may next feel anger: "Why do I have to be an alcoholic?" "Why can't I drink as he does?" or "This just isn't fair."

And then, the bargaining stage often follows: "I won't drink as much," "I will control my drinking," "I won't drink before sundown," "I'll only drink beer," or "I'll only drink on weekends." Finally, after a period of grief, they accept their alcoholism.

However, the alcoholic's entourage rarely experiences this grieving process. They don't feel the same loss. They can remain in denial without suffering the consequences the alcoholic suffers. So most of the entourage maintains their denial because nothing prompts them to make a 'life-saving' change by giving up something they 'need.' And if they escape denial, it's more an intellectual than an emotional acceptance because they don't suffer the alcoholic-craving.

Ignorance Isn't Always Bliss

Since none of us are all-knowing, we are all, more or less, unknowingly ignorant.

The most knowledgeable are those open-minded enough to embrace competing and alternative perspectives. The ignorant remain threatened by thinking that is unlike their own.

But denial isn't merely the lack of specific knowledge; it's the preference or seeming need to lack that knowledge—to remain ignorant. So we hear, "What I don't know can't hurt me."

The self-proclaimed intelligent alcoholic often has more difficulty escaping the darkness of denial. They're convinced they're in the light—convinced they are right, even in the face of indisputable evidence that they're not. We often hear, "He's too smart for his own good." So, denial is usually ignorance on demand.

Denial in the Alcoholic's Entourage

IRONICALLY, ALCOHOLICS ARE usually in much less denial than their entourage, although they rarely grasp the severity of their drinking problem. They're aware of their alcoholic thoughts, their compulsive need to drink, and the behavior they struggle to hide, which increase as alcoholism progresses.

One symptom of alcoholism is to remain undetected while persuading others to stay in denial. It's not an intentional scheme but reflexive, like recoiling our hand from fire. Alcoholics integrate this deceit much like their breathing, rarely giving it a thought. And the longer the entourage remains in denial, the longer alcoholism has to grow, like an unchecked cancerous cell.

Health Care Professionals

The American Medical Association said alcoholism was an illness in 1956 and a disease in 1965. All well-known and respected groups and institutions *slowly* followed. All federal and state laws now proclaim it a disease.

The American Society of Addiction Medicine, the nation's largest group of doctors treating and preventing alcoholism and other addictions (addiction specialists), claims alcoholism is a "chronic brain disease, not just bad behavior" or poor choices. It lists one sign of alcoholism as "distortions in thinking, *most notably denial.*"[1] [Italics added.]

Uncontrolled drinking is only one symptom of alcoholism. It's not bad conduct and lack of morals that cause alcoholism and need treatment. Instead, it's primarily a biological disease that must be treated.

The law and those that treat, research, or fund the study of alcoholism state that it should be treated like every other fatal disease.

Health care workers know this, but denial supports their misbelief that there isn't much they can do about it. Denial allows them to ignore alcoholism, 'unaware' that this is an irresponsible practice.

George E. Vaillant, MD, a professor of psychiatry at Harvard Medical School, disclosed during an interview that "...when it comes to treating alcoholism the medical profession feels so helpless, so without hope. And for a doctor, feeling powerless is reason enough to put his head in the sand."[2]

Health Care's Denial of Equal Treatment

Treating alcoholism like other illnesses means having the same concern for the alcoholic as the cancer patient. It means not treating the alcoholic as hopeless. It means all health workers get the same training in alcoholism as in other terminal diseases. Finally, it means doing a brief screening and, if needed, making a diagnosis or referral.

None of the many alcoholics I've interviewed who were medically managed while detoxing received an adequate referral when released. At most, some received an over-copied, illegible list of numbers they *could* call. Are oncology referrals this casual?

Treating alcoholism as a terminal illness requires referrals to be processed the same as for any terminally ill patient. This includes scheduling and informing the patient of the place, date, and time of the visit.

Practices that understand alcoholism realize it is essential to schedule the referral of alcoholics with a specialist because denial and fear of abstinence are symptoms that cause them to delay or dismiss any follow-up.

The hospital's unabashed and unwritten policy is to keep alcoholics alive during withdrawal and quickly release them while avoiding liability. Hospitals believe the likelihood that alcoholics will stop drinking is so low that treating them wastes time and money.

Further, several doctors I've spoken with confirmed the alcoholic's comfort is unimportant: "If we make them too comfortable, they'll want to return more often." Since most doctors only treat withdrawal symptoms, 90% *will* return.[3] It's an endless cycle. To ignore alcoholism by treating only the present physical complaints is denial and benefits no one.

The Health Care Disparity Fueled by Denial

If we view alcoholism as we do other diseases, where are all the flags, awareness ribbons, bumper stickers, balloons, and buttons?

As mentioned in Chapter 4, "The Alcoholic Stigma," I've never seen a walk raise funds to treat the 'hopeless' neighborhood drunk.

Why is one of the most deadly diseases that causes the most public harm the least and most poorly treated?

Patients receiving treatment for alcohol-related health issues occupy nearly 40% of all hospital beds in the United States.[4] These health problems include stroke, neuropathy, dementia, heart problems, high blood pressure, cancer, liver disease, stomach problems, and diabetes.[5]

Also treated are alcohol-related injuries from car accidents, falls, drownings, burns, suicide attempts, firearms, and alcohol-induced mood disorders like depression and anxiety.[6]

According to the CDC, between 2016 and 2021, excessive drinking caused 178,000 deaths and cost $249 billion yearly in the United States. Too much drinking shortens the lives of those who die prematurely by an average of 24 years, resulting in four million years of potential life lost each year.[7]

The money spent on alcoholism pales when compared with other illnesses. For example, the CDC reports that $237 billion was spent to treat 28.7 million with diabetes in 2017.[8] In contrast, only $28 billion was spent treating 15 million alcoholics.[9] Moreover, 95.6% of the money spent on alcoholism was to treat the results of drinking too much. Unfortunately, only 1.9%—or about $35 for each alcoholic treated—went to prevention and treatment.[10]

The *treatment* gap is also revealing. People with diabetes receive treatment at a much higher rate than alcoholics—73% of those with diabetes receive help, compared with 10.9% of all alcoholics.[11] These disparities are not unique to diabetes but exist across the board with all other similar conditions.

So, although we claim we treat alcoholism like every other deadly illness, the financial and treatment disparities prove we don't.

The Physician

Family and emergency doctors on the front lines are usually the first ones to hear the alcoholic's complaints. Patients expect instant relief, so doctors feel pushed to provide it. Alcoholics who are 'convinced' their drinking is unrelated to their health problems only want their symptoms removed so they can continue drinking with impunity.

Still, the doctor and the alcoholic patient view even a hint of alcoholism as accusatory.* The alcoholic's typical reaction to an alcoholic diagnosis is the doctor is incompetent. So, the physician prefers not to alienate patients by making such an 'accusation.'

Medical schools routinely teach about heart disease, hypertension, cancer, diabetes, and other life-threatening conditions as part of their required curriculum. After recent pressure from governmental and accreditation bodies, a few schools offer substance abuse courses as electives during residency. Still, they are not part of the general two-year classroom curriculum. Moreover, these courses don't provide adequate information about alcoholism.[12]

Physicians usually diagnose alcoholism in the advanced stages when it's obvious to everyone. Unfortunately, most doctors don't recognize the early and middle stages of alcoholism, so they don't see it brewing in their patients, friends, loved ones, or—themselves.

---

*However, skills acquired from brief training can soften this view.

I've heard of doctors flippantly boasting, "I diagnose alcoholism if my patient drinks more than I do."[13] This comment raises a sensitive statistic: about 30% of medical students meet the criteria for alcohol abuse and dependence,[14] and more than 26% of practicing physicians are problem drinkers.[15]

Reported problematic drinking among doctors rose from 16.3% in 2006 to 26.8% in 2020.[16] Still, these percentages are likely much higher since it is well-known that the medical community greatly underreports problem drinking.[17] Also, because the survey questioned drinking behavior during the past 12 months, it excluded many doctors who were only temporarily sober. Education can cure this denial.

According to the CDC, alcohol screening and brief counseling can reduce consumption by 25% in those who drink too much. But "only 1 in 6 adults talk with their doctor, nurse, or other health care worker about their drinking." Some suggest doctors are concerned that such a discussion can prompt an emotional flood that a busy practice can't absorb.

The National Center on Addiction and Substance Abuse at Columbia University (CASAColumbia) found not much progress was made between its 2000 report, *Missed Opportunity: National Survey of Primary Care Physicians and Patients on Substance Abuse*,[18] and its follow-up report in 2012, *Addiction Medicine: Closing the Gap between Science and Practice*.[19] Both reports cited these reasons for the physician's failure to diagnose alcoholism.

1. It's wasted time since most patients lie about their drinking and resist treatment.
2. Successful treatment is unlikely.
3. Time limits.
4. The concern they wouldn't be paid for discussing alcoholism with a patient and performing alcohol screenings.
5. The doctor's discomfort talking about alcoholism.

6. Fear of losing patients by upsetting them.

However, these 'reasons' are not evidence-based, which reveals health care's denial about alcoholism.

To illustrate, don't patients with other illnesses sometimes resist treatment? Are other patients refused treatment because the likelihood of a successful outcome is low? Do time restraints exclude diagnosing other diseases? Doesn't insurance cover discussing the patient's illness and conducting screenings? Shouldn't doctors overcome their discomfort about discussing a patient's disease with them? Finally, would the fear of losing patients stop doctors from diagnosing other diseases?

Proper training dilutes these reasons. Primary care doctors should know, at a minimum, *all* symptoms during *all* stages of alcoholism and must be able to discuss such things with their patients.

CASAColumbia stated family doctors should accurately diagnose alcoholism and encourage treatment. It further contends that this is the lowest standard of medical care acceptable, and anything less risks liability for "negligent failure to diagnose."

It's Not My Job!

Many doctors believe it's not their responsibility to care for an alcoholic beyond the current *physical* health consequences of drinking. Yet it's undisputed that our thoughts and emotions cause many physical complaints and illnesses, which is more noticeable with some physical complaints than with others.

Consider the cutter who copes with negative or numb emotions by cutting, burning, or injuring their skin.[20] The treating doctor selects the best way of closing the wounds to reduce the possibility of infection and scarring. Still, the doctor is likely frustrated treating what she sees as needless, repeated, self-inflicted injuries.

Or consider one who presents with symptoms of severe

weight loss or gain. After ruling out biological causes, the doctor diagnoses a psychiatric eating disorder. Moreover, mental disorders can cause or exacerbate other conditions, such as high blood pressure, heart disease, obesity, asthma, and diabetes.

Failing to address the emotional contribution to these illnesses allows them to continue. Fortunately, most doctors recognize this and will refer these patients to a mental health professional.

However, the symptoms of a cutter and an eating disorder are much more apparent than the symptoms of alcoholism. Doctors want to believe their patients, yet alcoholics hide their symptoms well, which includes (a) lying about how much they drink, (b) how they feel when not drinking, (c) how the alcoholic-craving affects them, (d) whether they hide any of their drinking, (e) if their drinking is getting worse, (f) if drinking is causing problems in their life, (g) how often they think about drinking, (h) whether they feel a need to drink, (i) how others view their drinking, and (j) if they feel guilt or remorse about their drinking.*

If the doctor suspects a drinking problem, ethics demand discussing it with the patient as with any other suspected illness. How the doctor approaches the defensive alcoholic must be thought about and practiced in advance, yet it need not be perfect. Any discussion with the alcoholic is better than ignoring it.

Alcoholics who successfully deny the extent of their drinking problem aren't referred to a specialist or for treatment. Instead, while in denial and not recognizing alcoholism, doctors often do more harm by masking these symptoms with sedatives, anti-depressants, sleeping pills,

---

*This is discussed in more detail below under "Internal Denial—The Early Statge of Denial;" Chapter 2, under "The Typical Alcoholic;" Chapter 3, under "The Importance of Recognizing the Alcoholic-Craving," "Research of the Alcoholic-Craving," and "The Neuroscience of Craving;" and all of Chapter 7, "Health Care, Alcoholism, and the DSM."

tranquilizers, and other drugs. So, patients feel less of a need to seek treatment for the cause—alcoholism—while receiving care for its symptoms.

This 'treatment' often results in alcoholics developing a need for these drugs in addition to alcohol. The doctor's denial enables alcoholics to continue drinking as their alcoholism worsens, increasing the risk of further injury or death.

Since most doctors are untrained in alcoholism, they see distress, worry, sleep disorders, fatigue, general unease, and sadness and believe marital, work, and financial problems cause them. They assume their patient's physical symptoms will improve when these 'temporary' problems settle.

So the doctor *may* send the alcoholic to a mental health professional to help cope with life—not for alcoholism—but not any professional will do. Only those well-trained in identifying and addressing a drinking problem will likely help.

The Mental Health Professional

Many mental health professionals are in denial, nurtured by their stereotypical view of the alcoholic, the alcoholic's ability to hide symptoms, and lack of adequate training, which contributes to the misdiagnosis of 90% of all alcoholics. Moreover, the therapist's denial is further encouraged by their concern that the alcoholic may abruptly end therapy if confronted too soon or aggressively about their drinking.[21]

Confrontation is the enemy of denial. James Baldwin said, "Not everything that is faced can be changed ... but nothing can be changed until it is faced." I would add, "We're not ready to face everything ... and nothing faced before we're ready to face it can change."

For example, confrontation stabs at piercing our veil of denial and telling us what we need to know. Confronting alcoholics who are in the depths of denial can be helpful or hurtful. If they're not ready to deal with their alcoholism, it can cause severe emotional distress, further reinforcing denial, which could extend the time before they are ready to "face" it.

For example, a bud naturally blooms into a beautiful flower. Yet, if we try accelerating this process by pulling, twisting, and creasing the petals, a withered flower will emerge. If we're eager for a sapling to grow into a tall tree, we may overwater and overfertilize it, slowing or stopping its growth ... forever. So it is when confronting the alcoholic's denial—timing and patience are critical.

It can be challenging for therapists to suspect a drinking problem because most alcoholics are practiced at concealing their symptoms of alcoholism behind their symptoms of depression, anxiety, and other mood disorders. Determining whether these disorders are caused by, contribute to, or exist independently of alcoholism is complicated.[22] (See Chapter 7, "Health Care, Alcoholism, and the DSM.")

Therapists must gently confront the drinker without provoking too much defensiveness. Striking this delicate balance is an artful skill that requires developing trust and rapport, which requires patience and time. Because alcoholics are prone to quitting therapy before seeing the extent of their drinking problem and the limited visits insurance covers, timing becomes more critical.

Many alcoholics spend much time, energy, and money for help in taking this brave journey, only to resign moments before the discovery.

Many often end therapy because it's taking too long, not working, too costly, no longer needed, a waste of time refreshing unimportant and uncomfortable memories, they're too busy, their therapist is ineffective, or other 'reasons' arise. Although sometimes valid, usually they're not, especially when they flee just before the breakthrough of finally seeing their alcoholism. Denial of alcoholism is most stubborn just before exposing it.

Those alcoholics who don't benefit from talk therapy may benefit more from an intervention skillfully prepared and facilitated by an experienced interventionist. An intervention is the most common way to unclog the spillway, allowing the

The Court-Ordered Alcohol Assessment

The courts are in denial, relying on the court-ordered alcohol assessment as reliable evidence and giving it undue weight when deciding one's fate. Most judges making alcohol-related decisions are clueless about alcoholism, except for the few in recovery. Most believe it's not an illness but misconduct, which punishment can cure.

This denial is made worse by court evaluators using a flawed screening. The most common screening used is the MAST, which was *not* designed for court-mandated screenings and relies on self-reporting. Unfortunately, this screening only identifies the rare alcoholic who admits their drinking problem.

The questions on this screening are so transparent that alcoholics can easily navigate them to avoid detection. Here are some questions appearing on the MAST:

- Can you stop drinking without difficulty after one or two drinks?
- Have you ever lost friends because of your drinking?
- Has your drinking ever resulted in your being hospitalized in a psychiatric ward?
- Do you feel you are a normal drinker ("normal" means drinks as much or less than most other people)?

As reflected, the answers to 'pass the test' are so obvious that any screening asking only, "Are you an alcoholic?" would be as effective and yield the same result. Even so, online sources preserve denial by teaching how to 'trick' this evaluation.

Since the evaluation is court-ordered, in the unlikely event one is found to have a drinking problem, 'punishment' results. The absence of doctor-patient privacy also encourages false responses. Nor does the court-ordered evaluation include a review of independent data such as medical records, blood tests, court records, or interviews with those close to the alcoholic. All of this contributes to invalid results and enhances denial.

Alcoholics can be clever and charming. During a court-ordered assessment, they're on their best behavior, and the evaluator understands the 'punitive' effect of finding a drinking problem. Undoubtedly, finding someone to be an alcoholic who isn't would be legally catastrophic. So, the reverse is almost always the case—the evaluator doesn't conclude alcoholism. Of the many alcoholics I've spoken with, *all* 'fooled' this evaluation.

The result is devastating since the alcoholic now has a 'certificate of nonalcoholic,' causing a government-supported rationalization to delay seeking sobriety: "The court evaluated me and found I don't have a drinking problem, so I'll have one more, ... please!"

Moreover, the courts are in denial, believing the assessment is valid. This denial survives because the court budget misallocates funds instead of paying for the solution: Effective screenings and adequately trained assessors who are given the required time to conduct meaningful evaluations.*

The Employer, Employee, and Co-worker

The employer is in denial, concerned about the loss or absence of an experienced employee and the costly expense of addressing a drinking problem. This expense includes the cost of inpatient treatment and paying substitute or current employees more to cover the alcoholic's duties while absent in

---

*However, the costs of not improving the process far outweigh the costs of improvement when considering the expenses of multiple arrests, incarceration, damage to property, personal injuries, deaths, and the court system's time.

treatment. If the employer terminates the alcoholic, it will have the added expense of training a new employee.

These potential expenses cause the employer to bury its head deeper in the sand, supporting the belief that the employee's drinking "isn't too bad." For example, if an employee is often late or has difficulty completing tasks timely, efficiently, and effectively, the employer may overlook this and attribute it to causes other than alcoholism. The employer *wants* to believe the drinker will cut back when the 'short-term' problems in their life disappear. This denial is often long-lasting, allowing the alcoholic employee to postpone sobriety while spiraling deeper.

Also, tolerating the alcoholic will cause the morale of co-workers to decline as they cover the employee's workload and deal with the alcoholic's behavior.

However, in time, the employer usually realizes that the employee's drinking problem will not disappear on its own, and the long-term expenses of retaining such an employee will exceed the short-term expenses of attending to it.

Moreover, employees may avoid confronting a boss suspected of having a drinking problem, fearing retaliation.

Loved Ones

Loved ones easily assume the alcoholic's denial. For example, the husband thinks he must be more patient because of the stress his alcoholic wife endures, to which he believes he has contributed.

The consequences of drinking, such as a DUI arrest, a job loss, an injury, or a car accident, also affect loved ones who naturally want to avoid them. They often depend heavily on the alcoholic, so when they enable continued drinking by stopping the natural flow of drinking's consequences, they are also protecting themselves.

Yet they're not only protecting their financial interests, they're also trying to avoid embarrassment. And the most common way to do this is through denial—denying that drinking is causing problems and their loved one is an alcoholic. This denial may reach a point where they refuse to talk or think about the alcoholic's drinking.

Since their denial comes effortlessly, they are encouraged to believe the alcoholic, who skillfully discounts the signs of alcoholism by claiming drinking hasn't caused these problems.

For a time, loved ones often believe the alcoholic who claims everything and everyone else is to blame: an envious co-worker caused their firing, they divorced because of their spouse's misconduct, the other driver's carelessness caused the accident and injuries, or merely bad luck. Denial convinces loved ones that most people would drink if they had the alcoholic's problems. Denial also allows loved ones to ignore the fact that if the alcoholic didn't drink, they wouldn't have these problems.

Unfortunately, those affected see the truth long after much of the damage the drinker has caused is irreparable, which is when most interventions occur.

Children experience their own denial. In addition to the shame of having an alcoholic parent, they 'enjoy' the freedom their parents' permissiveness allows, fueled by their obsession with alcohol rather than their children.

Finally, loved ones nurture their denial in many ways that are unknown to them. The solution is to make them aware of these, exposing their denial. (See Chapter 8, "The Affected.")

Friends

Friends soon realize their present bond is based solely on their past. They now have little in common. Everything the alcoholic does involves drinking. They're drifting apart.

Friends know the drinker has a problem but hope it's a phase that will soon end. They're also reluctant to label him an alcoholic, believing good friends don't do that. They may casually mention a concern about their friend's drinking, which causes the glue that once bound them to become brittle as their friendship falls apart.

The alcoholic senses the 'disapproval' of his friends, which causes him to hide his drinking. Still, these friendships magnify his drinking problem, so he decides his friends "just aren't much fun anymore," causing further discomfort during visits. Phone calls soon give way to curt text messaging. As time passes, the alcoholic slowly exchanges his long-time friends for new ones.

If a friend drinks like the alcoholic, they both have distorted views fueling their denial. If the friend confronted the alcoholic, it would be self-confrontation. And both worry about losing longtime drinking companions who encourage the other's denial.

Denial and the Stigmatized Alcoholic

The stigma of untreated alcoholics supports their denial. Active alcoholics believe their drinking is a secret—it's not. They fear seeking treatment will expose this secret, inviting stigmatization—it doesn't.

Alcoholics, like others, resist acting in ways that incite and invite moral condemnation. Yet denial prevents them from realizing they *are* stigmatized, and if they were sober, they'd be less stigmatized. Indeed, most people—who mistakenly believe that a weak will and a flawed character cause alcoholism—admire the sober alcoholic.

THE PROGRESSION OF DENIAL

NO ONE DISPUTES that alcoholism is progressive. Chapter 2, "A Description of the Alcoholic," details the stages of this progression. Yet it's not only the alcoholic's drinking that intensifies—all symptoms of alcoholism worsen, including denial.

Although alcoholics know they're getting worse, they misjudge how much worse, as they increasingly try convincing others and themselves that it appears worse than it is. This includes progressively comparing, rationalizing, justifying, hiding, blaming, deceiving, isolating, and resenting.

Just as alcoholism doesn't progress the same for every alcoholic, neither does its symptoms. The symptom of denial is dynamic—stronger at times, weaker at other times. Alcoholics often experience denial at various times and intensities, which I've separated into three types.

1. *Internal denial* is when alcoholics believe they don't have a drinking problem.
2. *Partial denial* is when alcoholics suspect they may have a drinking problem but think it's not too bad, and those worrying about their drinking are overreacting.
3. *External denial* is when alcoholics know they have a drinking problem but deny or minimize it to others.

It's not unusual for alcoholics to slide back and forth through the various types of denial as their alcoholism progresses—the stages are not as distinct as outlined.

Internal Denial—The Early Stage of Denial

Many of us have known someone reputed to be a pathological liar—a habitually "good" or "convincing" liar. And when Abraham Lincoln spoke this truth, "No man has a good enough memory to be a successful liar," he clearly wasn't including those alcoholics deepest in *internal* denial, who believe their own lies.

Initially, alcoholics hide nothing about their drinking because they see nothing to hide. They feel better when drinking, freely express how good they feel, and function well.

Their enjoyment of drinking is obvious as they become more obsessed with alcohol. Since they're developing an increasing tolerance for alcohol, they appear to manage their drinking without affecting their relationships or job performance, which further obscures their drinking problem.

Because much of the alcoholic's denial in the early stage is subtle, they and others are deep in *internal* denial—no one is concerned.

Examples of Internal Denial

- Alcoholics maintain their stereotypical view of the alcoholic as a skid-row resident. This view allows them to compare their functional lives with the dysfunctional lives of other alcoholics. Because they're employed, own a home and car, and are successful, they insist they can't be alcoholics. Still, a comparison to only 10% of all alcoholics doesn't help one self-diagnose alcoholism.
- They announce reasons for drinking, such as "I just need one or two to calm down."
- They claim, "I don't need to drink. I can take it or leave it. I drink because I want to."
- They insist that it's wasteful to leave an unfinished drink. But it's not wasteful to leave an unfinished glass of iced tea.
- They are irritated if anyone or anything interferes with their drinking.
- They say, "I'll have just one more," and believe it as they repeatedly drink 'one more.'
- They believe rejecting an offer to buy them a drink is rude. But it isn't rude to decline an offer to buy them coffee.
- They justify their loss of control when they drink too much.
- They become concerned about running out of liquor.
- They may inquire whether there will be drinking at a planned event.

Partial Denial—The Middle Stage of Denial

Denial surges in the middle stage. It is no longer internal

denial but partial denial. Alcoholics now *suspect* they *may* have a drinking problem, even though they're unaware of its severity, and contend any comment about their drinking is an overreaction.

Others are seeing them differently than they see themselves. By the time others notice a problem, alcoholism has progressed to a severe level.

Examples of Partial Denial

- They compare their drinking with others ("Did you see how much John drank? *He* clearly has a drinking problem").
- They *try* masking the smell of alcohol by drinking different types of liquors, using breath fresheners, and avoiding close contact with others.
- They usually say, "I only had a couple," when they've had more.
- They explain that drinking allows them to relax. Their need to relax causes their surrender to the alcoholic-craving, which initially caused the anxiety they now seek to escape.
- They insist they drink because of the growing problems in their lives and dismiss that drinking is worsening these problems.
- They assert that since they can hold their liquor and can drink "anyone under the table," they can't have a drinking problem. They see tolerance as a virtue rather than caused by a damaged brain and liver.
- They claim they drink to reduce pain or worry, boost creativity, or for any reason besides their need for alcohol.
- They explain they don't need to drink every day, unaware that most alcoholics are periodic drinkers and don't drink daily.

- They believe drinking water between drinks proves they can control their drinking and that they're not alcoholics.
- They order doubles because they get more for their money and deny it's related to their increasing tolerance for alcohol.
- They often attempt to justify their drinking through complex rationalizations and make rules about their drinking to convince themselves and others that they don't have a drinking problem ("I only drink on weekends" or "I never drink before sundown"). (See Chapter 2 under "Rationalization.")
- They focus on their socioeconomic status to support their denial. This applies to high-functioning professionals, who rely on what others think of them to maintain denial. If no one sees a problem, there must not be one.
- They may begin vanishing for brief periods to sneak a drink.
- They condemn the drinking of others who they believe are 'worse' drinkers.
- They focus on and seem concerned about another's drinking to avoid facing their own drinking problem and may even confront them about it.
- They claim they hide their drinking to keep loved ones from needlessly worrying. It's not their drinking they're trying to hide, but just sparing loved ones from overreacting and needlessly worrying.
- They may stop at a bar after work to drink without distractions, perhaps claiming it's work-related.
- They claim the reason they drink is because of relationship problems, difficulties at work, or financial troubles instead of their need to drink ("Anyone would drink like I do if they had my problems").
- They find 'reasons' to drink instead of eating, claiming,

"I'm skipping dinner. I need to lose a few pounds," ignoring that most lose weight when they stop drinking.

- They explain their drinking even when no one prompts or wants an explanation.
- They need to create reasons to drink. This doesn't suggest the reasons are fictional, but they focus on, magnify, and intensify these 'reasons' until they become a 'good' excuse to drink.
- They focus on the fact that they get less drunk than others who drink the same, ignoring their increasing need to drink more to feel how they once felt when drinking less—the alcoholic symptom of tolerance.
- They claim they're too young to be an alcoholic, ignoring that alcoholism afflicts those of all ages.
- They are often apologetic and even remorseful about their drinking, claiming they didn't intend to drink that much.
- They now drink with people who drink the same or more, so they can deny drinking too much if anyone suggests they cut back by claiming, "Everyone I know drinks like I do, or more, so why focus on me?"
- They nurture resentments, which enables them to drink guilt-free and feel entitled to drink.
- They make a point to mention and seek praise for the times they don't drink ("Did you notice I haven't had a drink all week?").
- They believe that drinking beer or wine instead of liquor indicates they don't have a drinking problem.
- They explain that any DUI arrests were merely bad luck. They were at the wrong place at the wrong time. They focus only on getting caught, overlooking that they were driving while drunk and that their previous arrests didn't deter them from becoming repeat offenders.

- They feel unique and misunderstood, allowing them to ignore and devalue the opinions of those confronting them about their drinking.

Alcoholics, *deep* in internal denial, don't even consider that they may be alcoholics. Yet, once they move from internal to partial denial, they usually devote most of their lives obsessively asking this question: *Am I an alcoholic?*

When asking themselves this question, they will answer in one of three ways.

1) **Yes.** *I'll quit now.* A "yes" answer means no more drinking starting now. This is a frightening choice when thinking about a life without alcohol.

2) **No.** *I'll never quit.* A "no" answer means nothing changes, which is just as terrifying when considering that if nothing changes, life goes on *with* drinking, accompanied by remorse and misery.

3) **Undecided.** *Maybe I'll stop someday if I need to, but not today.* This third answer of "undecided" is most attractive because it poses no immediate threat of abstinence and leaves drinkers with a glimmer of hope that they aren't doomed to live this way forever. However, accepting that most alcoholics won't choose to get sober, this is a cruel, self-imposed life sentence with intensifying suffering unless a life-changing event intervenes.

Further, since alcoholics repeatedly question whether they have a drinking problem, they will answer it differently as their alcoholism and denial progress. Still, this inquiry is a natural and necessary process to escape denial.

External Denial—The Late Stage of Denial

Alcoholics now *know* they abuse alcohol. So, to avoid anyone expressing concerns that could hamper their drinking, they try hiding it. Although they believe they're hiding it well, they're not. It's becoming clear that alcohol is controlling them more than they're controlling it.

Examples of External Denial

- They often sneak a few drinks before going to a bar, party, or event so it doesn't look like they're drinking too much after arriving.
- If they occasionally go to a bar after work, they may go more often and stay longer to avoid confrontation. Dinner is getting colder more often.
- They're often annoyed or irritated when someone casually mentions their drinking, and they give reasons and blame others for drinking so much. If pressed about it, they become defensive, claiming, "I haven't had as many as you think," or "These drinks are weak." They may be evasive, complaining, "Do you need to ruin everything by bringing that up now?" and hostile, shouting, "Give me a break. All you ever do is complain about my having a drink or two—it never stops!"
- They obsess about others who might think they have a drinking problem.
- They may occasionally and temporarily stop drinking to convince others they're not alcoholics and announce this by saying, "I'm on the wagon, just taking a break from drinking."
- They often announce a limit on the number of drinks they will have and then give reasons for exceeding it.
- They attempt to conceal their drinking by secretly drinking, hiding bottles, making quiet trips to and alternating liquor stores, paying cash for liquor, transporting liquor in a flask, trying to act sober, texting rather than slurring words, trying to hide the smell of alcohol, and lying to and avoiding those concerned.
- They agree that they need to cut back on their drinking someday, hoping to avoid more aggressive suggestions

that they quit drinking.
- They are angry if anyone drinks their alcohol.
- They go to great lengths to avoid discussing their drinking ("Not this again. If you'd quit harassing me, I wouldn't drink as much. I told you I'm cutting back").
- They may occasionally and surprisingly control their drinking by stopping after one or two, which further confuses observers.
- They avoid others and hide their drinking by isolating themselves so people can't see their worsening condition.

Finally Escaping Denial

During the final stage of alcoholism, alcoholics have mostly escaped denial, except for a few remnants, such as denying that they can stop drinking and denying that recovery is possible.

They no longer bother to hide their drinking since it's obvious they're drinking excessively. So they're less defensive when asked about their drinking, no longer explaining it. They concede their drinking problem is severe and they need to quit. Still, instead of entirely quitting, they usually only consider cutting back.

Although they may still deny the severity of their drinking, they and others know the truth. They have alcohol-related health problems and now drink because they believe they must and to avoid withdrawal symptoms. They are beginning to resemble the stereotypical alcoholic.

They no longer compare their drinking with others—less severe alcoholics compare their drinking to them.

The Story of Jim, Sue, and Bob

THIS STORY ILLUSTRATES the three dynamic stages of denial and how alcoholics alternate between these stages at various times as their alcoholism progresses. Although alcoholics experience them differently, common threads weave through them all. I'll let Jim tell it.

I'M FINALLY HERE. *I hope it doesn't look like I've been drinking, and I don't see anyone I know.*
"Hello, how's your day going?"
"Good, thanks," I reply.
"Can I help you find something?"
"No, thanks."
"If I can, just holler."
"Will do." As I walk toward the whiskey section, I see her out of the corner of my eye. *I can't believe this is happening.* I look down and move toward the wine section. Grabbing the closest bottle, I turn, lower my head, and pretend to concentrate on the label.
"Jim, ... hey, Jim! How's it goin'?"
I casually glance up. "Oh, Sue? How are you?"
"Great!"
I mumble, "What about this weather?"
"You can't ask for any better. I love it! Worked in my garden all morning!"
I nod. "Vegetable or Flow—"
"—Flower—it's a flower garden. It's beautiful! You know that—you've seen it!"
"Oh, yeah. It's—"
"Vegetable?" Sue shakes her head. "I don't live on a farm!"
"Of course, you don't. Anyways, I need to pick up some wine for a friend—dinner." I glance at my watch. "In fact, I'm running late, so I better—"
"You? Running late? Imagine that," Sue chides.
I half-smile, half-nod while staring at nothing. "Well, I better—"
"I know you're in a hurry, Jim, but can I ask you a quick question? I hate asking you here—"
"Sure. Go for it." *She could've called and asked me.*

"Well, a few of us have been a little worried about you lately. You haven't been looking or acting . . . like yourself and —"

What is this feeling? I feel like my skin could ignite. I could spontaneously combust, just like I've heard about. Poof! Just like that! I interrupt, "I appreciate your concern. I do. Where's a mirror? There's one. You're right. I do look a little . . . puffy. Too much salt and stress, the doctor recently told me. Maybe a slight blood pressure issue, too." *I do need to see a doctor—it's been years.*

"You need to take care of yourself!" Sue says.

"I will—you, too. Hey, great seeing you— I'm sure I'll see ya soon." I pause, waiting for her reply. *She looks as if she's seizing—maybe a stroke. I couldn't be so lucky.* She's frozen, with her mouth parted and an empty stare. She looks like she's getting ready to drool any second. *I sense she has more to say. I wish her mouth quit working.* Oh, no. It seems like she's coming to.

"Uh . . . I don't know how to say this, but . . . honestly, we've been a little worried about your . . . drinking."

"Worried about my . . . what?" *I wish she'd shut her mouth.* "Now, what are you worried about again?"

"We're a little concerned about your—"

"My drinking?"

"Just a little . . . concerned." Sue breaks eye contact. "Just a little, that's all."

"Who are *we*?"

"It doesn't matter."

"Well, yeah, it kind of does because I'd like to know who cares about me that much to be a . . . *little* . . . concerned."

"You know, just people we see at parties. It's no biggie. Just a little concerned, that's all."

"It's funny you say that because I've been worried about your drinking." *I wonder if people are really talking about my drinking. If so, Sue is causing this by spreading lies behind my back. Is she actually saying this in a liquor store? She irritates me so much, but if I show it, it'll be worse.*

"I shouldn't have said anything. I can see you're a little upset with—"

"Upset? No. A little amused, maybe. This is perfect." I laugh while rubbing my temples. Then, I look down, shake my head, and quip, "A mutual intervention in a liquor store?"

Sue looks at me, tilts her head, smirks, and says, "At least no one else is here."

"That's true, at least. Well, I appreciate your, or should I say, *everyone's* concern. But I drink maybe a couple a week, if that many. I know you saw me at those holiday parties when I was a little juiced, but I'm good. It's a New Year's resolution thing." *I feel a heat wave swirling throughout me. I hope she doesn't notice. I wonder if this is how it feels right before spontaneously combusting.* "Thanks again, though. I sincerely appreciate your *concern*. And please relay my thanks to everyone else concerned." *What a—I can't stand her! I can't believe I'm explaining my drinking to her in a liquor store!*

"Good! I'm glad to hear you've got it under control." Her voice sounds raspy, grating, irritating, and insincere.

"I guess I'll see you later." I squeeze out a smile and raise my open hand in front of me, which could be viewed as a gesture of waving goodbye or "stop, don't come any closer."

"See ya," she says.

Here I was, happy, and then Sue had to be here, walk over to me, open her stupid mouth, and ruin my day. Okay, Jim, be calm. Buy the wine and get out of here. I walk over to the clerk and hand her the bottle.

"Oh, this is an excellent wine. Have you tried it before?

"Nope."

"You will love it!"

"I'm looking forward to it. I'll tell you what I think the next time I see you," *which I hope is never. Why doesn't she shut up? How does she know what I'll love?*

"Let's see, that'll be $87.00."

"Eight . . . I'm sorry, 80 . . . what?"

"Seven . . . 87."

"Well, if it's as good as you say, it's worth every penny." *She must be kidding. Eighty-seven dollars? I hate wine—and Sue. Now, she's fumbling around with a stack of sacks stuck together. She'd better finish before Sue gets behind me. Oh, this is driving me crazy.* "I don't need a sack," I blurt.

"Sorry, I almost have it, and it's the law."

No, it's not the law, even though everyone thinks it is. But I'm not about to say anything that might delay this. I should make a run for it. I'll say I had an emergency or something. She places the bottle in the sack. *Well, it's too late to run. I could've if Sue weren't here.*

"Here you go. Sorry for the bag delay."

"No problem." I pay her. She hands me the bottle and says, "Thanks, see you next time."

"Thank you," I mumble. *No, there won't be a next time.*

"See ya," Sue shouts.

I wave goodbye and wonder what just happened. *Did I pay $87.00 for a bottle of wine I don't want because of Sue? I dislike her more and more as each second passes. Why does this walk to my car seem longer than the store? I had better look where I'm walking; this is the last place I want to trip and fall.*

Keys? Where are they? . . . I must've left them on the counter. That's just great. What a day this is turning into—because of Sue. I walk back to the store, crack the door, and quietly ask, "Did I leave my keys on the counter?"

"No, but . . ." She points to my right hand, covers her mouth, giggles, and says, "Oh, I do it all the time. In fact, last Saturday—"

I nod while half-smiling and walk away. *I don't care about her embarrassing moments. The walk to my car feels even longer the second time. What am I doing with this wine? I guess I could put it up in case of an emergency. Now, I have to go to another liquor store because the clerk probably heard everything we said. That Sue is such a waste of time.*

I'M FINALLY HOME. I don't think I've ever despised anyone as much as Sue.

I should've also bought a bottle of whiskey. I could've said I needed it for a friend. Oh, well. I bought some at another liquor store on the way home.

So people think I've got a drinking problem. What a nightmare. I'm going to slow down so no one else catches on. I just can't imagine life without drinking. I guess I'll have one more shot. "Aaah! So warm and soothing."

I wish I could find that spare bottle I tucked away. Where could it be? It makes no sense. I can remember hiding it, but not where I hid it. Oh, well. While tapping my fingers on the counter, I decide I need a better system.

What is Sue's problem? I want her to know how much I despise her. No one's concerned, and she isn't either. She just wanted to irritate and embarrass me. Why else would she say those things? She needs to look at herself, and that drunk she lives with. She's stupid or evil, or maybe she's both. That's it. It's people like her that cause me to drink.

Still, if I'm not careful, my drinking could get out of hand and become a problem. Well, I've got that problem solved—I'll slow down.

I couldn't even get help if I wanted to because more people would think I had a drinking problem. I wonder what people are thinking and saying. No wonder everyone's been acting a little strange lately. I just need to drink at home more. Where does Sue get off . . . ? Whatever.

I'm never talking to her again. I guess I'll have one more. Just my luck, I had to see her. But I was smooth. She didn't even know I'd been drinking. That's how stupid she is. And the wine confused her—what a brilliant idea!

—

COMMENT: Jim is weaving in and out of partial and external denial.

He is trying to conceal his drinking and hide other things about it, such as hoping no one he knows sees him in the liquor store. He's deceitful when moving to the wine section, telling Sue he's picking "up some wine for a friend" and then buying wine. Alcoholics believe if no one thinks they're an alcoholic, their drinking can't be that serious. So if they hide it, no one will ask about it. And if no one asks about it, they can avoid sobriety.

His thinking is distorted. He thinks he "was smooth. She didn't even know I'd been drinking," which we later learn is incorrect. Denial prevents alcoholics from realizing others know more about their drinking than they think they do. Living this lie includes hiding the nature of their drinking from those who don't care, such as trash collectors, liquor store clerks, or other strangers.

The more he deceives others, the more he deceives himself. He can't let anyone think he has a problem and considers isolating when he decides, "I just need to drink at home more." He suspects people are acting differently. He's rationalizing excuses for not getting help, concluding, "I couldn't even get help if I wanted to because more people would think I had a drinking problem," which shows he's at least somewhat aware of his drinking problem.

It's partial denial—denying and lying to others while believing his drinking is less severe than it is and external denial—knowing his drinking is severe and trying to hide it from others.

Jim is defensive when Sue confronts him, yet he discounts her concern by deciding, "No one's concerned." Still, he obsesses about "what people are thinking and saying," even people he doesn't know, including the clerk.

He tries to justify his recent drunkenness at parties with excuses and claims he made a New Year's drinking resolution, which nonalcoholics don't consider.

Jim's alcoholism fuels his impatience with the clerk and his resentment of Sue. His focus on Sue and the clerk blurs his problem and justifies his drinking. His anger also overshadows his guilt and doubt about drinking.

He's obsessed with possibly running out of liquor while trying to recall where he hid a bottle. He's also annoyed he didn't buy two bottles, even though he's holding a full one. He's keeping the wine for an "emergency," which means he would drink it if he ran out of whiskey.

He's isolating, comparing, justifying, concealing, blaming, lying, denying, deceiving, and resenting, which are characteristics of partial and external denial.

Sue is in internal and partial denial, comparing her drinking with Jim's and focusing on him.

Jim's internal debate illustrates the denial alcoholics struggle with, which is often a constant companion monopolizing their thinking. As denial evaporates, a feeling of terror usually erupts because many who finally accept their alcoholism take no action to treat it.

—

Let's drop in on Sue and meet Bob.

"**HEY, BOB! YOU'LL** never guess who I saw today?" Sue asks as if it's breaking news.

"Who, Sue?" He takes a swig. "I'm waiting."

"Guess."

"I'm not guessing." He takes another swig. "Who?"

"Jim!"

"Jim . . . Jim the drunk?"

"Yep."

"Where'd you see him?"

"It's ironic, but I saw him at the liquor store."

"Nothing ironic about that. You'd have a better chance of seeing him in a liquor store than anywhere else. Was he drunk?"

"Oh, yeah, he was so drunk he could hardly stand. He tried avoiding me by pretending to read the label on a wine bottle. He was mumbling and slurring his words. And I said something about his drinking, but, of course, he shrugged it off."

"Well, of course, he did." Bob smiles while nodding as if

he's further convinced of something. "In the liquor store, that's funny."

"I was discreet when I whispered it. We were the only ones in there except for the clerk, but she didn't hear us." Sue pauses. "I felt sorry for him."

"Sorry for him? Are you serious? Remember the last time we saw him at the Christmas party? He was so obnoxious he ran everyone off."

"Oh yeah, I remember. That was the night you thought you were so cute wearing that lampshade on your head." She shakes her head, takes a deep breath, and sighs, "Real original."

"It *was* funny. Everyone was laughing—except you." Then, turning his head in the other direction, he says, "That's what made it so funny, you know, the old lampshade on the head act we've all heard about. I know it was funny."

Bob finishes his drink. The rattling ice interrupts the silence, signaling the time for a refill.

"All this talk of Jim is making me thirsty; want one?"

"Well, today's been stressful. I guess I'll have a glass of wine to unwind. Any plans for lunch?"

"Nope. I'm drinking my lunch. . need to lose a few pounds. Why, hungry?"

"Oh, I don't know—"

"Here you go." He hands her the glass. "I can't believe you didn't think my lampshade act was funny."

"Okay. Both Jim and you were quite entertaining."

"Jim and I? Jim ruined the party. I was the funny one, and he was nothing but an ass. How can you use both our names in the same sentence? I hope I never see him again."

"Yeah, I know, I know. He's quite pathetic."

"He's pathetic, alright."

"Oh, and listen to this. He bought an $87.00 bottle of wine at the liquor store instead of whiskey, trying to fool me. Isn't that sad?"

"I'll tell you, Sue; he's a nut—a real nut. All I have to do is compare my drinking to his to know that my drinking is normal. They ought to drop every drunk like Jim on some deserted island."

"I'd miss you if they did that," Sue chortles.

"Funny, very funny. You're making me thirsty. I'm making *one* more. You want *one* more?"

"Well, since I haven't had a drink in a few days, I'll have *one* more. But please don't use those small glasses. They're more trouble than they're worth, and pour some in it this time . . . please. I'm not getting up and down, running back and forth, and pouring more wine every few minutes."

He mumbles, "You never do, I do," then walks off.

"Whatever!"

He returns a minute later. "Here you go."

"That's better. Thanks."

—

COMMENT: They discuss Sue seeing Jim at the liquor store, ignoring that Sue was also there. Sue and Bob never stop comparing Jim's drinking with theirs. Bob says, "All I have to do is compare my drinking to his to know I'm a normal drinker." Then, Sue discounts her drinking by comparing it to Jim's and Bob's. Alcoholics can deny their drinking problem when comparing it with someone who drinks more, even though the amount one drinks means little. Still, it's a common way to strengthen internal denial.

Sue's comment about Bob's drinking blunders and her quip that he would be among the drunks dropped off on a deserted island help discount her drinking and subtly confront his. Her grumbling about the small glasses, not stopping after "just one more," and making the excuse that it saves her from "getting up and down, running back and forth" all reveal her increasing tolerance and excuse-making, which is internal denial.

Both reveal their internal denial by giving reasons for their drinking: Bob says, "You're making me thirsty," and "All this talk of Jim is making me thirsty." Sue says, "Well, today's been stressful. I guess I'll have a glass of wine to unwind," and

"Well, since I haven't had a drink in a few days, I'll have *one* more."

Just as water seeks its own level, alcoholics seek others who drink like them. They support each other's denial by condemning the drinking of others. Still, they're defensive when one remarks the others' drinking. Bob insists, "I was the funny one, and he was nothing but an ass," all examples of partial denial.

If they disclosed their true thoughts, their armor of denial would shatter, exposing their alcoholism. Then their bond would begin to crumble, which neither is prepared to deal with—at the moment. They are both mostly in internal and partial denial.

Let's revisit Bob and Sue and see how they're doing.

THIRTY MINUTES LATER.

"I'm having one more; you want one?"

"Why not? It's Saturday. Here's my glass. I'll have just *one* more, too." Sue taps her foot. "And I mean it, just *one* more."

"Uh, . . . Sue, . . . bottle's empty."

"What? Check the cabinet. You'll find another one."

"I'll check." Bob opens and closes the cabinet doors quickly and routinely without looking inside. "Nope. Nothing."

"That's impossible. I had two bottles. Have you been drinking my wine?" Sue sighs. "Well, I guess I'll have one of yours. You know the routine."

"Yep, two ice cubes and a splash." He hands her the drink.

"Looks like you might've gotten it right this time."

"This time and every other time," he mumbles.

TWO DRINKS LATER.

"By the way, have you seen Cindy lately? It looks like her drinking is starting to take its toll," Sue comments.

"I was thinking that when I saw her last week." He

chuckles, shaking his head. "Maybe Cindy and Jim should get together."

"Oh yeah! They'd be the perfect couple." Sue runs her fingers through her hair, straightens her posture, and asks, "Have you noticed that most of our friends have drinking problems?"

"I was thinking that earlier today."

"Compared to them, we have nothing to worry about," Sue murmurs, then slumps and gazes at her drink. "How does that phrase go? But for the grace of God, I go, or something like that. You know what I mean."

"Well, Sue, we've done something right. You want *one* more?" He sways as he walks toward the bar. "And I mean it this time."

"Sure, I guess. Might as well. I only planned to drink wine, and I've already had more than I planned! I'll have just *one* more, and that's it, no more."

"Deal," he confirms.

—

COMMENT: Sue continues drinking her third "*one* more" by justifying, "It's Saturday." Bob knows the "routine." It's the repeating event of Sue running out of wine, Bob looking for her bottle expecting not to find it, and her drinking whiskey. This way, Sue can talk herself into believing she's a wine drinker and justify her drinking the fourth "*one* more" by claiming, "I only planned to drink wine." But it looks as if Sue may be a closet whiskey drinker. She was looking at the whiskeys in the liquor store, not the wines. Claiming one drinks only beer or wine, not the hard stuff, is common to support partial denial. But alcoholism doesn't discriminate between distilled and undistilled ethanol—drinking one instead of the other isn't more symptomatic.

Comparing their drinking to others continues to dominate their conversations. Sue mentions Cindy's "drinking is starting to take its toll," and Bob suggests, "Maybe Cindy and Jim should get together." Sue says, "Compared to them, we have nothing to worry about," and she even uses God to compare her drinking with others by asserting if God didn't grace her, her drinking would be similar to everyone she criticizes. They have two drinks after they agree to "just *one* more." They can't stop. Both are invested in internal and partial denial.

Their chances of admitting their drinking problem and seeking help soon seem unlikely unless one accepts their alcoholism and confronts the other or an intervention occurs. If that happens, they have a chance.

Now for the end of the story.

TWO DAYS LATER.

"Sue, you've been drinking my whiskey?"

"No, why?"

"Why? Bob is shaking the bottle above his head. "Because it's half empty, and it was full last night!"

"Half the time, you don't remember how much you drink." Her voice trails, "So don't blame me for your problem."

"Problem? What's that supposed to mean?"

"You heard me."

"Are you saying you didn't drink any of my whiskey? Because if you're— "

"Your whiskey? How is it *your* whiskey?" Sue sits rigidly with her fists clenched. "I bought it for us. It's *our* whiskey, and I can drink as much of it as I want, and if—"

"So, you did drink some, and you were lying to me."

Sue stands. "No, I wasn't lying. You asked me if I drank some of *your* whiskey, and I didn't." She walks to the window and looks out. "I drank some of *our* whiskey."

"You're the one with the problem, Sue." He glares at her as she gazes out the window. "A real problem."

"That may be, but I'm not as bad as you are," she says in a softer voice.

"I'm not the one sneaking my drinks and lying about it.

That's classic alcoholism."

They both stare in opposite directions, tears blurring their vision. Then, the dam of denial opens enough to let a gentle flow through the spillway, creating a moment of clarity. They make eye contact.

"Let's face it, Bob; we both have drinking problems." Sue slumps, drops her head, and uncrosses her arms. She takes a deep breath and exhales. "I think we might be—"

He looks down and mutters, "Alcoholics." Silence. "So . . . where do we go from here?"

—

COMMENT: Sue is hiding her drinking, and Bob is outraged that Sue is secretly drinking his whiskey. They blame and compare their drinking with each other: "But I'm not as bad as you are," says Sue, and "I'm not the one sneaking drinks and lying about it," says Bob—all examples of external denial.

Yet, in an unusual moment of clarity, they both finally escape denial and recognize their alcoholism.

—

SO, ALTHOUGH DENIAL can be helpful or harmful, the alcoholic's denial is a symptom of alcoholism and is always harmful. Denial, which often comes and goes, even in sobriety, is progressive and comes in various forms. Still, the entourage's denial is a significant barrier to recovery and lengthens the misery for *everyone*.

Various sources kindle the entourage's denial, including the alcoholic stigma and their vision of the stereotypical alcoholic.

Denial is the primary reason most alcoholics never seek sobriety and the reason for most relapses. One simple solution is better education.

QUESTIONS FOR DISCUSSION

1. What are your thoughts about the alcoholic's entourage?
2. What do you think about denial fueling the disparity of healthcare?
3. Did you know that healthcare is in denial?
4. Was the discussion about the three types of alcoholic denial helpful?
5. Did you relate to anything in the story of Jim, Sue, and Bob?
6. Before reading this, were you aware of the progression of denial?
7. Have you had or observed any of the symptoms of denial?
8. Do you agree that denial can be helpful?
9. Has this chapter affected you? How?
10. Has this chapter altered the way you view denial?
11. Can you identify with any of the listed characteristics of the alcoholic's denial in this chapter? If so, which ones?
12. If you're a sober alcoholic, what stage of denial did you reach before sobriety? Are you aware that denial is the primary reason for relapses?
13. Do you strongly agree or disagree with anything in this chapter? If so, what? Why?
14. Did this chapter persuade or dissuade you about any of your thoughts regarding denial?
15. Did you learn anything from this chapter? If yes, discuss.

THE PERIODIC ALCOHOLIC
(Binge or Episodic Drinker)

CHAPTER 6

*You're probably an alcoholic if
you've ever thought or said, "I'm
not an alcoholic—I don't have to drink
every day. But when I start, I don't stop."*
—

IT'S A COMMON myth that one must drink daily to be an alcoholic.* Most alcoholics are periodic drinkers—they don't drink every day.[1] Yet once they start, they often don't stop. Alcoholics who drink periodically (periodics) struggle more with denial than alcoholics who drink daily (chronics). Periodics focus on the days they don't drink to convince themselves and others they're not alcoholics. But periods of abstinence prove nothing. Normal drinkers don't focus on the times they don't drink.

Not all daily drinkers are alcoholics—most periodic alcoholics drink less than many normal drinkers. Moreover, to reemphasize, most alcoholics are not physically dependent on alcohol. So, alcoholics aren't identified by how much or often they drink. Instead, it's how alcohol affects them and their inability to always control how much they drink once they start drinking that defines alcoholism.

---

*For a more detailed discussion of this, see the section *The Typical Alcoholic* in Chapter 2, "The Description of the Alcoholic."

The Periodic Alcoholic's Denial

PERIODICS HAVE ETCHED in their minds a magnified view of the stereotypical alcoholic. Periodics zoom in on the differences between their occasional drinking and the daily drinker to support denial of their drinking problem.

The Periodic's Rationalization

Rationalization is denial's favorite tool. It lets us create 'reasons' for our actions, which make sense but obscure the truth.

The periodics' rationalizations enable them to deny their alcoholism and continue drinking without the burden or the benefit of knowing the truth.

The comparisons made by periodics also fuel their rationalization and strengthen their denial.

The Periodic's Comparisons

Periodics obsess about the differences between their drinking and chronic alcoholics to convince themselves and others they're not alcoholics. They indulge in these comparisons more than chronic alcoholics do because it's easier for periodics to find those who drink more often.

However, comparing the amount and frequency of drinking between periodics and chronics is pointless without comparing alcoholic symptoms. If they did, they would see that both have the following symptoms. They often:

1) lose control over how much they drink after the first drink;
2) drink at the worst times;
3) are unable to see or ignore how their drinking harms others;
4) claim the problems caused by their drinking aren't that bad;
5) intend to quit or reduce (control) drinking;

6) know others complain about their drinking;
7) hide some of their drinking; and,
8) have missed important events because of their drinking.

Although both have similar symptoms, the periodic's behavior is often more noticeable and offensive. For example, periodics usually ignore work, family, and other responsibilities during a spree.[2] Also, since they don't drink daily, they justify compressing more drinking in a shorter period. This causes most periodics to suffer more consequences during drinking episodes.

Also, because periodics may go long intervals without drinking, they're usually less prepared to resist the alcoholic-craving when it strikes without warning. And since it's easier for periodics to find 'supportive' differences between their drinking and chronic alcoholics, they have a more challenging time escaping denial. Further, because their bottom is slower to reach and less visible, periodics are more leisurely about accepting their alcoholism and seeking sobriety.

The supportive differences that periodics clutch to fuel their denial even further include the following. They:

1) rarely develop the same alcohol tolerance as chronic alcoholics—they don't need to drink more to get the same effect;
2) are not *physically* addicted to alcohol;
3) don't have physical withdrawal, although their psychological withdrawal may be worse;
4) don't need medically managed detox;
5) usually are high functioning since occasional drinking doesn't interfere with their lives as much as daily drinking; and
6) avoid many health problems that afflict chronic alcoholics.

Still, these differences don't reveal whether the periodic is an alcoholic.

Some alcoholics who drink periodically never become daily drinkers. Yet all alcoholics who drink daily once drank periodically.

Examples of the Periodics' Denial

Examples of the rationalizations, comparisons, and deceptive thinking periodic drinkers employ to strengthen their denial follow. They:

1) compare their 'occasional' glasses of wine or 'couple' of beers with the daily whiskey drinker;
2) refuse to compare their drinking to the average drinker;
3) don't see their comparisons as obsessive, irrational, and meaningless;
4) minimize the severity of their drinking and drunken behavior by focusing on others' conduct;
5) dismiss the concerns of loved ones;
6) claim they don't have a drinking problem because they don't *need* to drink daily;
7) claim they only continue drinking after the first one because they choose to and don't want to stop, but forget how much they regretted drinking after their last spree, vowing never to drink as much again;
8) blame their difficulties on others;
9) use their martyrdom as an excuse to drink and 'reason' that since they work so hard for long periods without drinking, they deserve to let loose every so often;
10) ignore the problems their drinking, thinking, and behavior cause their loved ones;
11) are excessively defensive about their drinking;
12) forget how they panic when they run out of alcohol during a spree;

13) invite superficial drinking companions into their lives;

14) don't see that drinking causes their despair and problems; and

15) fail to do anything about their drinking.

The periodic's drinking pattern makes it challenging to identify a problem. For example, periodics may go days, weeks, months, or even years without drinking and without the alcoholic-craving. These dry times become valuable when convincing themselves and others they're not alcoholics. Yet these times of abstinence become fewer as their alcoholism progresses.

The alcoholic-craving that periodics experience ebbs and flows. They would likely drink if alcohol were available when the craving struck. Still, before the severe symptoms of the later stage arise, they seem nonalcoholic except during a spree.

Although they realize their lack of control, they fortify their denial by comparing their drinking to those *they believe* have a worse drinking problem. They may do this by changing the 'friends' they drink with and the places they drink.

As discussed in Chapter 5, "The Darkness and Lightness of Denial," others also support their denial. For example, if charged with DUI, the court orders an alcohol evaluation. An undertrained evaluator doesn't see an alcohol problem since the periodic isn't a daily drinker. Instead, the assessor finds that their drunk driving was a one-time judgment error and it will probably never happen again. So, most alcoholics slip through the loosely strung net of the court assessment unless they self-report their alcoholism, which is unlikely.

Unfortunately, the results of these evaluations further strengthen the periodic's denial. If anyone mentions their drinking, they declare the court assessed them and found they don't have a drinking problem.* This assessment will support their denial and remain valid in their minds beyond any

---

*Few normal drinkers are ever evaluated.

reasonable period. They will view this pass to drink as a 'certificate of nonalcoholic' without any expiration date until their undeniable alcoholism results in a certificate of death, or worse.

PERIODIC OR CHRONIC: DOES IT MATTER?

MANY THINK BINGING is blackout drinking for days without sleeping or eating, but that's a *bender*. According to the NIAAA, a binge is four drinks for women and five for men over several hours.[3] That's a bottle of wine or less than a six-pack of beer.

Periodics don't need to drink between drinking episodes. During these intervals, they can take or leave it, so they often leave it—it looks better.

But when they drink, they have worse problems than chronic alcoholics. Studies show that binge drinkers account for 77% of the $249 billion that excessive drinking costs the U.S. each year, and they are at a higher risk of injury.[4] They provoke or are victims of violence more than daily drinkers.

For example, periodics often have blackouts, slurred speech, difficulty walking, rapid mood changes, poor judgment, and engage in risky and offensive behavior. They usually drink at the worst times, causing them to miss important events. They compulsively continue drinking after their first drink and usually endure severe hangovers. *This compulsion (the alcoholic-craving) separates the alcoholic from the nonalcoholic.*

Still, this pattern of drinking is confusing to everyone, including the periodic, who don't understand how they can go so long without a compulsion to drink but then don't stop once they start. Although they claim they don't *want* to stop once they start, it is apparent that they can't.

So, whether we drink daily or periodically, if drinking causes problems in our lives, we have a drinking problem.

Revisiting the Village Where It All Began

YOU MAY RECALL the story in Chapter 4 about Fred and Barney, who started the stigma. Well, there's more to that story. Let's travel back 7,000 years and revisit the small village of Jiahu, known for the origin of alcohol and, likely, the alcoholic stigma. We'll see how Fred is doing after losing his best friend, Barney.

This story illustrates how the periodic's alcoholism progresses. It also reveals the thinking, behavior, rationalizations, and comparisons periodics use to support their denial. Finally, it highlights some symptoms of periodic alcoholics and how these affect loved ones.

The Perfect Evening

FRED IS UPSET after the accidental death of his best friend, Barney. He not only misses him, but he feels responsible. Fred believes Barney would be alive if he hadn't introduced him to the fallen fruit.

His guilt is worsening, and his constant thoughts about Barney have reached a point where they're often disabling.

While searching for relief, he remembers the fermenting drink Barney left behind. So, he finally drinks some, and within minutes, he feels relief beyond his wildest imagination. Still remembering its effect on his best buddy, he knows this relief can be deadly. But he's sure he won't become like Barney.

A few days later, Fred is shopping at the village market. "Hi, Fred. I'm so sorry to hear about your friend. How are you doing?"

"Oh, thanks, Betty. I'm having a hard time with it. I feel like it's all my fault. It would've never happened if I hadn't taken Barney to the fallen fruit."

"Fred, that's not your fault. Many of us drank some, and that didn't happen to any of us. It was just bad luck. The same as if a falling rock struck him, a lion attacked him, or the fever got him. I know you miss him, but try to give yourself a break."

"Thanks, Betty. I know you're right."

"I've got an idea, Fred. Why don't you come with me to watch the stone-skipping finals tonight? It'll get your mind off Barney. It'll be fun!"

Fred pauses. He's had feelings for Betty, which he's ignored since Barney died. "I don't know, Betty . . . how far is it?"

"It's only eight stone throws away. It's on the lagoon side near Cove Hut. They say the Hard Rock team might break a record and skip one across the entire lagoon. But Rolling Stone is a great team, too. It'll be fun. Come on, Fred. Please!"

"Alright, Betty, when should I come for you?"

"Oh, how about when Crescent Stone Mountain is half-shaded? How's that sound?"

"Sounds good, Betty; see you then."

FRED'S A LITTLE nervous about his date with Betty. So, he drinks half a stone mug, and his worries are gone within minutes as he goes off to call on her.

He's outside her hut, shaking the door rattle and thinking about drinking one more so he'll feel even better. But he doesn't have time.

"Hi, Fred. How are you?" Betty eagerly asks.

"Oh, I'm great! And you sure look great, as usual!"

"Thanks, Fred. Well . . . you ready?"

"You bet I'm ready! I'm really ready! I'm really, really ready!" Fred answers with a chuckle and a wide grin.

Betty giggles. "What's gotten into you, Fred?"

Fred feels less shy than usual, so he holds her hand as they walk to the competition. Betty blushes.

"Hey, Betty, I've got an idea. Why don't you come back to my hut after the game, and we'll watch Shooting Stars? I bet it'll be a glorious show since the sky is so clear."

"Sounds like fun, Fred. Maybe we can do that."

Fred is trying to ignore the thoughts of another drink. After the competition, they lie on fine furs outside Fred's hut, gazing at the heavens. It's a clear night. Every so often, a star shoots across the village sky, and they *ooh* and *ahh*.

"You know, Betty, sometimes I look at our village sky and wonder if there's another village somewhere with its own sky and stars."

Betty giggles. "Don't be silly, Fred. There aren't other villages."

It's a romantic evening.

SIX MOONS LATER, Fred and Betty are watching shooting stars while calling out names for their baby, due in a few moons.

"If it's a boy, what should we call him, Fred?"

"I like Stone."

"I like that, Fred. That's a good, solid name! And if it's a girl, we'll call her Pebbles. What do you think, Fred?"

"Perfect name. . . . Oh, there's one! Did you see it? It shot all the way across the village. It's our lucky shooting, star!"

"You're so romantic, Fred." They kiss . . .

TWO MOONS LATER, Betty is waiting for Fred. He only drinks on Saturday night—perhaps a little on Friday night—but never before sunset. Betty waits all night and finally falls asleep. When she wakes up, she sees Fred lying on the floor near the door.

"Hey, Fred. When did you get home last night?"

"I don't remember, but it was earlier than you think. You had just fallen asleep; I could tell." Hoping to end the questions, Fred grumbles, "Sorry, it won't happen again."

"I think you've got a drinking problem, Fred."

"Oh, yeah? And I think you get on my back about drinking because you're pregnant, big, moody, and I'm having more fun than you . . . I didn't mean . . . too big! You're a perfect eight moons big."

"That big comment didn't help you at all, Fred. You're a

perfect 15 moons big—what's your excuse? But you've got to see—"

"No, Betty, you've got to see it! —"

"No, Fred, you've got to see it! —"

"I see that I don't drink every day like Barney did. I only drink on weekends. It's no big deal to me. I can take or leave it."

"So why don't you leave it?"

"Because . . . I choose to take it. I don't have to. I choose to leave it all week and take it on the weekend. Nothing wrong with that."

"If I'm so important to you, and if you can take it or leave it, and you know if you don't drink, I'll be happier, but you *choose* to drink—your message is clear." Betty walks toward the door. "And you know we get along much better when you're not drinking."

"You just don't get it, Betty. Will you listen to me for a minute?"

"Fred. I hate to say this, but you're acting more and more like Barney when you drink."

"That's a low blow, Betty," Fred says with a tone she's never heard. "And I'm not sure I like how you said, "choose." I only drink on weekends, and not long ago, I went a full moon without a drink. Barney drank every waking moment. And don't forget I work all week, but Barney was too drunk to work. We live in a beautiful, large new hut built with the finest mudbrick and a thatched roof with a modern slant that keeps you dry. Everyone knows poor Barney ended up hutless."

"By the way, the roof is leaking," Betty softly blurts.

"I spear the best fish for you, and Barney died trying to spear the moon. I provide you with fine furs and leather coverings, while other women wear fig leaves woven with itchy wool. You don't itch. And look at that large, clear, perfectly shaped stone I gave you, proving my endless love for you. No other woman has a stone like that. I don't do many of the bad things Barney did while drinking. The truth is I do many of the good things Barney never did."

"You don't remember much of what you do and say when you're drinking, Fred." She looks around with her arms wide open. "You know I appreciate everything you do for me, but my appreciation doesn't lessen my love and concern for you."

"Well, well! Aren't you smooth? But I don't believe I do all you say I do."

"What reason would I have to make it up, Fred?"

"I'm just saying. Maybe you're not making *all* of it up, but I think you're making it sound worse than it is to stop my drinking."

"You can ask Berry and Rose. They saw you holding that spear above your head, making jabbing motions, staggering, grinning, and slurring your words. And you kept repeating: 'I see a fish on everyone's face, and I'm in the mood to spearfish!' Fred, you're laughing at me, but it isn't funny."

"Well, that's something Barney said to me once about spearing fish, and I . . . I guess I'm dealing with the grief . . . and I—"

"Fred, I understand, but—"

"And I'm not laughing *at* you; I was just laughing at how you tried to sound like me. I don't sound like that," Fred says with a muted chuckle.

"You sound worse than that, Fred. You frightened and embarrassed me. Did you notice people put their heads down, covered their faces, and emptied out in seconds? And you thought it was funny when you cut Berry's ear."

"Oh, whatever! It hardly bled, and I didn't do it on purpose. I tripped on something and lost grip of the spear. Plus, Berry said something to me a while back that I can't ever forgive or forget. He's lucky it was just his ear. It could've been a lot worse."

"So, what did Berry say that was so bad?"

"I can't remember right now, but I remember it was bad."

"Well, if you can't remember what he said—"

"It comes back to me a little at a time." He mumbles,

"Thanks for your reminders."

"Fred, it's got to stop!"

"Okay! Okay, already! I'll quit... I mean... not quit, you know what I'm saying; it'll be as if I quit. You'll be happy. You'll see."

"Okay, Fred. Once again, I'm taking you at your word, but I don't know why."

Fred quickly tries to fix the problem. He first hides the jug in the outhut and decides only to drink out there. He figures that what she doesn't see can't hurt her. Betty notices Fred deep in thought and warns, "Don't think you can hide anything from me because you can't."

"Betty, I wasn't thinking anything like that. You want to know what I was thinking. You ready for some truth?"

"Sure, Fred, lay it on me."

"I was just thinking about how much I love you. And I'm wondering if there's any way I might express my timeless love for you—if you know what I mean. Betty? Where'd you go? Betty?... Betty?... Betty?..."

BUT IT HAPPENS again, and again, and again. Fred keeps focusing on the differences between Barney and himself and some similarities with a few villagers who drink normally. He always has an excuse and someone else to blame when acting up. And his conversation with Betty is making him thirsty even though it's only Thursday. So, he waits until Betty says she's going to bed before he mentions, "Well, pleasant dreams. I'm going to pitch a pebble or two to relax. Won't be long." After Betty falls asleep, he quietly makes his way to the outhut and grabs the jug.

IT'S THE NEXT morning, and Betty doesn't sound happy. "When did you get home last night, Fred?"

"Oh, please, Betty, not now. I'm not feeling very good."

"Well, you said you were going to pitch a few pebbles. Right after you left, I started going into labor. Our friends spent hours calling and looking for you. They finally gave up, and I gave birth to our new son, Stone."

"Yeah, I heard. I meant to come right back then, but I was so excited that I celebrated a little bit too much. Betty, I'm so sorry, but I don't remember much after that."

"And this is Friday morning. Next, you'll do this on Thursday morning, then Wednesday morning, then. . . . By the way, how many mugs did you drink?"

"A couple."

"A couple to you means you didn't stop once you started."

"Please, Betty, not now. I said I was sorry. I only planned to drink one or two. But I was winning at Pebble Pitch and so excited about our new baby. Before I knew it, the jug was almost empty. Please let me get some rest. I feel awful."

"Fred, I can't understand this. So much of what you're doing is just like Barney—but worse. I don't know how much more I can take."

"What are you saying? You want to roll our stone off the cliff? Are you seeing someone? That's it. You're seeing someone!" Fred takes a deep breath, looks the other way, and half-whispers, "I knew it wasn't my drinking."

"Fred! Don't be ridiculous! I just gave birth this morning, and I'm seeing someone?"

"Well, Barney started drinking the moment he woke up— I never drink before Crescent Stone Mountain is full shade, and—"

"Except on shady days," Betty interjects.

"—and Barney—"

"You just won't see it, Fred. I'm talking about the *same* way you and Barney acted when drunk. You talking about the differences between you and Barney doesn't change *your* actions."

"For God's sake, Betty, don't you realize? Barney had a problem, not me! *He* was the alcoholic!"

"That's right. And we're comparing your drinking to the one who started the stigma. That should tell you something. I notice you don't compare your drinking to those who didn't drink themselves to death!"

"Okay! Okay! Betty. If you didn't get on to me so much, I wouldn't drink as much. But I've already said it won't happen again. I promise. What more do you want from me?"

"Okay, Fred, once again, I'm taking you at your word, but I don't know why."

IT'S ANOTHER FRIDAY night. Fred has been feeling bad all day from drinking too much last night. He knows a drink will help. If he only drinks two, that will work. This time will be different. This time, he'll stop after two. This time, he'll pitch a few pebbles and then watch shooting stars with Betty and Stone. And this time it will be . . . the perfect evening.

The next morning, Betty sees Fred lying by the door and asks, "When did you get home last night, Fred?"

—

IS FRED A PERIODIC ALCOHOLIC?

DO THE SYMPTOMS related to Fred's drinking reveal alcoholism (alcohol use disorder)? Let's see. The symptoms displayed are criteria for alcohol use disorder in the DSM-5 (the parenthetical numbering links with the criteria numbering).

1. Fred cannot stop drinking once he starts. He often drinks more and longer than intended (*Criterion 1*).
2. He's tried and failed to control his drinking (*Criterion 2*).
3. He spends much time drinking, hiding his drinking, recovering from hangovers, and arguing with Betty about his drinking (*Criterion 3*).
4. After one or two drinks, the compulsion to drink more strikes. When the weekend comes, he develops the alcoholic-craving, compelling his drinking (*Criterion 4*).
5. His alcohol use interferes with fulfilling major duties at home. He missed plans to spend time with Betty and

wasn't there during the birth of their child (*Criterion 5*).

6. He continues to drink despite constant and repeated problems with Betty (*Criterion 6*).
7. He continues to drink despite repeated physical or psychological problems his drinking is causing, such as blackouts and hangovers (*Criterion 9*).

Fred has seven criteria present, which suggest *severe* alcohol use disorder (AUD) according to the DSM-5 and other sources.

Although not in the DSM-5 and most other diagnostic instruments, I contend the following should be recognized symptoms of alcoholism and are present with Fred's drinking:

1. He compares his drinking to those he thinks have a worse drinking problem (Barney).
2. He hides his drinking (the outhut).
3. He breaks his promises to drink less ("This time will be different").
4. He focuses on periods when he didn't drink ("I went an entire moon without drinking").
5. He always has an excuse and blames others for his drinking.
6. Since he only drinks sometimes, he doesn't think he can have a drinking problem ("I don't drink every day like Barney, who drank the minute he woke up").
7. He minimizes the severity of his drinking (tells Betty she exaggerates his drinking).
8. He lies about how much he drinks ("I only had a couple of mugs").
9. His condition is progressing—he's drinking on Thursdays (he initially only drank on Saturday nights, which progressed to Friday and then Thursday nights).
10. He's in denial.

THIS STORY ILLUMINATES the denial of Fred, who is a severe, periodic alcoholic. Fred believes that each time he drinks, it will be different, but it never is and will never be ("This time will be different").

Fred, Betty, and Stone will continue riding this roller coaster as it struggles to climb steep inclines into the light, then plunges deep into the darkness, speeding around terrorizing curves upside down on a track falling apart. They will do this for years until it derails them into the alcoholic abyss unless sobriety shuts the roller coaster down.

Millions of families experience this. And it's often more traumatic than the predictable spiraling descent of the *chronic* alcoholic.

For example, with the chronic alcoholic, everyone knows what to expect—it progressively worsens. But with the periodic, the trauma caused by constantly fearing the next bender takes its toll. It's well known that fearfully awaiting an event is usually more stressful than when the event finally occurs.

The periodic and their loved ones know the drinker could spin into a drinking episode anytime, with unknown results. And suppose those affected have learned the signs of an approaching spree. The anxiety of always looking out for these signs creates enormous stress.

So, just because the alcoholic drinks every so often, like Fred, doesn't make it any less severe than the alcoholic who drinks daily.

CONSUMPTION, FREQUENCY, AND dependency vary among alcoholics. Many alcoholics drink occasionally—much less than normal drinkers. But some don't drink and haven't for years, while others drink daily.

The main difference between alcoholics and normal drinkers is not how much or how often they drink. Instead, the difference is the periodics inability to foresee, with any reasonable certainty, when they will next drink and *how much they will drink once they start.*

Questions for Discussions

1. Did you know that one who drinks more than an alcoholic is not necessarily an alcoholic?
2. Did you know that most alcoholics are periodic alcoholics?
3. Are you or someone you know a periodic alcoholic?
4. Did this chapter cause you to reconsider whether you or someone you know may be a periodic alcoholic?
5. Have you ever compared your drinking to another drinker? If yes, did you think the target drinker had a worse problem than you? Discuss your reason for comparing.
6. Have you or someone you know ever acted similarly to the examples of the periodic's denial described in this chapter? How?
7. If you're a sober periodic alcoholic, how did you navigate out of denial?
8. If yes, did you consider the target drinker to have a worse problem than you? Discuss your reason for comparing.
9. Did or do you ever have an alcoholic-craving? If so, did or do you drink when it comes, or fight it off?
10. Do you agree with the author that the ten symptoms he listed are symptoms of alcoholism?
11. Have you or someone you know ever had these symptoms?

Contact Information

Suicide & Crisis Lifeline:
Call or text **988** or chat at **988lifeline.org**

Suicide Prevention Lifeline:
1-800-273-TALK (8255)

For confidential information about help for alcohol dependence, contact one or more of the following:

NIAAA ALCOHOL TREATMENT NAVIGATOR
"Pointing the way to evidence-based care"

A service of the U.S. federal government providing unbiased information for finding quality alcohol treatment through mutual support groups, therapists, doctors, and outpatient & inpatient care.

www.alcoholtreatment.niaaa.nih.gov

Mutual-Support Groups

(AA) Alcoholics Anonymous
www.aa.org | 212–870–3400
(or local phone directory)

Al-Anon Family Services/Alateen
For Those Affected by Another's Drinking
www.al-anon.org | 888-425-2666 for meetings

Adult Children of Alcoholics & Dysfunctional Families
www.adultchildren.org | 310–534–1815

AA Agnostica
A space for AA agnostics, atheists and freethinkers worldwide
www.aaagnostica.org | admin@aaagnostica.org.

Celebrate Recovery
A Christ-Centered Recovery Program
www.celebraterecovery.com | 800-723-3532

LifeRing
Secular (nonreligious) Recovery
www.LifeRing.org | 800-811-4142

Moderation Management
www.moderation.org | 212–871–0974

Secular Organizations for Sobriety
www.sossobriety.org | 314-353—3532

Secular Alcoholics Anonymous
AA meetings for agnostics, atheists and freethinkers
www.secularaa.org

SMART Recovery
An Alternative to AA, Al-Anon, and other 12-Step Programs
www.smartrecovery.org | 440-951-5357

Women for Sobriety
www.womenforsobriety.org | 215–536–8026

INFORMATION RESOURCES

The Alcohol and Drug Addiction Resource Center
(800) 390-4056

Alcohol and Drug Helpline
www.alcoholanddrughelpline.com | (800) 821-4357

Alcohol Hotline Support & Information
(800) 331-2900

American Council on Alcoholism (ACA)
www.recoverymonth.gov | (800) 527-5344

National Child Abuse Hotline
1-800-25-ABUSE

National Clearinghouse for Alcohol and Drug Information
www.ncadi.samhsa.gov | (800) 729–6686

National Council on Alcoholism & Drug Dependence, Inc.
www.ncadd.org | *HOPE LINE*: 800/NCA-CALL (24-hour)

National Domestic Abuse Hotline
1-800-799-SAFE

National Helpline
Treatment referral and information 24-7
www.samhsa.gov | 1-800-662-HELP (4357)

National Institute on Alcohol Abuse and Alcoholism
www.niaaa.nih.gov | (301) 443–3860

National Institute on Drug Abuse
www.nida.nih.gov | (301) 443–1124

National Institute of Mental Health
www.nimh.nih.gov | (866) 615–6464

HEALTH CARE, ALCOHOLISM* AND THE DSM
Problems and Solutions

CHAPTER 7

*You're probably an alcoholic if
you had a few to calm your nerves
before an alcohol assessment and convinced
your doctor that you don't have a drinking problem.*

—

IF DRINKING IS causing one problems, then one has a drinking problem. That's a simple and reasonable diagnosis and should be enough to realize a problem with alcohol.

But here's the snag. Denial prevents most problem drinkers from realizing that drinking is causing their problems. Conversely, they believe they drink to cope with their problems and see drinking as the solution.

Those who know they're dependent on alcohol don't need a diagnosis telling them what they already know. Still, few alcoholics will ever say, "What a beautiful day. I think I'll quit drinking for the rest of my life." Recovery from alcoholism doesn't work that way. It's almost always others who prompt the drinker to consider sobriety.

So, one symptom of alcoholism is hiding it from those who can and want to help. That's one of the differences between alcoholism and other illnesses and disorders.

To illustrate, those suspected of having cancer or

---

*The DSM-5 and many health care professionals no longer use the term alcoholism or alcoholic because of disagreement over its meaning and the associated stigma. It's no longer a diagnosis—alcohol use disorder (AUD) and alcohol dependence have replaced it. These terms are used interchangeably in this chapter.

depression will not obstruct the diagnostic exam. Instead, those with cancer or depression usually want to know and treat it quickly. In contrast, although the purpose of diagnosing alcoholism is to encourage treatment, most in the hopeless depths of alcoholism and denial can't even imagine sobriety. At the time, most would rather die than 'endure' the rest of their lives without any alcohol. So, they will go to great lengths to avoid a positive diagnosis, which would invite terrorizing thoughts of abstinence.

This avoidance includes skillfully and artfully deceiving the diagnostician and foiling an accurate diagnosis unless the clinician is skilled enough to penetrate this ploy. But, as we'll see, few are.

For example, a doctor who suspects her patient has alcoholism asks: "Do you think you might have a drinking problem?"

"I don't think so. Why do you ask?"

"Well, would you like to find out?"

"Sure, why not?" (Undoubtedly, answering "no" admits a drinking problem.)

"Good. I'll just ask you a few questions. Do you promise to be honest? If you're not, we're just wasting time."

"Sure! Of course, I do."

The doctor likely believes her patients are eager to discover if they have a drinking problem and will candidly answer a few simple questions. But patients in denial aren't eager at all.

Still, the *primary* problem isn't the flawed screening or diagnostic interview; it's failing to even suspect alcoholism and when suspected—ignoring it. These two failures prevent the diagnostic interview from ever occurring, contributing to 90% of alcoholics never receiving help.

However, this chapter doesn't only identify the problems afflicting health care. It also offers detailed, useful, and practical solutions, as seen by many on the outside looking in, including past subjects of the AUD diagnostic exam.

I have divided this chapter into six sections.

SECTION ONE — ALCOHOLISM AND MEDICINE discusses the contributions of psychiatry to sobriety from the 1930s to the present and health care's current understanding, view, and treatment of alcoholism. It presents an example of a general practitioner's effective six-minute screening/diagnostic interview with an alcoholic patient, including an analysis of symptoms and the physician's techniques. It also highlights how health care's stereotypical views and frustrations, coupled with the alcoholic's denial, affect the recognition and treatment of alcoholism, and it offers solutions.

SECTION TWO — THE SCREENING emphasizes the critical need for detecting alcoholism early, outlines various alcohol screenings, and examines the responsibility of health care to screen for alcoholism, the difficulties of and solutions for a practice integrating screenings, the public's overdependence on health care to identify alcoholism, and it provides alternative screening questions.

SECTION THREE — THE DIAGNOSIS explores the challenges in diagnosing alcoholism, including the critical importance of identifying comorbidity and recognizing which comorbid disorders are alcohol-induced and which ones are independent to avoid misdiagnoses. It also discusses the use of objective testing, the failures to diagnose, and the urgent need to educate the public and adequately educate the medical community about alcoholism.

SECTION FOUR — THE AUD SECTION OF THE DSM: LIMITATIONS AND IMPROVEMENTS illustrates five of the flaws in the AUD section of the DSM-5 and suggests solutions for curing and, alternatively, avoiding these flaws.

SECTION FIVE — EFFECTIVE USE OF THE DSM-5 AUD DIAGNOSTIC CRITERIA provides suggestions for using the DSM-5 AUD diagnostic criteria more effectively. It discusses methods of establishing rapport to soften the alcoholic's denial. This section lists the 11 DSM-5 and my five proposed criteria, with 200 optional diagnostic questions divided among the criteria for interviewers to conduct a fluid, flexible, accurate, and meaningful conversational evaluation, which encourages sobriety.

SECTION SIX — HEALTH CARE EDUCATION considers the status of alcoholism education in health care. It includes a suggested outline for a 2-day seminar that would educate health care professionals enough about alcoholism so they can better manage the alcoholic patient.

SECTION ONE

ALCOHOLISM AND MEDICINE

IN THE BEGINNING...

HEALTH CARE, ESPECIALLY psychiatry, has significantly contributed to sobriety and the understanding and treatment of alcoholism, beginning with psychiatrists Dr. Carl Jung, Dr. William Silkworth, and Dr. Harry M. Tiebout.

Carl Jung, MD (1875–1961) was a Swiss psychiatrist who set the ball of victory rolling by admitting defeat. In 1931, after unsuccessfully treating his hopeless alcoholic patient, Roland Hazard,* he gave him his dim prognosis. Jung conceded he didn't know of any medical or psychiatric treatment that could help him. But Jung also said he had heard of a few rare cases where an extraordinary "conversion experience" causing an entire psychic change had released an alcoholic from the compulsion to drink.

Hazard then shared Jung's view with another alcoholic who was considered hopeless, Ebby Thatcher. Then, in 1934, Thatcher shared the doctor's view with his drinking companion, another alcoholic who was also considered hopeless, William Griffith Wilson (Bill Wilson).

Jung's treatment of Hazard had the ripple effect of parting the waters for Bill Wilson to co-found Alcoholics Anonymous in 1935, resulting in millions of hopeless alcoholics living sober lives.[1,2,3] In a letter to Dr. Jung, dated January 23, 1961, Bill Wilson wrote:

> You frankly told him [Hazard] of his hopelessness, so far as any further medical or psychiatric treatment might be concerned. This candid and humble statement of yours was beyond doubt the first foun-

---

*Rowland Hazard, an investment banker and former Rhode Island state senator, traveled to Zurich, Switzerland, to see Jung in the hope of solving his drinking problem. He saw Jung daily for several months, quit drinking, and then relapsed.

dation stone upon which our society [Alcoholics Anonymous] has since been built.⁴

Around the same time, William D. Silkworth, MD (1873–1951), a neuropsychiatrist, was treating alcoholics at Towns Hospital in New York City. Bill Wilson was one of his patients. Silkworth treated over 40,000 alcoholics during his career.

Silkworth wrote the foreword in the book *Alcoholics Anonymous* (referred to as the *"Big Book"* by AA members) entitled "The Doctor's Opinion."⁵ In this foreword, Silkworth detailed his observations of alcoholics, introducing and coining the "Phenomenon of Craving," now a widely accepted concept. He explained this phenomenon as a physical allergy causing a reaction that compels the alcoholic to continue drinking insatiably after the first one.

Additionally, Harry M. Tiebout, MD (1896–1966) was an outstanding psychiatrist and pioneer in addictions. He also treated many alcoholics in the 1930s and was influential and contributed to countless alcoholics becoming sober by explaining Alcoholics Anonymous to the public, his patients, and other psychiatrists. One of his patients was Margaret "Marty" Mann,* who was the first woman to become sober in AA.⁶ She made many contributions related to alcoholism, including the founding of the National Council on Alcoholism (NCA) with Tiebout's support.

Dr. Tiebout also supported the disease concept of alcoholism, which was much more unpopular then. He noticed a common thread woven through the fabric of *every* alcoholic he met. Tiebout introduced this as an inflated ego characterized by feelings of omnipotence, self-absorption, and grandiosity

---

*Marty Mann's other contributions *included* (1) defining "alcoholism" as a disease and persuading the AMA to adopt the disease concept; (2) forming the American Society of Addiction Medicine (ASAM); (3) creating the first employee assistance program; (4) fighting stigma; (5) establishing Alcohol Awareness Month; (6) successfully campaigning for the 21-year old Minimum Drinking Age Act; (7) successfully promoting the alcohol container warning label; and (8) successfully advocating insurance coverage for treatment.

and believed this ego would safeguard itself at all costs. He wrote and spoke about this often between 1944 and 1966, and the *American Journal of Psychiatry* published these writings.

He said: "The alcoholic is typically resistant to the point of being unreasonable and stubborn about seeking help or being able to accept help even when he or she seeks it." He believed the alcoholic had to deflate this ego to become sober. He also asserted that the alcoholic's deflated ego remains inflatable and does inflate before a relapse.

Dr. Tiebout persuaded the New York State Medical Society to invite Bill Wilson to speak about Alcoholics Anonymous at an American Psychiatric Association (APA) meeting, and the *American Journal of Psychiatry* published his talk.[7] Wilson spoke two more times at these meetings, which the *Journal* also published.

Tiebout served as president of the National Council on Alcoholism from 1951 to 1953 and as a nonalcoholic trustee on the AA General Service Board from 1957 to 1966.

According to Bill Wilson, Alcoholics Anonymous would not exist had these doctors not cleared the path for its founding.[8, 9]

Finally, and more recently, George E. Vaillant, MD (born 1934), a psychiatrist and professor of psychiatry at Harvard Medical School, has done much to bridge the gulf between alcoholism and medicine. He has lectured worldwide and is known as a top researcher.

Vaillant has received many awards, including the Foundations Fund Prize for Research in Psychiatry from the APA and the Jellinek Award for research on alcoholism.

According to Vaillant, "Alcohol abuse is not black and white; it is gray." With this in mind, he assumed the daunting task of examining "the different shades of gray expressed through [the] drinking behavior" of over 600 alcoholics for more than 40 years. In 1983, he published the results in his book, *The Natural History of Alcoholism*,[10] which the press widely praised as the most influential book on alcoholism in the 40 years since the book *Alcoholics Anonymous*.

Remarkably, after publishing this book, he studied the same 600 alcoholics for another 15 years. His purpose for doing so was to answer specific questions. He opined that this prospective study of alcoholics for 15 years might answer the following "seven controversial questions" that brief clinical studies probably could not.

> 1) Is alcoholism a symptom or a disease?
> 2) Does alcoholism usually get progressively worse?
> 3) Are alcoholics, before they begin to abuse alcohol, different from nonalcoholics?
> 4) Is abstinence a necessary treatment, or can insisting on abstinence sometimes be counterproductive?
> 5) Is returning to safe social drinking possible for some alcoholics?
> 6) Does treatment alter the natural history of alcohol?
> 7) How helpful is Alcoholics Anonymous in the treatment of alcoholism?[11]

In 1995, he published the answers to these questions in his updated book, *The Natural History of Alcoholism Revisited*.[12] What he learned from this follow-up led him to reassess the nature of alcoholism and discover, assess, and support new treatment theories.

Vaillant has been a strong proponent of teaching doctors about alcoholism. He wrote: "Such a serious and widespread problem demands to be studied, yet our lack of knowledge about alcoholism is astonishing."

Vaillant joined the AA General Service Board as a Class A (nonalcoholic) trustee in 1998.

Any sober alcoholic who grasps the impact of psychiatry

and health care in general on sobriety would feel timeless gratitude. Bill Wilson often voiced this appreciation.[13] He wrote, "We owe our very lives to the men and women of medicine."[14]

And Currently . . .

Most health care providers freely admit that they have little or no training in alcoholism, hold the stereotypical view of the alcoholic, and see alcoholism as a sin, not a sickness. This view foils a competent diagnosis unless the one examined fits the stereotype.

Even though many know their opinion is a problem, the medical community's unashamed contempt for drinking alcoholics runs rampant.[15] Another problem is the denial of those physicians who believe they hold no negative or stereotypical views of alcoholism.

One such doctor wrote an article about her enlightened attitude towards alcoholics. However, even this doctor included a sentence that read, "...but at some point, the alcoholic *voluntarily* took a drink of alcohol." [Italics added]

This standard thinking ignores that no one knows if they'll develop alcoholism before their first drink of alcohol. Moreover, judging an act as voluntary or involuntary concludes responsibility and casts blame. When doctors blame a patient for having an illness, they risk infecting their treatment of that patient.

Undoubtedly, it's natural to feel frustration when treating excessively drunk alcoholics, who are often offensive. Health care providers have optimistically seen alcoholics endure detox, remorsefully admit and regret the emotional pain they've caused loved ones, and commit to never drinking again. They appear so genuine because, at the moment, they *are* so genuine, and they're just as genuine every time the hospital readmits them for detoxing. Moreover, it doesn't help when doctors learn the relapse rate after inpatient detox hovers around 90%.[16]

The doctor's early disappointment and frustration often transform into cynicism, contempt, scorn, and sarcasm. These negative emotions are infectious, and they mix with science, as well as oil mixes with vinegar.

Still, it's important to recognize that chronic relapsers wish they weren't and know they're slowly suiciding while miserably existing. They feel bad enough about themselves without the caregiver's disapproval.

A Psychiatrist Speaks Out

Professor George E. Vaillant, MD, disclosed this during an interview:

> Probably 50% of all the people brought into emergency rooms had blood-alcohol levels over .25— which is enough to make any non-dependent person comatose, not just prone to accidents. And even though this is a clear biochemical fact staring doctors in the face, no referral is made—nothing is done about it—because when it comes to treating alcoholism the medical profession feels so helpless, so without hope. And for a doctor, feeling powerless is reason enough to put his head in the sand.
>
> [M]edical students learn how to be doctors ... on hospital wards and in the emergency rooms... And ... *for very good reasons, hate active alcoholics with a passion.* Therefore, the educational program has to begin again after residency.[17] [Italics added]

A Nurse Speaks Out

My conversation with an emergency nurse that I know was revealing. Having recently completed nursing school and now working in hospital emergency, she was candid and eager to discuss her experiences.

I asked about her training in alcoholism, and she said there was some about managing intoxicated patients. She believed it was adequate, claiming, "I really don't need to learn more about it. It's not very complicated."

I asked if she learned any of the signs of alcoholism, and she insisted: "Everyone knows what an alcoholic looks like."

So I asked her what alcoholics look like, and she said, "It's easy," and described the stereotypical alcoholic who is homeless, unbathed, unemployed, stumbling, smelling of alcohol, slurring words, wearing tattered clothes, and is "obnoxious and repulsive."

I questioned if she was aware that reliable studies show only 10% of all alcoholics fit her description, to which she responded all the alcoholics she sees fit her description.

When I mentioned those alcoholics who are successful professionals, own upscale houses and cars, dress well, and pay their bills, she stopped me, "No way!" She insisted that no alcoholic could function that well. "They may drink quite a bit, but we all drink too much at times, even me. But alcoholic, no."

While inquiring about alcoholics who have been sober for years that don't fit her description, she interrupted, "Then they're not alcoholic anymore if they ever really were."

As we were discussing the disease concept, that is, alcoholics have a disease that removes their choice to drink, making it a compulsive need, she said it may be called a disease, but to her and others, "it just looks like rude and disruptive behavior."

I asked if she had heard anything about neuroimaging that shows the alcoholic brain differs from the nonalcoholic brain, to which she had not.

I mentioned that the ER is in a unique position to identify and help alcoholics get treatment and asked if an alcoholism expert is on staff who can help these patients. She smiled, shrugged, and said, "Oh, I've heard we do, but I've never seen them. We just don't have time for that." She further explained that it's an emergency room, and the job is to treat the emergency and move on to the next one. She believed if alcoholics don't want to drink, they won't, and said, "To be honest, we just let them sleep it off."

When I asked if patients ever came in experiencing alcohol withdrawal, she said, "Regulars just show up for a warm bed and a few hot meals, especially if it's cold." She added that they get them in and out quickly, believing they can't do much for them.

I asked if intoxicated patients are treated the same as other patients, to which she answered, "Probably not. We're only human, and they've done it to themselves."

I asked her if she thought that *any* education about alcoholism could be helpful, to which she chuckled, "Honestly, I think I would be offended if someone tried forcing me to attend some class on alcoholism. If someone wants an education, let them walk my shift."

While smiling, she interjected that my inquiry had been "interesting but has little to do with reality."

I ended by asking if most of the nurses she knows share her views about alcoholics, and she replied: "They all do. And doctors do, too."

Although admittedly, this casual conversation was not a peer-reviewed study, sometimes anecdotal research is more candid and reliable than empirical research.

Moreover, this doesn't suggest that all nurses lack adequate or any training in alcoholism, just most. A study revealed nurses and nursing students often stigmatize alcoholics and don't feel trained enough to care for them.[18] This study also found nursing students were less tolerant of alcoholics than those students studying psychology, social work, health, and social care.[19] In 1994, a nursing professor at New York University and director of Substance Abuse Education in Nursing (SAEN) published an article stating: "Basic knowledge about alcohol abuse and its related problems has not been included in general nursing education in any consistent manner."[20] Unfortunately, not much has changed in the 30 years since then.

THE GENERAL PRACTITIONER AND THE ALCOHOLIC PATIENT

BECAUSE OF DENIAL and inadequate training, doctors are quick to diagnose depression, anxiety, and other conditions instead of alcoholism.[21] For example, Judy visits her doctor with high blood pressure. She's also a closet alcoholic, but that's not why she's here. The doctor doesn't see any signs of alcoholism because Judy dresses well, is clean, speaks without a slur, walks without a stagger, and is a successful professional, not a skid row resident. The doctor casually makes a comment disguised as a question: "You're not much of a drinker, are you?" Judy raises her eyebrows. "Well, I had to ask," the doctor says apologetically, sure that drinking doesn't contribute to Judy's hypertension.

So, she treats Judy with medication, unaware that too much drinking is the culprit. A doctor without training doesn't even know how to approach a patient about drinking, much less know the symptoms of alcoholism, or as medicine now calls it, Alcohol Use Disorder (AUD).

Had the doctor used her stethoscope, she would have smelled alcohol. Had she tested Judy's blood, it would have revealed a .23 blood-alcohol level, which is incongruent with Judy's clear speech and coordination, disclosing an alcohol tolerance.

However, the doctor prejudged her patient by comparing Judy to the stereotypical alcoholic. This comparison prevented her from suspecting that Judy's drinking may be raising her blood pressure.

Most doctors believe their patient's answer of "a couple" or "none" to this question on their intake sheet: "*On average, how many alcoholic drinks do you consume weekly?*" They're unaware that giving a false answer is a symptom of alcoholism, and they should expect most problem drinkers to respond deceitfully. Although deceit about one's drinking doesn't make a diagnosis, it compels further examination.

Years ago, in trying to shatter this stereotypical view, the American Medical Association (AMA) published the pamphlet *The Illness Called Alcoholism.* It stated:

> Some alcoholics actually drink less than some social drinkers.... The key factor is loss of control and craving.... Drinking by one's self or drinking early in the morning, may be signs of alcoholism, but they are not always present. Similarly, living on skid row, being irresponsible and other behavior commonly regarded as fundamental to alcoholism, are neither limited to the disorder nor necessarily part of it. In fact, the class of alcoholics made up of financially successful professional persons may well be one of the largest, and certainly one of the most seriously neglected, groups in this country.

SAME DOCTOR AND PATIENT— DIFFERENT TRAINING AND RESULTS

THE FOLLOWING ILLUSTRATES Judy's visit with the same doctor, who takes a different approach after training.

"You know diet affects our blood pressure, right?"

"Of course."

"And salt is *one* of the worst offenders."

"Right."

"Do you use much salt?"

"Well, I rarely add salt to my food, if that's what you mean."

"Okay. That's good. But did you know that other things in our diet can affect our blood pressure?"

"Like—"

"Well, like, and I'm not suggesting anything, but even small amounts of alcohol can be a problem. Do you mind if I ask you a few questions about drinking?"

"Sure. My drinking isn't a problem, but have at it."

Note: *Judy answered, "A **couple** glasses of wine sometimes with dinner," to this question on the intake sheet: "On average, how many alcoholic drinks do you drink each week?" Alcoholics aren't likely to answer "seven bottles of wine" or "67 drinks." Instead, alcoholics give unasked information that is vague and irrelevant.*

The intake question doesn't ask what she drinks or what she's doing when she drinks. Still, most people think wine and beer are less alcoholic than mixed drinks, and wine with dinner is more acceptable than drinking alone. Also, in 'alcoholicese,' a "couple" means three or more, and "sometimes" means often. The answer to the trained clinician is explanatory and defensive, prompting more discussion.

The doctor rolls her stool over, sits, leans slightly toward Judy, and, while making eye contact, gently and caringly asks, "When was the last time you had anything to drink?"

"Anything?"

"Anything."

"Well . . . uh . . . let me think."

"Anything, Judy," whispers the doctor.

"Well, come to think of it, I had a glass of wine last night . . . *with dinner*. That's not a problem, is it? I've heard wine can be healthy. I don't drink the hard stuff unless I'm having cocktails with friends. And I never drink beer and never drink in the morning."

"Well, researchers are now questioning whether a daily glass of wine is healthy, but you know how that goes. So, how much wine did you drink last night?"

"Oh, let's see. I had a glass with dinner or, actually, maybe two, to be perfectly honest. Is that a problem?"

"And how much did you drink after dinner?"

"After dinner? Oh, I don't know . . . maybe another one."

"Did you finish the bottle?"

"It's interesting you ask that because last night I did."

"Would you say you drink a bottle nightly?"

"I don't know about every night. Some nights, I fall asleep before I finish the bottle. But I have a stressful job. It's not easy being a judge, a wife, and a mother. It's a balancing act, and wine keeps me balanced. A bottle of wine helps me relax and sleep better. It's not like I'm drinking from a bottle wrapped in a brown paper sack."

"Oh, believe me, I know. As a mother and a wife, I understand balancing a career and a family is hard. But your blood pressure is way too high. And you won't be balancing anything if it kills you. Did you know drinking one bottle of wine within four hours is binge drinking?"

"So now I'm a binge drinker? Next, you'll be calling me an alcoholic!"

"There's no labeling here. I'm just trying to help you. Do you always get your wine at the same place?"

"It just depends. It depends on where I am, but I usually get it at four or five places. Why?"

"Does anyone in your family or friends ever suggest you could cut back a little?"

"Oh, you know how people are—constantly overreacting."

"How difficult would it be for you to cut back?"

"Well, if I had to, I guess . . . I could *try*."

"Have you ever tried to cut back?"

"Oh, sure I have, but I gave up trying because I think I was using the wrong method."

"So you're saying you've tried, but it didn't work for whatever reason?"

"Yes, but it didn't work because I didn't do it right."

"How long have you been drinking a bottle a night? I mean, you didn't start off drinking a bottle a night?"

"Of course not. I used to drink a glass or two, maybe a couple nights a week."

"How long ago was that?"

"Oh, I'd say, about five years ago. It was before I sat on the bench. I know that."

"And then, did you increase to a bottle twice a week, or did your "glass or two" occur more often?"

"I don't really remember when it happened. I started drinking a couple at night more often. Then, I would drink a bottle on weekend nights. And then, eventually, before I knew it, I was drinking a bottle every . . . or most nights. So it hasn't been that long."

"Do you become more intoxicated now than five years ago?"

"No, if anything, I'd say less now. I just don't feel it as much as I used to. I guess that's good."

"Do you eat dinner every night?"

"No, not every night. Sometimes, I just snack. I'm often held up at work, so it's not the same every night."

"So, do you ever open a second bottle on the weekends?"

"No, not every weekend."

"Do you drink more than you intended?"

"Oh, all the time. I don't start the evening thinking I will drink a bottle. But I figure it's no big deal after one or two. The bottle's already open, so I might as well finish it."

"Judy, I'd like to refer you to someone who only deals with this type of thing. She's outstanding and could help you. Would you consider it?"

"Refer me to someone? Like who and for what?"

"She's a doctor specializing in diagnosing and evaluating alcohol use disorder and a member of ASAM.*[22] She may not identify any problem, but at least you'll know. And she can only make a recommendation, so it's up to you. No one is going to force you to quit drinking wine. You have nothing to lose. And in this case, I think she's an excellent choice instead of an alcohol counselor because she's a medical doctor and you have hypertension. You know I wouldn't waste your time."

---

*The American Society of Addiction Medicine.

"Look, I appreciate it, but I'm getting ready to launch my campaign for senator. If any of this got out, it would be disastrous. This isn't a good time for me."

"Judy. No time will ever be good for you. You're career-driven, and you're only getting busier and more public. So I assure you this *is* the best time and the earlier, the better. I'm not saying you need to quit drinking wine. I'm just asking you to have a slightly open mind. I'm on your team. And, as you know, everything we talk about is, by law, just between us. You can rest assured nothing's going to leak out." The doctor smiles and touches Judy's shoulder. "You won't regret this. Can you give me a moment? I'll be right back."

Judy looks out the window, slight tears blurring her vision as she stares at nothing. She inhales deeply, turns toward the doctor, and exhales, "Sure."

The doctor returns. "Okay, Judy. Your blood pressure medicine will be ready in 30 minutes. And here's some info on diet and hypertension. It's brief, and I'd like for you to read it. And here's a card with the date, time, place, and name of the doctor you'll be meeting. Everyone loves her, and I'm sure you will, too. And here's my card with the date and time of our next follow-up appointment two days after you visit the specialist. This way, we can check your blood pressure, and you can tell me how your visit went."

"Thanks, doctor."

"Sure. And if you have any questions, second thoughts, or just want to talk, *please* call me. I mean that."

The doctor's office scheduled a call to remind Judy of her specialist appointment the day before her visit. But more than a reminder, Judy will feel more obligated to attend. If she misses the referral, the doctor will reset it at their follow-up appointment. The doctor doesn't give up. It can't get much better.

And the reason it can't get much better is because it's a fairytale. Its purpose is to show how quick and easy it is, with proper knowledge and training, to assess if it's likely that a patient has a drinking problem. This assessment took only six minutes.

Analysis of the Six Minutes

During that brief six-minute interview, the doctor identified seven symptoms: (1) loss of control with failed efforts to cut down; (2) craving; (3) drinks despite health problems (hypertension); (4) developed tolerance (progression); (5) causing problems with those concerned; (6) *concealing, defensive and misleading about her drinking,* and (7) *denial.* The first five are in the DSM-5, and I propose that the remaining two symptoms (6 & 7) should be in an updated DSM.

A Look at Judy's Symptoms

1) **Loss of control with failed efforts to reduce drinking.** Judy says she doesn't open a bottle, intending to drink it all. But then, she drinks the entire bottle. She also loses control every night. So, Judy's doubt about cutting back is relevant. Why would she hesitate unless she's tried? Still, if it wasn't a problem, she could easily quit and wouldn't need a referral.

2) **Craving.** Judy has the *alcoholic-craving*,* although she doesn't see it because she drinks before it's recognizable. Still, she needs to drink to cope with her busy life. Drinking keeps her "balanced," and a bottle of wine helps her "relax and sleep better." Also, her inability to stop at just one or two glasses shows that the alcoholic-craving controls her.

3) **Drinks despite health problems (hypertension).** Even though drinking worsens her blood pressure, she drinks every night.

4) **Developed tolerance (progression).** In five years, Judy's two glasses of wine two nights a week progressed to a bottle most nights. Also, she feels less intoxicated than five years ago despite drinking more now, which is a sign of tolerance and

---

*See Chapter 3, "The Alcoholic-Craving" for an explanation of this word.

dependence.

5) *Causing interpersonal problems with those concerned.* If another worries about Judy's drinking, yet she continues to drink, troubles are brewing.

6) *Concealing (defensive and misleading).* Judy claims she's being "perfectly honest," admitting she had two glasses of wine with dinner. Then, she discloses she doesn't eat dinner every night but admits to drinking a bottle on weekday nights and often two on weekends.

After being asked when she last drank, Judy evasively says, "A glass of wine with dinner." Yet she knows she drank the last glass of wine when she emptied the bottle. She implies that she had only two drinks all evening while claiming to be "perfectly honest."

Judy admits to buying wine "at four or five places," which is typical for alcoholics trying to hide the amount they drink, even from store clerks and others who don't care.

Judy's defensiveness appears when she says, "Next, you'll be calling me an alcoholic," and "That's not a problem, is it?" Her hesitation and dodging are also revealing. Almost every answer she gives is misleading.

7) *In denial.* This is a clear case of denial. For example, her comment, "Next, you'll be calling me an alcoholic," shows she denies her drinking problem despite having severe AUD, according to the DSM-5 and other sources.

An Analysis of the Doctor's Techniques

The doctor is confident, reassuring, not arrogant, judgmental, or demeaning.

Focused. The doctor knows alcoholics minimize their drinking. So, if Judy has alcoholism, it's safe for the doctor to assume her drinking exceeds her admissions. Judy thinks the questioning will end after disclosing she "drinks two glasses of wine *with dinner*," which would have ended with most doctors. But while focusing on Judy's drinking, she never loses focus on her hypertension—she mentions it 11 times. And that's because alcoholics are less defensive about drinking when talking with the doctor treating their physical complaints.

Hesitation is admission. The doctor considers hesitation to be an admission when forming her follow-up questions. Whether it *is* an admission doesn't disrupt her inquiry. Judy then admits to drinking another glass of wine after dinner, again hoping the inquiry will end.

Doesn't appear too organized. The doctor's questions aren't anticipatory. Instead, she jumbles and returns to the questions Judy thought she had evaded and isn't now prepared to dodge.

Flexible anticipation. The doctor remains flexible instead of rigidly adhering to a script, thwarting Judy's anticipation of the next question. For instance, rather than asking if she had another glass after dinner, the doctor takes a surprising leap by asking if she drank the entire bottle, which results in Judy confessing she did.

Then the doctor asks if she drinks a bottle every night since the chances of that being the only night she drinks a bottle are slim. Judy's first response is, "I don't know about every night." Yet she doesn't dispute it when later asked, "How long have you been drinking a bottle a night?" Judy is caught off guard by the doctor skillfully asking questions that trigger her candid answers.

Expresses urgency, not hysteria. The doctor advises Judy that addressing her drinking is a priority without sounding judgmental, hysterical, or self-righteous. The doctor preserves the seriousness of their meeting by reminding Judy she will have nothing left to balance if her drinking and blood pressure kill her.

Expects and handles objections well. She manages Judy's objections well with a firm and logical response. For instance,

Judy mentions her work and political ambitions as reasons for her to delay following her doctor's advice. However, the doctor uses Judy's excuses to persuade her not to postpone. At other times, she ignores her objections rather than giving them credibility by addressing them.

Communicates care with body language. Nonverbal communication of our body language is often heard more than our verbal communication. Studies show that 93% of our communication comes from slight body motions. It's so potent that it's usually impossible to talk our way out of it. Thus, the phrase, "Actions speak louder than words."

The doctor sitting at eye level with Judy, not 'looking down on her,' allows them to connect. This connection encourages Judy's candor. Touching her shoulder and leaning forward expresses concern rather than appearing judgmental from an elevated position of self-righteousness.

Compassionate and empathetic. The doctor is compassionate yet efficient, expressing compassion and empathy when agreeing that "it's hard to balance a career and a family."

Confidential. The doctor reaffirms everything is confidential, lowering Judy's fear of information leaks.

Expresses concern. The doctor inviting Judy to call if she has any "second thoughts" further shows her concern. She knows Judy may think twice before the appointment and miss it.

Some may think this is too much to offer every patient. But not every patient will need this, and few will call. This also increases patient accountability and trust in their doctor, leading to more following their doctor's advice. Further, the effect of this invitation to call is so valuable that a practice unable to integrate it might consider limiting new patients. Finally, insurance covers telemedicine.

She takes charge. Scheduling the specialist's appointment, the reminder call, and the follow-up appointment after Judy's visit with the specialist shows her commitment and compassionate care.

The doctor scheduling the appointments without Judy's input prevents Judy from claiming a fictitious scheduling conflict to delay hearing the truth.

She's on the same side. She reminds Judy that she's on her team and only wants to help, which lessens Judy's defensiveness, reinforcing trust in her doctor. Also, the doctor telling Judy that "no one is going to force you to quit drinking wine" lowers her fear and defiance. Alcoholics often distrust anyone who threatens their drinking, so these reassurances are essential.

She takes nothing personally. Although Judy tries to provoke a confrontation to avoid looking at her drinking, it doesn't work; the doctor knows that alcoholics are defensive when confronted about their drinking. For instance, when Judy says, "It's not as if I'm drinking out of a bottle wrapped in a brown paper sack," the doctor could remark, "Not yet." Instead, she expresses her understanding of Judy's difficulties balancing work and family.

When Judy asks, "Is that a problem?" and "That's not a problem, is it?" the doctor doesn't answer. Nor is the doctor provoked when Judy exclaims, "So now I'm a binge drinker? Next, you'll be calling me an alcoholic!" This only prompts the doctor to reassure her: "I'm here to help you." The doctor expresses care, not contempt, knowing that arguing with her would strain their rapport.

Regardless of how or if Judy addresses her alcoholism, the doctor knows she has at least softened the soil of denial when she planted the seed so deep that it can't ever wash away. The doctor also knows that sobriety rarely follows a one-time suggestion.

Having this perspective encourages the doctor to continue this style of practice rather than becoming callused, bitter, uncaring, and adopting the prevalent health care belief that caring for alcoholics is a waste of time.

Section Two

The Screening

LIKE MANY OTHER diseases, the early signs of alcoholism almost always go unnoticed for years before the obvious signs surface. The progression of these signs and symptoms is subtle—it's as noticeable as an hour hand progressing. By the time alcoholics are showing *clear* signs of alcoholism, it has reached a severe level.

At this stage, alcoholics may experience alcohol-induced anxiety and depression or worse. Brain damage is likely, with some damage worsening and some becoming more irreversible with each drink.

The simple things in life no longer produce pleasure. A general malaise shrouds the alcoholic. The beautiful days aren't as beautiful or as often. Now, whether drinking or briefly sober, an emptiness expands. If it hasn't already, the time will finally come when drinking no longer fills this void, no matter how often or how much the alcoholic drinks. Sadness, remorse, guilt, helplessness, and shame increasingly devour the alcoholic, who now feels hopeless.

However, this isn't only devastating and fatal for alcoholics. AUD is unique in that, unlike other diseases, allowing it to progress undetected is also disastrous for many innocent victims, including children and loved ones affected by the alcoholic's affliction. (See Chapter 8, "The Affected.") This also includes those who are the casualties of drunk drivers (drunk driving causes 55% of all traffic deaths),[23, 24] the victims of violence that intoxication encourages, and the billions it costs the public yearly.

Early detection can prevent much of this and reduce the odds of this harm occurring. Early detection is also vital because achieving lasting sobriety can take "8 or 9 years after one *first* seeks formal help."[25] Undoubtedly, the best way to detect AUD early is to screen for it.

The Alcohol Screening

It's common and easy to confuse alcohol screenings with diagnostic testing—they often overlap. As we saw with Judy and her doctor, a screening can blend with a diagnostic exam.

Screenings aim to detect if one *might* have a drinking problem, not to conclude that one does. The broadly framed questions of a screening lower the threshold, increasing its sensitivity to identifying those who *likely* have a drinking problem, but it also includes those who don't. Unfortunately, time restraints and costs prevent increasing the screening's accuracy—assessing 80% with no problem would be impractical and wasteful. Conversely, a negative screening identifies those who *probably* don't have a drinking problem while missing some who do. If the screening is positive, a diagnostic exam presumably follows.

According to all prominent professional organizations, including the AMA,[*] all health care should screen for alcohol abuse, especially primary, urgent, psychiatric, and emergency care. These organizations also recommend universal and continuing screening for adults and teens. Further, the risk of fetal alcohol syndrome demands screening all women of childbearing years.

Additionally, the NIAAA, CDC, and most medical associations recommend that all health care include brief interventions as part of their routine practice. (See Chapter 10, "The Intervention.")

The National Center on Addiction and Substance Abuse at Columbia University (CASAColumbia) suggests this is becoming the lowest standard of acceptable medical care.[26] It also suggests doctors should be cautious and understand that falling below this standard could expose them to liability for "failure to diagnose."[27]

According to the National Institute on Alcohol Abuse and

---

[*] This also includes the American College of Obstetricians and Gynecologists, the American Academy of Family Physicians, the American Academy of Pediatrics, and many others.

Alcoholism (NIAAA), alcoholics are more likely to seek care from their primary care physician for an alcohol-related medical problem than for a drinking problem. However, CASA-Columbia reported: "The vast majority (94%) of primary care physicians ... failed to diagnose substance abuse when presented with early symptoms of it in an adult patient."[28] This study also revealed that "Most patients said their primary care physician did nothing about their addiction."[29]

Screening Types

Some screenings are simple, and others complex. Ideally, a screening only asking, "Are you an alcoholic?" would identify everyone with an alcohol problem and exclude those without one. However, that would depend on accurate self-reporting, which denial, stigma, and lack of knowledge discourage.

An example of a screening in its simplest form is the common question on the typical medical intake sheet: "On average, how many alcoholic drinks do you consume weekly?" Still, it's important to remember that heavy drinking alone doesn't make a positive diagnosis, which the AMA and others support with findings that many nonalcoholics drink daily, while some drink more than many alcoholics do.

Various alcohol screening types exist, from the simple one-question SASQ* to the 25-question MAST.° Other popular screenings are the AUDIT[30] (consisting of the 3-question AUDIT-C and the 10-question AUDIT), the 8-question ASSIST[31] developed by the World Health Organization (WHO), the 4-question CAGE (two "yes" answers are positive), and the 5-question TWEAK.

I suggest a two-tier screening. The first question on the first tier asks, "Have you drunk any alcohol in the past year?"

---

*The NIAAA's *Single Alcohol Screening Question* asks, "How many times in the past year have you had (4 for women, 5 for men) or more drinks in a day?"
°The *Michigan Alcoholism Screening Test* (1971), which also has revisions and updates, including the 13-question Short-MAST and the 10-question brief MAST.

A "no" answer concludes a negative screening, completing the screening for one-third of the participants.[32] Those answering "yes" would answer the second question on this first tier: "Have you ever set a limit on the number of drinks you intend to drink?" A "yes" answer prompts a second tier of more detailed questions, which the intake nurse could ask.

As with heredity inquiries about other health issues, the following question should also be on the intake sheet: "Does any blood-related family member drink alcoholically?" Since most are willing, almost eager, to discuss a relative's drinking, this question opens the door for asking, "What about you?" without arousing too much defensiveness.

Early intervention screenings have become more prevalent. These screenings identify *pre-alcoholics*—those at a high risk of developing alcoholism—looking at genetic and environmental factors to assess this risk. For example, an alcoholic ancestry is a high-risk genetic factor; past traumas and a social circle comprising heavy drinkers are high-risk environmental factors.

For those assessed to be pre-alcoholics, the clinician conducts a brief intervention, which briefly counsels and advises how to prevent alcoholism from developing. (See Chapter 10, "The Intervention.")

Health Care's Accommodation of Screenings

Ignoring alcoholism by only treating its physical symptoms is no longer acceptable. However, the physician's dilemma is not simple to resolve at first glance.

Initially, a six-minute alcohol screening sounds reasonable. Surely, a practice can seamlessly integrate that time. Yet a closer look reveals more of a problem than first thought: Six minutes a patient turns into two hours daily, 40 hours monthly, and three months yearly. Moreover, this doesn't include the doctor's apprehension about opening a can of assorted problems that could be difficult to contain. This, coupled with the time constraints when allotted an average of 15-20 minutes per patient and reminded every few minutes that other patients are restlessly waiting, further increases the doctor's apprehension.

To illustrate, Sandy visits her doctor for a few unexplained cuts and abrasions. The doctor surprises Sandy with an alcohol screening. The screening is positive, which shocks and traumatizes her. Most alcoholics live their entire lives avoiding this moment.

The doctor hands her a sheet with phone numbers she *can* call and wishes her good luck. Sandy remains alone in the cold, sterile examining room, with her world shattered. The doctor's office is bustling, and they didn't schedule more than 15 minutes for her. They need the exam room, but she remains seated in despair.

Understandably, Sandy insists on talking with the doctor before leaving. Despite the tight schedule, the doctor steps in and escapes after 10 minutes of trying to reassure her. The doctor tells her she could do something or nothing about it—it's her choice.

So the 'six-minute screening' turned into a much longer event. Replacing the 'assorted problems' back in the can could be difficult. The doctor will think twice before screening the next patient suspected of alcohol abuse because of an inadequately prepared practice.

This, coupled with the doctor's stereotypical view and the knowledge that a successful recovery is unlikely, further taints the physician's thinking. It becomes easier to overlook the signs of alcoholism in the next patient.

But what if the patient showed signs of cancer with a 10% survival rate? Would the doctor dismiss the patient without an oncology referral?

Not every patient will need screening. But those presenting with typical signs of abusive drinking will, and the primary and emergency doctor can no longer avoid this. Many resources exist outlining how to incorporate this responsibility into a medical practice with minimal disruption.[33] An excellent health care resource is www.niaaa.nih.gov. It offers many articles and information to help clinicians arrange practices to accommodate examining patients suspected of alcohol abuse. Also, insurers cover the cost of alcohol screening.

Undoubtedly, it wouldn't be enough for some patients if the doctor spent a lifetime with them. Still, it's usually not the quantity but the quality of time that matters.

Alternative Screening Questions

When the DSM-5 was released, the same publisher released *The Pocket Guide to the DSM-5 Diagnostic Exam*.[34] The Alcohol Use Disorder section of the *Guide* begins with four screening questions. The author suggests that affirmative answers to the screening questions prompt further diagnosis using the criteria (although the first two questions can't be affirmatively answered). However, while this may work with other mental disorders, it's unlikely to work as well with alcoholism. To illustrate, I have recited them with answers I suspect alcoholics, who are hoping to avoid detection, would likely answer. I follow this with my proposed screening questions and notes.

1. How often do you drink alcohol?
   Likely Answer: *Not very often.*
2. On the average day, when you have at least one drink, how many drinks do you have?
   Likely Answer: *It just depends. Sometimes one, sometimes a couple.*
3. Have you had any problems because of drinking?
   Likely Answer: *No, not because of drinking.**
4. When you stop drinking, do you go through with-

---

*The alcoholic is convinced drinking soothes the impact of problems, but it certainly doesn't cause them.

drawals?

Likely Answer: *Withdrawals? Like DTs? Are you kidding?*

The following suggested screening includes questions about experiences most normal drinkers haven't had and will likely result in more reliable answers.

1. Have you ever quit or reduced your drinking? (**Note:** *Normal drinkers rarely decide to reduce or quit drinking.*)
2. Have you ever set a limit on the number of drinks you intend to have? (**Note:** *Normal drinkers don't—they only want one or two.*)
3. Although you don't think you have a drinking problem, has anyone ever talked with you about your drinking? (**Note:** *No one is concerned about the normal drinker.*)
4. Do you hold your alcohol better now than you did three years ago? (**Note:** *Answering "yes" indicates tolerance has developed.*)
5. Have you ever felt remorseful or apologized to anyone about your drinking? (**Note:** *Normal drinkers haven't—they've had no reason to.*)

Too Dependent on Health Care?

OUR EXPECTATIONS ARE unreasonable when we rely too much on health care to identify alcoholism. Unfortunately, most doctors lack the training and time to spot alcoholism in patients who are doing their best to hide the signs. It's even more challenging when those in the early stage and deep in denial hide the symptoms and signs from themselves. It's like expecting doctors to suspect arthritis without observing the painful joint movements of their patients who don't mention any pain.

With more and better education, training, and experience, correctly screening for alcoholism or even suspecting the need to diagnose it would surge. Still, it's unlikely doctors will perform a screening interview on every patient suspected of abusing alcohol.

Without discounting the doctor's valuable role in recognizing and addressing alcoholism, it's more practical for those close to the alcoholic to detect a drinking problem. They have what the doctor will never have—more time to observe.

Although the differences between normal and abnormal drinking may appear subtle, they are not minor. Still, discerning them is more likely with adequate knowledge.

As detailed in Chapter 5, "The Lightness and Darkness of Denial," teaching students in grades 1 through 12 about the early signs of alcoholism and addressing the alcoholic stigma would provide some of this required knowledge. Removing the secrecy that shrouds alcoholism should be its primary goal.

Public service announcements only encourage those in the middle and late stages of alcoholism who have drunk excessively for years to seek treatment. Yet, more focus must be on prevention instead of the consequences of alcoholism by targeting pre-alcoholics and those in the early stages, including their loved ones.

Additionally, the general public, particularly employers, should understand the common symptoms and signs of the early and middle stages and how genetics, environment, and culture may increase the risk of developing alcoholism. This knowledge would alert those at risk and help them prepare to manage it should it arise.

Moreover, one would learn to recognize alcoholism in loved ones and the best ways to approach it. This would enable doctors to be more efficient rather than getting bogged down in the time-intensive battle of trying to pierce the alcoholic's armor of denial. Nevertheless, the medical community must always provide a needed line of defense.

Section Three

The Diagnosis

The diagnostic exam follows a positive screening, ideally confirming if AUD is present. The diagnostician typically uses the DSM-5 to conduct this exam. Depending on the accuracy of self-reporting, a diagnosis could be made in minutes or may take several visits, especially if a coexisting disorder (comorbidity) is suspected. However, the time restraints of practitioners and the alcoholic's resistance often thwart a diagnosis.

It's widely recognized that the responses given by an active alcoholic are unreliable. Providing false answers is denial—a symptom of alcoholism. Additionally, the one accompanying the alcoholic may also be unreliable since they're often caught up in the denial scheme. All this and more further hampers an accurate diagnosis.

Alcoholics don't usually seek help with a drinking problem but typically seek treatment for a physical complaint or general emotional distress.[35] However, untrained clinicians usually miss that alcohol abuse is the underlying cause of their patients' complaints.[36]

Most emergency and family doctors, social workers, therapists, and counselors, who are usually the first to see the alcoholic, lack suitable training to diagnose alcoholism. This is especially true if the patient is in the early stages of AUD and presents with milder signs and symptoms.

Still, psychiatrists and psychologists are not immune to missing AUD and often do, according to psychiatrists and *all* the many sober alcoholics I've interviewed. Moreover, deferring to a previous diagnosis or giving it undue weight is standard practice.

For example, consider John, who seeks help with severe depression and suicidal feelings. He lost his job two months ago, and his wife left him. He claims his depression has worsened over the past year or two. The undertrained clinician doesn't suspect alcohol abuse but diagnoses John with a depressive disorder and treats him accordingly.

However, an adequately trained clinician would have likely discovered that John was fired for drinking on the job and his wife left him because of his abusive drunken behavior.

The 2016 Surgeon General's Report echoed these serious concerns about this "shortage of skills" in health care regarding alcohol use disorder.[37]

Diagnosing Alcoholism is Challenging

In a paper published by the NIAAA entitled "Alcoholism and Psychiatric Disorders, Diagnostic Challenges," the authors discuss the complexities of diagnosing the alcoholic.

> *The evaluation of psychiatric complaints in patients with ... alcoholism can sometimes be challenging.* Heavy drinking associated with alcoholism can co-exist with, contribute to, or result from several different psychiatric syndromes. As a result, alcoholism can complicate or mimic practically any psychiatric syndrome seen in the mental health setting, at times *making it difficult to accurately diagnose the nature of the psychiatric complaints.*
>
> Prematurely labeling these conditions as major depression, panic disorder, schizophrenia, or ASPD *can lead to a misdiagnosis and inattention to a patient's principal problem—the alcohol abuse or dependence. With knowledge* of the different courses and prognoses of alcohol-induced psychiatric disorders, *an understanding of the comorbid independent disorders one needs to rule out,* an organized approach to diagnosis, ample collateral information, and practice; however, the clinician can improve diagnostic accuracy in this challenging patient population.[38] [Italics added]

Therefore, it is *essential* that clinicians not rush to judgment but thoroughly explore the possibility of comorbidity.

Comorbidity and Misdiagnoses

Alcoholic comorbidity means that another disorder in addition to alcoholism is present. Estimates are that about 40% of alcoholics have comorbid disorders.[39,40,41,42]

The most common alcoholic comorbid disorders are anxiety and depression.[43] Other less common comorbidities exist, such as psychotic, bipolar, sleep/wake, sexual dysfunction, and neurocognitive disorders.[44] All of these disorders have symptoms that can be present when drunk, sober, or during withdrawal.

So, although recognizing comorbidity is often challenging, training and experience can greatly reduce this challenge.

Alcohol-Induced Disorder or Independent Disorder

After identifying comorbidity, the next task is to determine if the AUD or the comorbid disorder came first. Without knowing this, the clinician is unable to target treatment.

For example, the treatment is less successful if treating only the anxiety without treating the underlying AUD. However, discovering which disorder first arose is often tricky since simply asking if anxiety symptoms occurred before or after drinking began is a question many can't answer. Nevertheless, an accurate diagnosis is more probable if the clinician has reviewed past medical records, interviewed others, and completed a physical exam.[45]

If the AUD was first, the comorbid disorder is likely alcohol induced.[46] Conversely, if the comorbid disorder was first, it is likely an independent disorder that may have caused or contributed to the AUD.[47]

Moreover, if the alcoholic is abstinent for longer than a month and the comorbid disorder persists, then it's probably independent. If independent, it's likely causing or contributing to the AUD and should be treated.[48] Those symptoms disappearing within 30 days of abstinence are usually alcohol-induced.[49]

For example, consider Jim, an alcoholic who has major depressive disorder and drinks to self-medicate his depression. If the clinician is unaware that Jim's depression preceded his drinking and doesn't treat his depression, his compulsion to self-medicate with alcohol will likely continue. Therefore, treating only his AUD may be less effective because depression often provokes a relapse.

Consider Sue, an alcoholic with alcohol-induced anxiety. She presents with severe anxiety, claiming she drinks to lessen her anxiety. So, the doctor only treats her anxiety, unaware that her drinking causes it. Unfortunately, Sue is treated for a condition that would have resolved without treatment if the doctor recognized that AUD induces her anxiety *and* if Sue quit drinking.

So, a prescription to treat Sue's anxiety will likely follow without a referral for AUD treatment. One adequately trained would have known that anxiety is a typical alcoholic comorbid disorder and would have treated it.

These complications often result in a flood of misdiagnoses fueling inadequate treatment, assuming a diagnosis even occurs.

Objective Testing

If the clinician suspects alcohol abuse, then objective testing, including several blood tests, can be helpful.

For instance, high blood-alcohol concentration and a sober-appearing patient reveal a high tolerance, which reveals probable alcohol dependence. This is much more reliable than answers to questions such as "Do you drink too much?"

One can see objective criteria, like legal problems, which leave a record trail, compared to less observable and verifiable subjective criteria, such as craving.

Blood tests can also reveal excessive alcohol consumption.*
Gastritis, hepatomegaly, esophageal varices, and hemorrhoids
may reflect alcohol-induced changes in the liver. Other physical signs of heavy drinking include tremors, unsteady gait,
insomnia, and erectile dysfunction. These are only a few of the
many revealing signs. They don't alone conclude alcoholism,
but they suggest a problem that should nudge the doctor to
counsel their patient about possible alcoholism and make a
referral.

---

*Elevations of gamma-glutamyl transferase (GGT) and carbohydrate-deficient transferrin (CDT) can indicate heavy drinking. Liver function tests, elevations in blood levels or lipids (e.g., triglycerides and high-density lipoprotein cholesterol), and high-normal uric acid levels can be helpful.

SECTION FOUR

THE AUD SECTION OF THE DSM:
LIMITATIONS AND IMPROVEMENTS

THE DIAGNOSTIC AND Statistical Manual of Mental Disorders (DSM) lists the symptoms (criteria) of all known mental disorders. The DSM has been the source of most screenings and diagnostic tools for decades.[50, 51] It has been known as the "Bible of Psychiatry."[*]

The DSM-5 is the latest edition,[°] which is mainly used in the United States to diagnose or classify psychiatric disorders, including Alcohol Use Disorder (AUD).[**]

DSM-5 combines alcohol use disorder with nicotine, caffeine, gambling, and other substances in the Substance-Related and Addictive Disorders section. The common thread of these disorders is that they affect the brain's reward center, producing "pleasure" or a "high."

Using the DSM-5, the diagnostician interviews the patient to discover the number of criteria present that reflect the extent to which symptoms of a suspected disorder impair and distress one's life. At least two criteria must be present for an AUD diagnosis. Although its use seems simple to the untrained, it's more complex than it first appears.

Most lack training to use the DSM effectively for diagnosing alcoholism. Those relying on the DSM-5 often rush to the diagnostic criteria, ignoring the 22 pages of detailed text

---

[*]According to the preface of the DSM-5, "the information [in the DSM-5] is of value to all professionals associated with various aspects of mental health care, including psychiatrists, other physicians, psychologists, social workers, nurses, counselors, forensic and legal specialists, occupational and rehabilitation therapists, and other health professionals to classify and diagnose mental disorders."

[°]The DSM-5 was published on May 18, 2013. The DSM-5-TR is the latest text revision published September 2022. None of the revisions apply herein.

[**]The International Classification of Diseases (ICD), published by the WHO, is also a diagnostic tool and counterpart to the DSM, used mainly outside the U.S.

explaining the use of the diagnostic criteria and AUD generally.

However, the American Psychiatric Association (APA) doesn't seem to discourage this practice, as implied by the publication of *Desk Reference To The Diagnostic Criteria From DSM-5*. This "convenient manual" only includes the diagnostic criteria for each disorder. It omits the text, although it claims it is "meant to be used in conjunction with the full DSM-5. Its proper use requires familiarity with the text descriptions ... that accompany the criteria sets."

PROBLEMS WITH THE AUD SECTION OF THE DSM-5

MY OBSERVATIONS FOCUS on the AUD section of the DSM-5 and DSM-IV. AUD is one of the most prevalent disorders afflicting 12.4% of men and 4.9% of women, according to the DSM-5.[52] Based on reliable evidence and the reasons mentioned in this book, I suggest the prevalence is much higher.

The DSM-5 section on alcoholism is lacking and flawed:

1) The craving criterion is incorrect;

2) The diagnostic criteria are incomplete;

3) The 12-month period is too restrictive;

4) The severity rating is inaccurate;

5) The special exception for prescribed drugs is unreasonable and suspect.

1. The Craving Criterion is Incorrect

The fourth criterion in the DSM-5 is "Craving, a strong *desire* or *urge* to use alcohol." [Italics added] As discussed in Chapter 3, "The *Alcoholic-Craving*," this description is incorrect. It is the generic definition in Merriam-Webster of any *satiable* craving, with the word "alcohol" merely added.

Seeing the alcoholic-craving as a *desire* or an *urge*—not a *need*—is a critical error, and using "strong" doesn't modify a desire or urge into a need.

Alcoholics who drink when they have an *urge* to or *desire* a drink are drinking voluntarily—it's misconduct. But those who drink when they *need* a drink are drinking involuntarily—it's a conditioned need to survive. *The DSM-5 supports the alcoholic stereotype by misunderstanding craving, and it needs revision.*

Another critical error is in the explanatory text of craving: "*Craving for alcohol* is indicated by a strong *desire* to drink that makes it difficult to think of anything else, and that often results in the onset of drinking."[53]

This bland definition misses the mark. It defines obsession more than craving. Again, a "craving for alcohol" is not the issue—the alcoholic-craving is. Further, "difficult to think of anything else" is an obsession. So, the DSM-5 implies that the craving for alcohol is a strong *obsessive desire* to drink.

However, a simple craving for anything could be similarly defined by substituting any word for "alcohol," such as chocolate milk. Yet unlike the alcoholic drinking alcohol, drinking enough chocolate milk *will* satisfy the craving for it.

One problem with the currently flawed definitions of craving is their failure to recognize that the alcoholic-craving is insatiable—the alcoholic can't drink enough alcohol to satisfy the alcoholic-craving. That's because it's never satisfied—the more the alcoholic drinks, the stronger the craving and the compulsion to drink more. The diagnostician must understand the *alcoholic-craving*.

INCREDIBLY, AT ONE point, the DSM-5 AUD Work Group decided to exclude craving. But first, to support their proposed exclusion, they studied whether including craving would identify more alcoholics. The result: "only marginally."[54]

How could this be if craving is a key symptom of alcoholism? It is because the study's participants, who were all emergency room patients, were asked: "In the last 12 months, did you feel such a strong desire to drink that you couldn't resist it or think of anything else?"[55]

First, alcohol-related problems cause *at least* 20% of emergency visits,[56] with studies finding it's nearly 55% on weekends, so the study's population is suspect. Alcoholics who are sick or injured *and* intoxicated differ from alcoholics in the general population, with most never needing alcohol-related emergency treatment.[57] Therefore, it's logical to assume that the research subjects would answer the question differently. So, those studied were not a representative sample of the general alcoholic population.

Second, it excluded periodic alcoholics who had not drunk in the past year. It also excluded alcoholics who were more than a year sober pending a relapse.*

Finally, the ones who answered "yes" to this transparent question would have had to have a blinding light experience and accept their alcoholism at the moment they answered. Still, in that unlikely event, the question might as well have been, "Are you an alcoholic?"

Therefore, one could expect the positive diagnoses from the questionnaire with the craving criterion to be slight compared to the one without it. Still, even slight differences are significant when considering millions of diagnoses.

Despite the study's result, the APA admirably included 'craving' in the DSM-5.

REMARKABLY, THE DSM-IV (1994-2013) omitted craving. This manual was referenced for 19 years, and some still use it.

The APA omitted it for two reasons: 1) The experts believed there wasn't enough reliable scientific data to prove that craving was a symptom of alcoholism, and 2) The experts could not agree on what craving meant.

The Work Group's attempt to agree on the meaning of craving implies that they believed craving existed. Why else

---

*According to the NIAAA, 90% of sober alcoholics will relapse at least once during the first four years of sobriety, and 50% of those sober a year or more will relapse.

would defining a non-symptom even be an issue? So, their inability to compromise on the meaning of craving must have been the only reason for its exclusion.

The six-member Work Group spent eight years working on the "alcoholism" section of the DSM-IV.[58] They had between 50 and 100 advisers critiquing their work. Yet they could not compromise on the meaning of craving enough to include it nor see reliable scientific findings proving craving is a symptom of alcoholism.

It's known that the alcoholic-craving existed before biblical times. In the 1930s, Dr. Carl Jung recognized craving, and Dr. William D. Silkworth wrote about and coined the "phenomenon of craving," convinced it's the driving force behind alcoholism and the primary difference between the alcoholic and the nonalcoholic.

Sixty years elapsed between Jung and Silkworth's observations and the DSM-IV's publication. Yet during those 60 years, a hypothesis that craving is a symptom of alcoholism wasn't proven enough to include it in the DSM-IV.

Even those who view alcoholics as morally flawed and weak-willed recognize craving by believing that giving in to it reveals these character flaws. Moreover, no authority on alcoholism fails to recognize craving other than the DSM-IV.

Craving is progressively present during all stages of alcoholism. To exclude this symptom of alcoholism from the DSM-IV for 19 years casts more doubt on the APA's grasp of alcoholism.

And why mention the revised DSM-IV? Because when the DSM-5 was released in 2013, not every copy of the DSM-IV was recycled or deleted. Many bookshelves still only contain the DSM-IV, and some shelve the DSM-III. Also, it's well known that the DSM-IV was the source used to create most alcohol screenings in use today.

Finally, an evolutionary view of the differences between the DSM versions allows for a more comprehensive evaluation.

2. The Diagnostic Criteria are Incomplete

Diagnostic nets need a finer mesh to capture symptoms earlier. This mesh is too large, allowing many alcoholics to avoid the sweep, resulting in excessive false negatives. For this to change, the diagnostic criteria must be inclusive, not exclusive.

The incomplete DSM-5 AUD diagnostic criteria exclude the following: (a) denial, (b) concealment, (c) remorse and guilt, (d) resentment and anger, and (e) legal problems.

However, despite the DSM-5's exclusion, the alcohol research and treatment community considers these five proposed criteria significantly relevant. Moreover, several screening and diagnostic instruments, widely regarded as reliable, also list most of them—*other than the DSM-5*.

a) Denial

The AUD section of the DSM-5 includes nothing about denial. Yet no authority disputes denial as a primary *symptom* of alcoholism (AUD). "Distortions in thinking, *most notably denial,*"[59] is a characterization of alcoholism, according to The American Society of Addiction Medicine (ASAM). [Italics added] The World Health Organization also adopts this view of denial.

It's disconcerting that clinicians will conduct diagnostic exams without first deciding if patients are in denial and, if they are, whether they're in denial about their alcoholism or if they're primarily denying it to others.

As shown in Chapter 5, "The Lightness and Darkness of Denial," denial progresses in tandem with alcoholism. Alcoholics spend much time fortifying denial throughout their drinking. If the diagnostician is unaware that the alcoholic is in denial, the examination is meaningless or nearly so. Moreover, getting helpful information from those closest to the alcoholic is questionable since they're often in denial themselves.

Alcoholics in denial won't candidly self-report. It's not stressed enough that despite the questionable research suggesting that self-reporting is often reliable, it is not. Ironically, this research uses the *self-reporting* of their research subjects to reach a conclusion. Moreover, the tested population is suspect: patients in treatment. Undoubtedly, these patients are much less in denial and are more likely to accurately self-report than the general untreated alcoholic population.

Therefore, if the alcoholic is in denial, alternative diagnostic methods must be used. Although objective testing is more reliable than subjective testing, well-framed and skillfully asked questions can ensure better reliability during a diagnostic interview. (Questions to discover the extent of denial appear under Criterion 16 in Section Five of this chapter.)

b) Concealment

Over time, alcoholics must control when and how much they drink to support their denial. But eventually, they can't. So, they hide their lack of control by hiding alcohol, drinking alone, sneaking to and switching liquor stores, paying cash for alcohol, never admitting to drinking more than a couple, and progressively and secretly drinking earlier in the day.

Alcoholics use many methods to convince others they drink normally, and they fine-tune these methods as alcoholism progresses.

A drinker hiding a drinking pattern would alone indicate a drinking problem, yet the DSM-5 omitted this. Concealment is more relevant than other criteria. Normal drinkers don't hide their drinking nor isolate while drinking to prevent others from detecting their condition.

c) Remorse and Guilt

The DSM-5 criteria contain nothing about feelings. All the criteria relate only to facts susceptible to skilled manipulation by alcoholics who will do anything to avoid abstinence, which they see as misery.

AUD is a feelings disorder. The alcoholic-craving that compels drinking is a cluster of feelings proportioned and blended to create a dysphoria reduced 'only' by alcohol, or so the reward network believes. (See Chapter 3, "The Alcoholic-craving," for a detailed discussion.)

Several popular screenings include questions about guilt. For instance, one of the four questions on the CAGE is, "Have you ever felt guilty about drinking?"

The well-known MAST asks, "Do you feel guilt [sic] about your drinking?"

Question 7 of the popular and reliable AUDIT screening asks, "How often during the last year have you had a feeling of guilt or remorse after drinking?"

Alcoholics, unlike ordinary drinkers, typically feel remorse and guilt about their drinking. They feel shame when they drink more than they intended, and guilt often prompts their drinking. Repeatedly apologizing for drinking suggests a chronic loss of control and indicates a drinking problem.

d) Resentment and Anger

Anger and resentment cause more drinking than other feelings. For example, during and after a dispute, alcoholics often feel compelled to drink.

It's not unusual for alcoholics to create feelings of anger to feel entitled to drink. Guilt-free drinking is preferable to guilt-induced drinking. Since anger reduces guilt, alcoholics quickly transform guilt into anger by convincing themselves that someone else is to blame. This rationalization is common for alcoholics.

It has been widely recognized for years that anger and resentment compel alcoholics to drink and are primary components of alcoholism.

An article in the Journal of Substance Abuse Treatment

states:

> Anger and alcohol use and dependence have been linked in both theory and empirical studies for several decades. Anger and related emotions (irritability, frustration, annoyance) are positively associated with alcohol consumption and adverse alcohol consequences in the general population.[60]

The book *Alcoholics Anonymous*, published in 1939, states, "Resentment is the 'number one' offender. It destroys more alcoholics than anything else."[61]

Determining whether anger and resentment often prompt one's drinking should be a part of the diagnostic interview and listed as a diagnostic criterion.

e) Legal Problems

The NIAAA contends that "run-ins with the law (arrests or other legal problems)" in the past 12 months related to drinking will *alone* trigger a finding of alcohol abuse.[62] Notably, the *"recurrent substance-related legal problems"* criterion appeared in the previous DSM-IV, although it isn't in the current DSM-5.[63]

The APA claims the Work Group excluded it "because of cultural considerations that make the criteria difficult to apply internationally."[64] However, it's hard to grasp that the DSM-5 Work Group believed the relevance of a fifth DUI did not outweigh "cultural considerations."

The popular MAST asks about DUIs, and even the briefMAST, with 10 questions, asks about legal involvement.

—

Adding these five criteria (i.e., denial, concealment, remorse and guilt, resentment and anger, and legal problems) would increase the accuracy of AUD diagnoses.

3. The 12-month Period is Too Restrictive

An AUD diagnosis requires meeting the criteria within the past 12 months.[65] Unfortunately, this 12-month period excludes millions of alcoholics.

With a relapse rate near 90% during the first four years of abstinence,[66] alcoholics who are *temporarily* sober for at least one year and the drinking patterns of many periodic alcoholics would dodge an AUD diagnosis.

The following example further illustrates the irrationality of this 12-month period. Suppose one was previously diagnosed with AUD but hasn't triggered any of the criteria for 366 days. In that case, they had AUD one day before the diagnosis but not one day later.

If the APA subscribed to the widely-held belief that "once an alcoholic, always an alcoholic," or, put another way, an alcoholic can't ever drink normally, that would support omitting any time limit. Nevertheless, a longer time frame, such as five years, would tighten the mesh.

Indeed, the DSM-5 also seems to tangentially support this by stating AUD is "characterized by remission and relapse" and that once the alcoholic relapses, "it is highly likely that consumption will rapidly escalate and that severe problems will once again develop."[67] It further acknowledges that if the alcoholic meets none of the criteria, except craving, for 12 months, the alcoholic is in "sustained *remission*."[68] This correctly suggests AUD is incurable. Therefore, after 12 months of meeting none of the criteria, AUD is merely in remission—present but not cured.

Although questionable studies here and there suggest that 10% of 'alcoholics' may resume normal drinking, the risk to the 90% is high enough to remove the 12-month limit. Finally, it could be harmful for an alcoholic 13 months sober to seek treatment for anxiety and receive a misdiagnosis as nonalcoholic. The alcoholic could easily treat this misdiagnosis as a pass to drink.

This 12-month period also ignores the evidence that AUD is an involuntary, *incurable*, chronic, progressive, metabolic, biochemical, central nervous system disease needing continued care and that the abstinent alcoholic's disease is merely in remission.

Simply put, the potential harm of the 12-month limit outweighs the likely benefits of a longer period.

4. The Severity Rating is Inaccurate

The DSM-5 provides a severity rating scale for AUD (and other disorders). Of the 11 AUD criteria (summarily listed in the next table and more fully listed later in this section):

2-3 = Mild AUD
4-5 = Moderate AUD
6 or more = Severe AUD[69]

The following illustrates some flaws with the rating scale. John goes to the bar once a month after work for an hour, drinks two beers with coworkers, and then drives home (Criterion 8: *hazardous activity*). He has no thought about drinking at any other time. Still, his wife is *unhappy* about his social hour with coworkers (Criterion 6: *continues drinking despite causing interpersonal problems*). According to the DSM-5, John is an alcoholic.

Consider Jane, who always carries a vodka-filled flask hidden in her purse because she can't go long without withdrawals. She also has four DUI convictions. She doesn't drink more than intended because she doesn't limit her drinking (excludes Criterion 1). Nor has she tried to control her drinking—she drinks as much as she 'wants' (excludes Criterion 2). She doesn't believe she spends a lot of time in "activities necessary to obtain alcohol, use alcohol, or recover from its effects" since she drinks continuously (excludes Criterion 3).

She denies any craving because she doesn't stop drinking

long enough to recognize it (excludes Criterion 4). Nor does she neglect major activities because she no longer has any to neglect. And since she's unemployed, drinking doesn't cause problems at work (excludes Criterion 5 & 7).

Her drinking isn't causing her any social problems because she started isolating years ago and has no social life (excludes Criterion 6). She never engages in "physically hazardous activities" (excludes Criterion 8).

She is *unaware* of any physical or psychological problems caused or worsened by her drinking (excludes Criterion 9). Additionally, tolerance is immeasurable since she can't drink much more than she does or measure the effects (excludes Criterion 10).

However, she does feel withdrawal symptoms when she briefly delays drinking (Criterion 11 is present). But since "concealing alcohol" and "legal problems" aren't diagnostic criteria, she only triggers Criterion 11 (withdrawal). So, according to the DSM-5, Jane can't be diagnosed with AUD.

One might argue that this example is absurd and that other criteria must be present if withdrawal occurs. But not according to the DSM-5: "Withdrawal is *usually*, but *not always*, associated with a substance use disorder."[70] [Italics added] However, this bold statement is unsupported by science.

Conversely, all the research indisputably supports that if one has physical withdrawal symptoms, that person is physically addicted to alcohol, which is a severe form of AUD. This is especially true since many alcoholics are *not* physically addicted but are psychologically addicted (dependent) to alcohol and would not be aware of or suffer Criterion 11 withdrawal.[71]

Additionally, according to the DSM-5, the presence of Criterion 11 (withdrawal) does not make an AUD diagnosis if drinking doesn't cause "clinically significant distress or impairment in social, occupational, or other important areas of functioning."[72]

This boilerplate phrase requiring a finding that the

symptoms are causing "clinically significant distress or impairment" before a diagnosis can be made appears under nearly every listed and unspecified disorder in the DSM-5. Mental health routinely applies this when considering any disorder. Its purpose is to determine whether the condition is disabling, which purportedly assists in deciding whether it's a disorder requiring treatment.[73] The number of triggered AUD criteria measures how much functional impairment or distress the suspected disorder causes.

So the DSM-5 claims a person physically addicted to alcohol, suffering severe withdrawal symptoms, doesn't have AUD if drinking doesn't cause other substantial problems in their lives. But how could that be? Doesn't addiction to alcohol, which is confirmed by hospitalization for detoxing and medical management of alcohol withdrawal, demand concluding drinking *is* causing functional impairment?

Interestingly, the DSM-5 seems to contradict itself, and 15 pages later, it supports my conclusion:

> Symptoms of withdrawal may serve to perpetuate drinking behaviors and contribute to relapse, resulting in persistently impaired social and occupational functioning. Symptoms requiring medically supervised detoxification result in hospital utilization and loss of work productivity. *Overall, the presence of withdrawal is associated with greater functional impairment and poor prognosis.*[74] [Italics added]

No evidence finds if one is drinking enough to have withdrawals, they have not developed a tolerance—but to the contrary. So, if Criterion 11 (Withdrawal) is present, one can conclude Criterion 10 (Tolerance) is also present. Moreover, wouldn't drinking enough to cause withdrawal also trigger Criterion 4 (Craving) and Criterion 9 ("Alcohol use is continued *despite knowledge* of having a persistent or recurrent physical or psychological problem that is likely to have been caused or exacerbated by alcohol")? Still, if the drinker doesn't have "knowledge" that their drinking is harmful (a rarity) or recognize their craving, then Criterion 9 doesn't apply, and they don't have AUD.

Therefore, the determination of whether those withdrawing from alcohol have AUD *could* pivot on whether they *knew* their drinking caused or worsened a physical or psychological problem. If they don't know, then no AUD. But the moment they know, they're instantly alcoholics—according to the DSM-5—although no research supports this faulty reasoning.

One is or is not an alcoholic. It is unreasonable to suggest that one suffering from delirium tremens may not be an alcoholic because their drinking doesn't cause dysfunction. It's as irrational as deciding one with an allergic reaction doesn't have an allergy because the symptoms aren't severe enough to cause "significant distress or impairment ... in important areas of functioning."

To further illustrate these flaws, assume a patient enduring withdrawal (Criterion 11) is found to have a tolerance to alcohol (Criterion 10) and a craving for alcohol (Criterion 4). In that case, the diagnosis would be *mild* AUD—the same diagnosis for John, who has a couple of beers after work with co-workers once a month.

All of this illustrates just a few of the defects in the AUD section of the DSM-5.

ONE SIMPLE SOLUTION to cure these diagnostic flaws is to weight the criteria on the severity rating scale, with each criterion having an assigned value.

Some criteria are symptoms, which are subjectively reported, and others are signs, which are objectively observed. Although signs are usually considered more reliable than symptoms, both can create the diagnosis.

This system gives the objective criteria more weight—the more objectively apparent and severe criteria are assigned higher values. These criteria relate to physical dependence or compulsive drinking, like tolerance and withdrawal, which are symptoms and signs easily observed with a high indication of late-stage AUD.

In contrast, the more subjectively less apparent and less severe criteria are assigned lower values. These criteria relate more to an obsessive, psychological dependence, like spending excessive time linked to drinking, neglecting important obligations, and causing social problems, which are symptoms that the drinker reports and less likely observed, which alone may not indicate alcohol abuse.

The criteria in the middle are less conclusive standing alone and require accurate self-reporting.

The following illustrates (*The **bold**, **italicized** criteria are those I propose and are not yet in the DSM-5*):

Proposed Value	Criterion Number	Description of Criterion
12	10	Tolerance
	11	Withdrawal
9	1	Drinking more than planned
	2	Impaired control (unable to reduce)
	4	***Alcoholic**-Craving*
	14	*Legal Issues (2 DUIs or public drunk)*
	15	*Hiding anything about alcohol use*
6	12	*Guilt or Remorse*
	13	*Resentment or Anger*
	16	*Denial*
3	3	Much time spent related to drinking
	5	Neglecting major activities
2	6	Causing social problems
	9	Drinks despite health problems
1	8	Drinking during hazardous activities

An example of the suggested scoring with this proposed weighted system is:

0-3 = No AUD
4-7 = Mild AUD
8-11 = Moderate AUD
12 or more = Severe AUD.

This system assigns a value of 12 to Criterion 11 (*withdrawal*) and Criterion 10 (*Tolerance*), which *instantly* diagnoses anyone having alcohol withdrawal, or alcohol tolerance, with severe AUD without triggering other criteria. Both criteria can be objectively observed and are signs of physical dependence; tolerance is seen when one has drunk heavily, has a high BAC, and appears sober or touts how well they can hold their alcohol.

Criterion 14 (*Legal Issues*) is assigned a value of 9 because it can also be objectively observed by reviewing court records, and two DUIs reveal that the first one wasn't a deterrent—a clear sign of AUD. However, it isn't valued higher because it doesn't clearly indicate *severe* AUD.

Several reasons could explain the lower-valued subjective criteria. For example, Criterion 9 (Drinks despite health problems) is assigned a lower value of 3 because some people are less health-conscious and are unaware that their drinking is causing health problems. Another example is Criterion 8 (Drinking during hazardous activities), which is assigned a value of 1. This is because some people are more reckless and risk-taking than others who never engage in hazardous activities, whether drinking or not. Therefore, engaging in dangerous activities while drinking isn't alone indicative of AUD. Moreover, Criterion 6 (*social problems*) is assigned a value of 2 because various reasons can explain it, such as that previously shown with John's wife, who is unhappy about his monthly social hour with coworkers. Also, social problems can emerge when the drinker is close to anyone who is against any alcohol use. It doesn't conclude AUD by itself.

So, the clinician using the currently flawed system would incorrectly diagnose John with mild AUD and Jane with no

AUD, whereas using the proposed system would correctly find John does not have AUD and Jane has severe AUD.

As demonstrated, weighting the diagnostic criteria would yield more accurate diagnoses.

5. The Special Exception for Prescribed Drugs is Unreasonable and Suspect

This special exception for drugs taken as prescribed also taints the credibility of the DSM-5,[75] which states:

> Symptoms of tolerance and withdrawal occurring during appropriate medical treatment with prescribed medications ... are specifically *not* counted when diagnosing a substance use disorder. The appearance of normal, expected pharmacological tolerance and withdrawal during ... medical treatment has ... [led] to an *erroneous diagnosis of "addiction"* even when these were the only symptoms present. Individuals ... should not receive a diagnosis solely on the basis of these symptoms.[76] [Italics added]

I doubt the brain's reward system knows or functions differently when one depends on drugs obtained by prescription or on the college campus. Most know someone with a substance use disorder resulting from taking medication as prescribed. Discounting medicine's role in this and its prescription method is disingenuous.

Considering the well-publicized concerns about the influence of drug manufacturers on health care, the disclaimer above is irresponsible and contributes to the *appearance* of impropriety.

During the development of the DSM-5, some raised concerns about potential bias, lack of evidence-based research, and conflicts of interest.[77] The flood of concerns about financial conflicts of interest prompted the APA to establish a written disclosure policy for those working on the DSM-5.[78]

This policy required panel members to file a disclosure reporting their associations with pharmaceutical companies.[79] Nevertheless, this disclosure requirement didn't create the intended transparency—the policy doesn't require disclosure of the amount received from these interested companies. Additionally, the policy allows panel members to receive a fee of $10,000 per year from these companies and own $50,000 worth of their stock.[80]

Still, transparency alone doesn't prevent potential bias. Indeed, before the disclosure requirement, 57% of DSM-IV task force members had financial connections to the pharmaceutical industry, with some receiving over $100,000 annually. After the disclosure requirement, this number increased to 69%. Moreover, the number of Work Group members working on Substance-related Disorders who were receiving financial benefits from drug companies rose from 17% to 58%.[81]

Years of research show that even small gifts will create "obligations to reciprocate."[82] A popular paper published the data from an extensive analysis of this issue.[83] This paper suggests that most Work Group members connected to pharmaceuticals worked on disorders or established new ones usually treated first with medication, demonstrating a "reciprocation."

Intensive analysis conclusively reveals that the pharmaceutical industry has extensively influenced the DSM-5. This analysis remains undisputed.

Still, the pharmaceutical industry has undoubtedly benefited health care and improved the lives of billions by discovering, developing, producing, and marketing products that save lives, prevent and treat illnesses, and relieve symptoms.

Nonetheless, this trillion-dollar industry remains potent. Even with numerous regulatory laws enacted to protect the public, big pharma still has a powerful influence on lawmakers and the practice of medicine. This influence has not always been in the patient's best interest.

The APA's practice of allowing the fox to guard the hen house is questionable and doesn't diminish the *appearance* of impropriety. Therefore, the APA should provide for an independent watchdog committee to oversee and mitigate the influence of pharmaceutical companies on the DSM's development. The primary purpose of any influence must be to benefit the public, not shareholders.

Section Five

Effective Use of the DSM-5 AUD Diagnostic Criteria

FEW ALCOHOLICS WILL voluntarily present for an AUD diagnosis without 'persuasion.' Therefore, it's helpful to determine their motivation for appearing—their state of mind. For example, a court-ordered assessment differs from a 'voluntary' assessment.

Usually, the first sign of the need for a diagnosis will arise when an emergency or family doctor sees the drinker for a physical injury or illness. Or, it may be others who prompt the drinker to seek a diagnosis, such as loved ones, friends, and employers.

Still, others will see a therapist for some distress in their lives, such as anxiety, depression, or other disorders, which are often unknowingly alcohol induced. Unfortunately, most alcoholics I've known and interviewed who were in counseling for months and years were never asked about their drinking—the subject never arose.

Nevertheless, it seems that the primary culprit causing most problem drinkers to deny their drinking problem is the common misunderstanding of alcoholism and alcohol-related terms. For example, the widespread misconception that alcoholics must drink daily, have withdrawals, financial difficulties, and other stereotypical characteristics prevents most from recognizing their drinking problem, causing them to remain in denial.

As mentioned, if drinking is causing one problems, then one has a drinking problem. However, a smooth transition is usually necessary for alcoholics in denial to open their minds enough to consider that drinking may be causing the problems they complain of.

Throughout this evaluation, it's essential to remember that the primary purpose of a diagnosis is to motivate the alcoholic to consider recovery. Although a diagnosis without treatment doesn't heal, even if the diagnosed alcoholic doesn't agree to immediate treatment, this discussion will likely help those in denial recognize that drinking is significantly impairing and distressing their lives and the lives of others.

Alcoholics must know their drinking is causing significant problems before they become open-minded enough to self-diagnose their drinking problem. So, the diagnostic interview is an excellent time—and may be the only time—for prodding alcoholics to explore recovery. One thing is sure: it will plant or nurture the seed already planted.

Therefore, before exploring the problems that drinking may be causing, measured by the number of AUD symptoms (criteria) triggered, it will likely be helpful to determine the type and extent of the drinker's denial.

The Drinker's Type of Denial

As discussed in Chapter 5, "The Lightness and Darkness of Denial," there are three types of denial, which generate the three main reasons for diagnosing alcoholism.

First, a positive diagnosis of alcoholics who are in *internal denial*—those who don't think they have a drinking problem—may prompt them to consider treatment.

Second, a positive diagnosis of alcoholics who are in *external denial*—those who know they have a drinking problem yet try hiding it—will allow them to realize they haven't hidden it, and they may be more likely to seek sobriety if they're no longer worried about others knowing.

Third, a positive diagnosis of alcoholics who are in *partial denial*—who have denied the severity of their alcoholism to themselves and others—will reveal that their alcoholism is worse than they thought, which may persuade them to seek treatment now instead of waiting.

The Drinker's Extent of Denial

A discussion to discover the extent of the drinker's denial will also help establish rapport and diminish defensiveness if alcoholics learn that they don't have to be Skid Row residents to have a drinking problem. So, the diagnostic exam will need a form of skilled 'cross-examination,' fashioned as a casual conversation, to unveil the truth. This conversation can begin by exploring one or more of these questions.

1) How do you define an alcoholic or problem drinker?
2) Have you ever thought, or now think, you might have a drinking problem?
3) If you don't think you have a drinking problem, how did you reach that conclusion?
4) Do you believe one must drink daily to be an alcoholic? (**Note:** *The answer is: No.*)
5) Did either of your parents drink alcoholically during your childhood? (**Note:** *The consensus is that children of alcoholic parents are at a high risk of developing alcoholism.*)
6) How old were you when you first got drunk? (**Note:** *Drinking around the age of 15 substantially increases the chances of developing alcoholism.*)

SUGGESTIONS FOR USING THE DSM-5 AUD DIAGNOSTIC CRITERIA MORE EFFECTIVELY

When the DSM-5 was released, the same publisher released *The Pocket Guide to the DSM-5 Diagnostic Exam.*[84] The book's back cover describes it as:

> ... the clinician's companion for using DSM-5 in diagnostic interviews... [and] walks the reader through a complete diagnostic exam that includes the follow-up questions for each of the DSM-5 diagnostic classes.... [It] is a pragmatic and concise resource for diagnosing mental distress ...

Although it has some helpful information about diagnostic interviews generally, the follow-up questions under the alcohol use disorder section are not as helpful. This is because diagnosing AUD is nearly always more challenging than diagnosing other disorders since alcoholics don't accurately self-report. Those with other disorders, such as depression and anxiety, are quick to divulge their symptoms in hopes of feeling better. But the alcoholic is convinced alcohol helps them feel better—they believe they need it to survive.

The AUD Criteria in the DSM-5

The following are the 11 criteria under Alcohol Use Disorder in the DSM-5, followed by the original question italicized for each criterion from *The Pocket Guide*. Following this is the alcoholic's *Likely Response* and my *Suggested Questions*, with some *Notes* trailing. My five proposed criteria (12-16) are included, also followed by *Suggested Questions* and *Notes*.

The suggested questions shouldn't be read verbatim; they are guidelines, not a script. Nor does every question need asking, only those contextually appropriate. Also, a flexible and fluid interview prevents exploring the applicable criteria in their presented order. Some questions are rephrased or repeated under various criteria. Additionally, once an answer triggers a criterion, every following question need not be asked. Still, one should ask those that may aid in further exploration, confirmation, identifying comorbidity, and seamlessly transitioning into discussing another criterion. The following illustrates.

> So, I see on your intake sheet you're married. How long have you been married? *Going on 12 years.* Do you get along well? *No, we've been having problems lately.* When did these problems start? *Oh, they've gotten worse in the last couple of years.* What seems to be causing them? *He's always complaining about things.* Like what? *Oh, he says I'm not taking care of*

things around the house like I used to (Criterion 5—failing to fulfill obligations at home), *spending too much time going out with my friends, drinking, ignoring the children, you know, things like that.* Do you ever complain to him about things he does? *Sure I do.* What are your complaints? *He's always starting arguments, especially when he's drinking.* So he drinks? *Yes, too much.* Have you ever confronted him about his drinking? *I've mentioned it several times.* What does he say? *He always turns it around, saying I drink too much.*

Alcoholics are often eager to discuss another's drinking. This is a good time to discuss the drinker's drinking and the effect drinking has had on the marriage relating to Criterion 6 (causing interpersonal problems) such as:

So, would you say drinking makes the marriage worse? (This will lead to a Criterion 5 discussion and inquiries about other criteria.) *Yes.* How do these arguments with him affect you? *I get mad, and it puts me in a bad mood.* Do you drink during these times? *Sometimes.* Does drinking make you feel better or allow you to deal with him better? *Yes.* (Criterion 4).

The drinker will often discuss many issues if allowed a few minutes to do so, which will prompt—after a pause—further questions.

So, you said your spouse thinks it's your fault because you're drinking too much (someone else concerned about the drinker—Criterion 16 and drinking more than intended—Criterion 1). This will also lead to questions about whether they've developed tolerance (Criterion 10), quit or tried to quit (Criterion 2), and most other criteria.

In other words, it shouldn't be a question-and-answer session resembling an interrogation with a checklist. The process should allow the drinker to discuss their situation with questions asked to clarify what they're saying, like a casual conversation. The questions asked will show interest, prompting answers pointing to other criteria if a problem exists.

Although some questions seek answers that appear obvious, and most are yes or no questions, they are designed to elicit conversation that further develops rapport, inviting light, casual conversation fashioned to fit the interviewer's style and the drinker's personality.

Allowing the drinker to explain answers may reduce defensiveness. These explanations, especially if uninterrupted by questions, will often reveal more than the answers. A flexible interview will create many questions itself that will flow naturally. If the drinker initiates a narrative, questions should be framed around it.

Understanding the drinker's distress may help both realize a joint alliance. The earlier illustration of Judy and her doctor is an excellent example of how to use these questions in an interview.

According to the DSM-5, if two or more of the following criteria are triggered, alcohol use disorder is indicated.

> **Criterion 1. Alcohol is often taken in larger amounts or over a longer period than was intended.**
> *When drinking, do you find you drink more, or for a longer time, than you planned to?*

Likely Response: "No." (**Note:** *A "yes" answer obviously admits a drinking problem.*)

Suggested questions: (Unless otherwise noted, if the answer is yes to any of the following, Criterion 1 applies):

a) Have you ever set a limit on the number of drinks you intend to have? (**Note:** *Normal drinkers don't set limits because they only want one or two. This question is rephrased under Criterion 4.*)

b) (*If the last answer is yes, ask this question:*) Have you exceeded that limit in the past year?

c) Do you monitor how much you drink, or do you drink freely? (**Note:** *Alcoholics will fear answering "no" to monitoring indicates uncontrolled problem drinking, so they will likely answer yes to monitoring and no to drinking freely, which reveals they try to control their drinking and don't get enough to drink—Criterion 1 applies. Normal drinkers don't monitor their drinking but drink freely because they have no reason to control their drinking.*)

d) Have you continued drinking after two drinks more times than not in the past year?

e) Do you ever control or try to control your drinking? (**Note:** *Nonalcoholics don't need to control drinking since it's not out of control.*)

f) Have you more than twice in the past year told anyone you were only drinking a couple but ended up drinking more?

g) After two drinks, have you continued drinking instead of eating more than twice in the past year?

h) If you've heard "last call" announced in the past year, were you surprised by how quickly the time had passed?

i) Has a bartender ever refused to serve you?

j) Have you tried convincing anyone to have "one more" drink despite their resistance?

k) Have you felt like you drank too much the night before more than once in the past year?

l) Do you believe you had a good reason for the times you lost control and drank too much?

m) Have you left an unfinished drink behind in the past year? (**Note:** *If "no," Criterion 1 applies.*)

n) Are you irritated if anyone or anything interferes with your drinking?

o) Within the past year, have you said you only wanted "one more" but changed your mind and continued drinking?

p) If you've heard "last call" announced, did you order another drink even if you hadn't yet finished the one you were drinking?

q) How many drinks does it usually take until you're satisfied and don't want anymore? (**Note:** *Alcoholics don't feel satisfied, so they will have difficulty answering. If there is much hesitation or they can't answer, Criterion 1 applies.*)

r) More than once in the past year, have you told anyone you were only drinking a couple but ended up drinking more?

s) After a couple of drinks, do you continue drinking when you're feeling good?

t) Can you hold your liquor better now than three years ago? (**Note:** *Alcoholics think they are controlling their drinking by not acting as drunk as others while drinking similar amounts. Answering "yes" indicates tolerance, and Criteria 1 and 11 apply.*)

u) Have you ordered a "double" more than once in the past year?

v) Have you felt satisfied enough when drinking that you switched to a non-alcoholic drink in the past year?

Criterion 2. There is a persistent desire or unsuccessful efforts to cut down or control alcohol use.
Do you want to cut back or stop drinking? Have you ever tried and failed to cut back or stop drinking?

Likely Response: "No, I could stop anytime; I just don't want to."

Suggested Questions: (Unless otherwise noted, if the answer is yes to any of the following, Criterion 2 applies):

a) Do you think you can stop drinking any time you want? (**Note:** *If no, Criterion 2 applies.*)

b) Would you be willing to go one year without a drink—starting now—to see how it affects you? (**Note:** *If hesitation or no, Criterion 2 applies.*)

c) Do you think your life would change much if you never drank alcohol again?

d) Have you ever thought about or told anyone you planned to quit or drink less? (**Note:** *Explore if they followed through with their plans to quit or drink less and, if not, why.*)

e) Have you ever thought you might quit drinking someday?

f) Have you ever quit or reduced your drinking?

g) Have you ever kept track of your drinking? (**Note:** *Normal drinkers don't because 1 or 2 drinks don't require tracking.*)

h) Have you ever made a New Year's resolution to stop or reduce your drinking? (**Note:** *Normal drinkers don't need to resolve a drinking problem, so they don't make drinking resolutions.*)

i) Do you ever try to delay drinking? (**Note:** *Normal drinkers don't endure the process of delaying their drinking, which is usually caused by struggling with the compulsion to drink. If they delay, ask about their thoughts and feelings during this delay.*)

j) If you drink less now than you did three years ago, why are you drinking less now? (**Note:** *If a response such as "was drinking too much," "drinking was causing problems," or "no longer enjoy drinking as much,"*

Criterion 2 applies.)

k) On a scale from one to five (1=easy and 5=hard), how easy would it be for you never to drink again? (**Note:** *If the answer is 2-5, Criterion 2 applies.*)

l) How easy would it be to cut your drinking in half using the same scale above? (**Note:** *If the answer is 2-5, Criterion 2 applies.*)

m) More than twice within the past three years, have you claimed you're never drinking again after a night of drinking too much but drank again?

n) Have you ever tried different methods to reduce your drinking, such as switching from liquor to beer, reducing how much or how fast you drink, changing drinking companions, eating before or during drinking, or drinking water while drinking? (**Note:** *Nonalcoholics don't use methods to reduce their drinking. If they want to cut back, they just do.*)

Criterion 3. A great deal of time is spent in activities necessary to obtain alcohol, use alcohol, or recover from its effects.

Do you spend much of your time obtaining alcohol, drinking alcohol, or recovering from alcohol?

Likely Response: "No, not really."

Suggested questions:

a) On average, how often and how much do you drink in a week? (**Note:** *This answer provides information for the following questions and doesn't trigger Criterion 3.*)

b) How much time do you spend acquiring alcohol each week? (**Note:** *Determine how many alcohol purchases are made and the time each purchase takes, including travel, each week. This answer doesn't trigger Criterion 3.*)

c) How much time do you spend drinking each week? (**Note**: *Determine the time spent drinking, including travel to and time spent in bars, each week. This answer doesn't trigger Criterion 3.*)

d) How much time do you spend nursing hangovers each week? (**Note**: *Determine the time spent nursing hangovers each week. This answer doesn't trigger Criterion 3.*)

e) What is the total time you spend each week related to drinking? (**Note**: *If the total weekly time exceeds 5 hours, Criterion 3 applies.*)

> **Criterion 4.** *Craving*, or a strong desire or urge to use alcohol.
> *Has there ever been a time when you had such strong urges to drink that you could not think of anything else?"*

Likely Response: "No." (**Note**: *The alcoholic knows a "yes" answer admits an alcoholic obsession and compulsion. Alcoholics safeguard their craving experience. However, the nonalcoholic may answer yes for reasons discussed below.*)

> **This criterion is incorrect.** (See Chapter 3, "The *Alcoholic-Craving*.") The normal drinker could have "a strong *desire* or *urge* to" drink a cold, frothy beer after mowing on a hot summer day. I propose this replacement:

> *Proposed Criterion 4.* Alcoholic-craving: an uncontrollable, obsessive, compulsive, *insatiable need* to change feelings by drinking and continuing to drink.

Suggested questions (If the answer is yes to any of the following, Criterion 5 applies):

a) Do you drink to change how you're feeling more often

than not?

b) Do you feel relief after your first drink? (**Note:** *The alcoholic feels relief—the nonalcoholic may feel relaxed.*)

c) Does drinking make you feel better when you're feeling down? (**Note:** *Nonalcoholics usually can't answer because their feelings don't dictate whether they drink. If the answer is feeling down when not drinking, explore.*)

d) Do you sometimes drink to remove thoughts about drinking?

e) Have you ever tried to stop your thoughts about drinking?

f) Have you ever owned any clothing imprinted with a brewery or distillery logo? (**Note:** *If 2 or more items, this indicates an obsession with alcohol, and Criterion 4 applies.*)

g) When you first think about drinking, do you try waiting before you drink? (**Note:** *Any waiting before drinking reveals one is trying to control drinking. Most ordinary drinkers don't delay drinking when they want a drink unless they have a good reason to, such as planning to drive, health reasons, commitments, etc.*)

h) When postponing drinking, do you tell yourself things such as "I can wait; I don't need one right now," etc.? (**Note:** *Delaying when needing a drink is a struggle for the alcoholic, whereas the typical drinker will have a drink if they want—it's no big deal.*)

i) Does anger, resentment, guilt, remorse, sadness, or stress prompt your drinking more times than not?

j) Do you think of drinking more during or after an argument than at other times?

k) In the past year, have you watched the clock until you get off work and can have a drink?

l) Have you had anything to drink while working in the past three years?

m) When you feel tired, nervous, or tense, do a couple of drinks help you feel better?

n) Do you drink more when you're feeling down?

o) Have you drunk more than twice in the past year to improve your mood?

p) Have you needed a few drinks to calm down after a rough day more than three times in the past year?

q) Do various people, places, or things ever trigger your thoughts about drinking, such as specific songs, scents, etc.?

r) If your drinking has ever caused any problems, just before you drink, do you ever tell yourself that you won't have these problems this time?

s) Have you had any traumatic events in your life causing uncomfortable feelings that drinking makes better?

t) When deciding whether to attend an event, do you find out if alcohol will be present?

u) Have you drunk at times that you later decided wasn't a good time to drink?

> **Criterion 5. Recurrent alcohol use resulting in a failure to fulfill major role obligations at work, school, or home.**
> *Have you repeatedly failed to fulfill major obligations at work, home, or school because of your alcohol use?*

Likely Response: "No." (**Note:** *Not a good question. The only portion of the question the alcoholic will hear is, "Have you repeatedly failed?" Answering "yes" is admitting failure.*)

Suggested Questions: (If the answer is yes to any of the following, Criterion 5 applies):

a) Have you chosen to drink more than twice within the past year instead of attending to an obligation at home like cleaning, lawn care, eating or spending other time with family, paying bills, preparing dinner, laundry, etc.?

b) Have you missed or been late to work or school, including doing homework or studying, because of drinking or a hangover two or more times in the past three years?

c) Have you attended work or school after drinking or with a hangover that affected your performance more than twice in the past three years?

d) Have you canceled or postponed any commitment, obligation, or appointment because of drinking or a hangover at least once in the past year?

Criterion 6. Continued alcohol use despite having persistent or recurrent social or interpersonal problems caused or exacerbated by the effects of alcohol.
Do you drink alcohol even though you suspect, or even know, that it creates or worsens interpersonal or social problems?

Likely Response: "No." (**Note**: *This question would put most on the defensive—it's accusatory. It suggests the drinker is to blame for arguments with their spouse, problems with a coworker, etc. Most people have interpersonal or social issues to some extent, so the answer will be "no."*)

Suggested Questions (Unless otherwise noted, if the answer is yes to any of the following, Criterion 6 applies):

a) Are you getting along better or worse with your spouse, parents, children, friends, coworkers, boss, or neighbors than you did three years ago? (**Note**: *If worse, determine if alcohol is likely causing this. If it is, Criterion 6 applies.*)

b) Has a friend, loved one, employer, or anyone ever mentioned your drinking?

c) Has a loved one, employer, or court ever given you a

choice to stop drinking or face a divorce, separation, job termination, or imprisonment?

d) Have you felt the urge to apologize for anything related to your drinking in the past year?

e) Do you argue more with certain people after drinking?

f) Have you ever promised anyone you would stop or slow down your drinking?

g) Do you drink because of the problems in your life?

h) Do you think your drinking has caused you or anyone any problems?

i) Have you argued with anyone to have an excuse for drinking within the past year?

j) Has your behavior when drinking embarrassed you more than once in the past year?

k) Have you discussed or argued about your drinking with anyone in the past year?

l) Have you ever told anyone you don't have a drinking problem? (**Note:** *Nonalcoholics wouldn't have a reason to.*)

m) Even though you don't think you have a drinking problem, does anyone else think you do?

n) Are you becoming more irritated by anyone thinking you have a drinking problem? (**Note:** *Any irritation suggests one or more people have expressed concerns more than once. Even if not irritated but doesn't dispute others are concerned, Criterion 6 applies.*)

o) Have you said or done anything while drinking that you later regretted more than once in the past year?

p) Has anyone ever claimed your drinking is causing problems between the two of you, even though you might disagree?

q) Have you ended any friendships in the past three years? (*If yes, ask the following question.*) Was the reason related to drinking, such as an argument while drinking, a complaint about your drinking, etc.?

r) Have you been in a physical fight with anyone after drinking in the past three years?

s) Have you ever caused physical damage to property or harm to anyone, including your property or yourself, while drinking?

t) If you've ever divorced or separated, did your partner claim your drinking was the reason, even if you disagree?

u) Has anyone you know ever sought help for the way your drinking has affected them, such as counseling or Al-Anon?

Criterion 7. Important social, occupational, or recreational activities are given up or reduced because of alcohol use.
Are there important social, occupational, or recreational activities that you have given up or reduced because of your alcohol use?

Likely Response: "No." (**Note**: *Alcoholics won't admit drinking caused them to stop anything.*)

Suggested Questions (Unless otherwise noted, if the answer is yes to any of the following, Criterion 7 applies):

a) If you have any hobbies, are you less interested in them now than three years ago? (**Note:** *Determine if the reason is alcohol-related. If so, Criterion 7 applies.*)

b) Are you less interested in activities at work or with friends than you were three years ago? (**Note:** *Determine if the reason is alcohol-related. If so, Criterion 7 applies.*)

c) Have you lost interest at work or school because of any activity? (*If yes, ask the following question.*) Does that activity involve drinking?

d) Have you become more involved in any new activities in the past three years? (*If yes, ask the following question.*) What are they, and do any of these new activities involve drinking?

e) Have you given up any activities in the past 3 years? (*If yes, ask the following question.*) What were they, and did any of these activities involve drinking?

Criterion 8. Recurrent alcohol use in situations in which it is physically hazardous.
Have you repeatedly used alcohol in conditions in which it was physically dangerous, such as driving a car or operating a machine while intoxicated?

Likely Response: "No." (**Note:** *Admitting to repeatedly driving while intoxicated is admitting an obvious problem.*)

Suggested Questions (If the answer is yes to any of the following, Criterion 8 applies):

a) Do you believe you do anything better after a drink or two that could accidentally result in harm to you or others?

b) In the past year, have you more than once done anything while drinking that could accidentally result in harm to you or others, such as boating, driving a car, swimming,* surfing, snow, water, or jet skiing, using a hot tub, sauna, bathtub, shower, or firearm, hiking, working, caring for others, operating lawn equipment or a machine, carrying heavy objects, or supervising anyone doing any of the above?

c) Have you driven after drinking with a passenger in the past year?

d) Have you driven while drinking and later regretted it in the past year?

---

*According to the CDC (2022), 31% of all U.S. drowning deaths involve a BAC of .10% or higher, which is over the legal limit to drive.

e) Have you had sex while drinking that you later regretted in the past three years?
f) Have you had unprotected, risk-taking sex after drinking in the past three years?
g) Have you caused or been the victim of a personal injury while drinking, such as from a car accident, fall, fight, etc., within the past three years?
h) Has anyone at work ever mentioned your drinking?
i) Have you transported an open container of alcohol in your vehicle in the past year?
j) Have you chased drinks or beers with shots more than once in the past year?
k) Have you gone with an unknown person to an unknown place while drinking in the past 3 years, which you would not have done if sober?

Criterion 9. Alcohol use is continued despite knowledge of having a persistent or recurrent physical or psychological problem likely to have been caused or exacerbated by alcohol.

Do you drink alcohol even though you suspect or know it creates or worsens problems with your mind and body?

Likely Response: "No."

Suggested Questions (Unless otherwise noted, if the answer is yes to any of the following, Criterion 9 applies):

a) Have you had more than three blackouts in the past year? (**Note:** *Although nonalcoholics can also have blackouts, it's a sign of excessive drinking and should be explored.*)
b) More than twice in the past year, has anyone mentioned anything you said or did while drinking that you recalled after being reminded (brownout)?
c) Have you had three or more hangovers in the past

year?

d) In the past two years, have you drunk alcohol to reduce the discomfort of a hangover?

e) Are your hangovers worse now than three years ago?

f) Has anyone ever suggested getting help with your drinking, like attending an AA meeting?

g) Have you ever attended an AA meeting or received any help for drinking?

h) How much do you think you can drink before it is unhealthy? (**Note:** *This prefaces the following question, prompts brief discussion, and doesn't trigger this criterion.*)

i) Do you drink more than you think is healthy for you?

j) Have you had more than 4 drinks within two hours more than twice in the past year? (**Note:** *Binge drinking is 4 drinks for women and 5 for men within 2 hours and cause for concern.*)

k) Have you had more than 4 drinks within a day more than twice in the past year? (**Note:** *Heavy drinking is 4 drinks for women and 5 for men within 1 day and cause for concern and follow-up.*)

l) Have you had more than [8 drinks for women or 15 drinks for men] within one week more than twice in the past year? (**Note:** *Heavy drinking is 8 drinks for women and 15 for men within 1 week and cause for concern and follow-up.*)

m) Have you ever gone to a hospital or urgent care for anything caused by or related to your drinking?

n) Have you ever sought help for your drinking?

Criterion 10. Tolerance, as defined by either of the following:

Criterion 10a. A need for markedly increased amounts of alcohol to achieve intoxication or desired effect.

Do you find to get intoxicated or achieve the desired effect of drinking, you need to consume much more alcohol than you used to?

Likely Response: "No."

Suggested Questions (If the answer is yes to any of the following, Criterion 10a applies):

a) Has anyone ever said anything positive about your drinking, such as "I see you've cut back" or "You handle your drinking well?"

b) Have you ever thought drinking isn't working as well as it once did?

c) Would you have to drink more now to feel how you felt in the past?

d) If you drink more now than three years ago, do you become just as drunk or less drunk?

Criterion 10b. A markedly diminished effect with continued use of the same amount of alcohol.

If you drink the same amount of alcohol as you used to, do you find it has a lot less effect on you than it used to?

Likely Response: "No."

Suggested Questions (If the answer is yes to any of the following, Criterion 10b applies):

a) Can you hold your liquor better now than you could three years ago? (**Note:** *Alcoholics often boast about how well they can hold liquor. Most don't realize it's tolerance, a symptom of physical alcohol dependence.*)

b) When drinking with others, do they usually act more drunk? (**Note:** *Nonalcoholics will reply neither act drunk because they rarely drink with alcoholics, or they* *don't compare because it's unimportant.*)

c) Can you drink the same as you drank three years ago and not get as drunk?

d) When you're not drinking, do you get as much enjoyment from life as you once did? (**Note**: *If the answer is "no," Criterion 10b applies.*)

e) Do you enjoy drinking less now than three years ago?

f) Do you ever seek the same feeling you once had when you first began drinking?

Criterion 11. Withdrawal, as manifested by either of the following:

Criterion 11a. The characteristic withdrawal syndrome for alcohol (refer to Criteria A and B of the criteria set for alcohol withdrawal, pp. 499-500).
When you stop drinking, do you undergo withdrawal?

Likely Response: "No." (**Note**: *A "yes" answer admits alcoholism. Also, this question assumes the alcoholic has previously stopped drinking. If withdrawal is an issue, most alcoholics drink enough to avoid it.*)

Suggested Questions (Unless otherwise noted, if the answer is yes to any of the following, Criterion 11a applies):

a) Do you drink daily or periodically (not drinking for several days between drinking episodes)? (**Note**: *If periodically, physical withdrawal symptoms will likely not apply. This answer doesn't trigger Criterion 11a.*)

b) Do you ever drink when you really don't want to?

c) Do you mostly drink to calm yourself, relieve anxiety, or help you sleep better?

d) Have you ever quit drinking for more than one day? (*If yes, ask the following question.*) Did you have two or more of the following: 1) trouble sleeping, 2) shaky hands, 3) agitation, restlessness, pacing, fidgeting, irritability, anger, distress, outbursts, nail-biting, pulling at clothes or hair, tapping fingers or feet, moving things around, taking clothes off and on, excessive talking with racing thoughts, inability to get in a comfortable position, 4) anxiety, 5) excessive sweating, 6) nausea or vomiting, 7) hallucinations or illusions, 8) seizures? (**Note:** *Less than 10% who have alcohol withdrawal will experience severe symptoms (i.e., tremors, increased heart rate and blood pressure, perspiration, alcohol withdrawal delirium), and less than 3% will have withdrawal seizures.*)

Criterion 11b. Alcohol (or a closely related substance, such as a benzodiazepine) is taken to relieve or avoid withdrawal symptoms.
Have you ever drunk alcohol or taken another substance to prevent alcohol withdrawal?

Likely Response: "No." (**Note**: *If they had and were inclined to answer "yes," they would have admitted their alcoholism long before the clinician asked the first question.*)

Suggested Questions (If the answer is yes to any of the following, Criterion 11b applies):

a) Do you have a flask or similar item to carry alcohol? (**Note**: *Carrying a flask indicates maintenance drinking to avoid withdrawal symptoms, and Criterion 11b applies.*)

b) Have you drunk within two hours of awakening two or more times in the past year?

c) Do you drink earlier in the day now compared to three years ago?

d) Have you had a drink to reduce the discomfort of a hangover in the past three years?

e) Have you ever had a drink or taken any drug (prescribed, over-the-counter, or otherwise) to minimize any emotional or physical discomfort, such as sleep problems, anxiety, headache, shaking hands, restlessness, irritability, sadness, etc., when you stopped drinking for three days or more?

ADDITIONAL INQUIRY FOR PROPOSED CRITERIA 12-16

I suggest including the following criteria in the diagnostic interview.

> **Proposed Criterion 12.** Any guilt or remorse prompting drinking or felt after drinking.

Proposed questions (If the answer is yes to any of the following, Criterion 12 applies):

a. Have you felt any guilt or remorse before, during, or after drinking for anything about your drinking in the past year?

b. Have you wanted to apologize for anything about your drinking within the past year?

c. Does guilt, remorse, or sadness prompt your drinking more times than not?

d. Have you apologized for anything about your drinking more than once in the past year?

e. Have you felt remorse or guilt because you drank more than you planned more than once within the past year?

f. Have you felt bad about your drinking in the past year?

> **Proposed Criterion 13.** Any resentment or anger prompting drinking.

Proposed questions (If the answer is yes to any of the following, Criterion 13 applies):

a. Has resentment, annoyance, irritation, or anger toward anyone, including a loved one, friend, boss, or coworker, prompted you to start or continue drinking in the past

year?
b. Do you drink more when you're angry?
c. Do you want to drink after someone has irritated you?
d. When you drink, do you drink more after someone has irritated or annoyed you?
e. When you're frustrated, does drinking help you feel calmer?
f. Does anger, resentment, annoyance, or irritation prompt your drinking more times than not?
g. Do you think of drinking more during or after an argument than at other times?
h. Do you think that if people would just leave you alone about your drinking, you wouldn't drink so much?

Proposed Criterion 14. Any alcohol-related legal problems.

(**Note:** *Court records will reveal legal matters related to drinking unless expunged or sealed.*)

Proposed questions (If the answer is yes to any of the following, Criterion 14 applies):

a) Have you been arrested for DUI or Public Intoxication more than once within the past three years?
b) Have you been arrested for anything else while drinking within the past three years?
c) Have you ever been involved in a legal civil matter where your drinking was raised, such as divorce, custody, personal injury, property damage claim, etc
d) Have you had any contact with the police when drinking in the past three years?
e) Have you had an alcohol ignition interlock device installed in your vehicle in the past three years?
f) Have you ever worn an alcohol monitor bracelet?

g) Has your driver's license or any license ever been suspended because of drinking?

Proposed Criterion 15. Concealing drinking, alcohol, or anything related to alcohol.

Proposed questions (Unless otherwise noted, if the answer is yes to any of the following, Criterion 15 applies):

a) Do you think that if you had a drinking problem and it became known to others, it would cause you any difficulties?
b) Have you ever secretly bought alcohol?
c) Do you usually pay for alcohol with cash?
d) Do you regularly purchase alcohol from more than two liquor stores? (**Note:** *Many alcoholics purchase alcohol from various stores to avoid anyone thinking they have a drinking problem.*)
e) Have you ever tried hiding the sound of making a drink to avoid anyone hearing it?
f) Has anyone ever asked you how many drinks you've had? (**Note:** *No one asks the normal drinker this question.*)
g) Have you tried to act sober in the past year?
h) Have you ever drunk alone to avoid arousing concern and confrontation about your drinking?
i) Have you ever hidden any thoughts or feelings about your drinking?
j) Have you ever avoided disclosing the time of day you had your first drink?
k) Have you ever hidden any personal injuries, property damage, or other problems caused by your drinking or asked someone else to keep quiet about it?
l) Do you drink alone more times than not?

m) More than two times in the past year, have you said you only had a couple when you had drunk three or more?
n) Have you concealed anything you did while drinking, including any indiscretions, in the past year?
o) Have you ever answered any questions about your drinking falsely?
p) Have you ever hidden alcohol?
q) Have you ever carried a flask or anything containing and disguising alcohol?
r) Have you ever falsely claimed you didn't do something while drinking?
s) Have you ever had a drink before going to a bar, party, or event where alcohol is present? (**Note:** *Alcoholics often 'pre-drink' before going where alcohol is available, so it doesn't appear they're drinking too much when they arrive.*)
t) Have you changed the places where you store alcohol within the past three years? (**Note:** *If changing more than one place and replying hesitantly without a reasonable explanation, Criterion 15 applies.*)
u) Have you, more than once in the past year, ever avoided anyone to prevent them from suspecting you had been drinking?
v) In the past year, after drinking, have you tried to mask the smell of alcohol when with someone or at an event where the smell of alcohol would have been inappropriate?
w) Have you ever concealed anything about your drinking to prevent people from forming the wrong impression, worrying unnecessarily, using it against you, or for any other reason? (**Note:** *Any hesitancy reveals an issue likely exists.*)

Proposed Criterion 16. Denial of a drinking problem or denial to others.

Proposed questions (Unless otherwise noted, if the answer is yes to any of the following, Criterion 16 applies):

a) Have you ever wondered if you might have a drinking problem or drink too much at times?

b) Have you ever limited or quit drinking temporarily to prove to yourself or others that you don't have a drinking problem?

c) Do you think you must drink daily to be an alcoholic?

d) Have you received any alcohol-related gifts, such as alcohol, a flask, accessories, clothing, novelty items, or shot glasses, in the past three years? (**Note:** *If yes, this indicates the drinker is so obsessed with alcohol that even others know it. If two or more gifts, Criterion 16 applies.*)

e) Do you believe you drink because of problems with work, finances, or a relationship? (Note: *Reference "o" for consistency.*)

f) Have you ever compared your drinking to another drinker and decided you don't have a drinking problem?

g) Even though you don't think you have a drinking problem, does anyone else think you do?

h) (If the answer to the previous question is "no," ask:) Would it surprise you that someone else thinks you have a drinking problem? (**Note:** *If no, Criterion 16 applies. Any hesitancy reveals that an issue probably exists. Both problem and normal drinkers may say "yes," but a "no" answer is clear.*)

i) To reduce the concern of anyone worrying about your drinking, have you ever made sure they know when you've cut back or aren't drinking? (**Note:** *If "no,"* *determine if anyone worries about the drinker. If anyone does, Criterion 16 applies.)*

j) Have you ever made any drinking rules, like not drinking before a specific time, not exceeding a certain number of drinks in an hour, not keeping alcohol at home, or drinking only on weekends? (**Note:** *Normal drinkers don't need to make drinking rules, but alcoholics often do to support their denial. In time, they relax or abolish these rules to accommodate their progressing alcoholism. See Chapter 2, under the section, The Alcoholic's Rules.)*

k) Have you ever talked with anyone about your drinking that you thought was needless? (**Note:** *Any hesitancy reveals an issue. The normal drinker doesn't have people concerned about their drinking.)*

l) Have you ever told anyone anything like: "I don't need to drink. I can take it or leave it. I drink because I want to?"

m) Have you made any new friends in the last year? (*If yes, ask the following question.*) Do they drink more than or the same as you do? (**Note:** *If more or the same, Criterion 16 applies.)*

n) Do you think anyone troubled by your drinking is overreacting?

o) Do you believe people, events, or situations contribute to your drinking?

p) Have you ever tried explaining to anyone that your drinking isn't as bad as it might appear or they think?

q) Do you believe you once had a drinking problem but no longer do?

r) Do you think you might have a slight problem with drinking, but it's not severe like alcoholism?

s) Do you now drink out of habit more than any other reason?

If these sound like trick questions, some are. Yet they're designed to 'trick' the affliction, not the alcoholic. Transparent questions will not identify an alcoholic who is compelled by alcoholism to avoid detection.

Section Six

Health Care Education

ONLY EIGHT PERCENT of medical schools have a *required* course on addiction medicine.[85] During their residency, psychiatrists receive, on average, only eight hours of substance use disorder training.[86] Additionally, schools teaching social work and psychology require little or no substance use disorder courses.[87] Nor do board exams test on alcoholism. This lack of adequate education doesn't appear to be improving.[88]

The consensus is that the medical school curricula should include alcoholism. However, replacing a course with a curriculum already saturated with information the medical student must know is unlikely. Although the obvious solution is to add an alcoholism course, educators can't agree on whether or how to adopt and integrate this solution.

For years, this has been an issue. And the many studies assuring that an alcoholism course would be effective and efficient have changed nothing.

Sometimes, science and logic must give way to common sense. Unfortunately, each year that educators fail to resolve this problem, about 180,000 alcoholics die, and each alcoholic affects at least 10 people who suffer—sometimes in brutal and horrific ways. So, the time for educators to build an 'evidence-based effective curriculum' has long past expired.

Now is the time to move forward. Anything is better than nothing when understanding and treating alcoholism. Reducing health care's negative attitude toward the alcoholic would be a good start.

For example, a required two-day seminar in the first year of medical school and a Continuing Medical Education (CME) seminar for practicing doctors would move health care closer to the solution. The general goals of the seminar follow (each numbered goal is a one-hour session):

1. *Dilute the stereotypical view of alcoholics with evidence-based facts that alcoholism is a progressive, relapsing, chronic disease.*

   Provide statistics showing that only 10% of alcoholics fit the stereotype. Most alcoholics are high-functioning, and many are professionals.

   This session will show alcoholism is not a blameful condition caused by a lack of morals and explain how to treat it like any other illness.

2. *Explain the basics of neurobiology and the effect alcohol has on the reward network of the alcoholic brain.*

   This segment will explain that drinking is a symptom of an underlying biological disorder. In the past decade, neuroscience has shown that alcoholism does not result from poor moral character and a lack of willpower. A neurobiologist will illustrate this with neuroimages of the alcoholic's brain and explain its functioning compared with the nonalcoholic brain.

3. *Managing intoxicated patients effectively.*

   Emergency rooms often serve as 'drunk tanks,' and Urgent Care has its share of intoxicated patients. This is a high-risk event, and doctors must protect themselves, their patients, and the intoxicated patient. These patients are often present against their will, so understanding how to manage them is essential.

4. *AUD and psychiatric comorbidity.*

   This session will explain the high prevalence of alcoholic comorbidity, the common comorbid disorders, and how to approach a comorbid diagnosis.

5. *Discuss the screening instruments available.*

   This session will describe the various AUD screenings and how to use them in all health care settings without negatively affecting a practice. It will highlight the strengths and weaknesses of these screenings and explain when a screening prompts a diagnostic exam. It will also emphasize the differences between an alcohol screening and a diagnostic exam.

6. *Enlighten the participant's understanding of recovery by attending several open AA meetings.*

Those health care professionals who have attended open AA meetings have said their thinking about alcoholism changed remarkably. According to George Vaillant, MD, a professor of psychiatry at Harvard Medical School:

> Few doctors have ever seen a recovered alcoholic.... Doctors overcount the failures and have no knowledge of the successes.... A doctor should go to open meetings ... [to] see for themselves these well-dressed people ... who look like anybody else and have been in recovery for years. It was terribly important for me to ... see sober alcoholics ... because they're terribly inspiring.

7. *Teach the signs and symptoms of AUD.*

Describe *all* the symptoms of alcoholism, especially during the early and middle stages of the disease.

8. *Teach how to communicate with alcoholics reassuringly and caringly, reducing defensiveness and denial.*

This session will explain how the alcoholic patient will be more receptive to the doctor's advice by developing an effective rapport and the most efficient way to do this.

This will also show how recovery from alcoholism is a process, not an event. Merely because the alcoholic doesn't initially follow the physician's advice doesn't mean the doctor failed. Instead, it means the patient is one step closer to sobriety.

Participants will learn that patients tend to follow the advice of doctors who treat their physical health complaints, such as hypertension, diabetes, and gastrointestinal issues, and the importance of relating their AUD advice to these complaints.

This session will also feature several skits showing a skilled diagnostician conducting a five-minute screening/diagnostic interview with students participating.

9. *Explain the objective tests and observations that reveal the probability of AUD.*

This hour will stress the importance of reviewing medical records, physically examining the patient for conditions that may reflect alcohol-induced changes in the liver (e.g., gastritis, hepatomegaly, esophageal varices, hemorrhoids, etc.), briefly interviewing those affected by the alcoholic with two simple questions (e.g., "Do you believe [patient] has a drinking problem?" and "Are you concerned about [patient's] drinking?"), and conducting other objective tests if AUD is suspected.

This segment could also highlight those blood tests that may indicate AUD. For instance, a high BAC in a sober-appearing patient is clearly indicative of tolerance, and high tolerance conclusively indicates alcohol dependence.

10. *Outline the methods available to treat AUD, including behavioral and pharmacological therapies.*

Historically, the go-to referral has been Alcoholics Anonymous. However, health care and the courts don't know that although AA seems to be the most effective treatment, it isn't the only treatment and isn't for everyone. Also, no research has found reliable predictors of who will become and remain sober attending AA. This session will describe other treatment methods available, including medications that have proven effective for treating AUD.

11. *Teach all the alcohol withdrawal symptoms.*

This session will explain how to identify withdrawal symptoms and which ones are mild and which are life-threatening. This hour will also describe methods of stabilizing the alcoholic who is having withdrawal symptoms.

12. *Teach the effectiveness and methods of alcoholic interventions.*

An interventionist will describe the intervention methods that work best with certain alcoholics, what to ask and look for in an interventionist, and how to find the right one.

13. *Explain the training and credentials of an AUD specialist and the best way to find and effectively refer a patient to one.*

This hour will explain the importance of not simply handing the patient a list of phone numbers to call because denial—a key symptom of AUD—reduces the probability of the patient calling.

This session will stress the importance of scheduling and providing the patient with the place, date, and time of the referral appointment. It will also include other procedures for an effective referral and follow-up.

14. *Approach the sensitive subject that one-third of medical students drink alcoholically, especially during their residency, and 10-15% of practicing doctors and 20-25% of nurses are drinking alcoholics.*[89]

The consensus is these percentages are higher. And they don't include the alcoholic doctors, nurses, and students who are *currently* sober but will relapse.

This session will feature a sober alcoholic doctor who explains the recovery process and how alcoholism often goes unnoticed in health care settings.

This will also explain the best way of approaching a health care worker who is suspected of abusing alcohol and how to get confidential help for a dependency problem.

It will discuss how doctors struggling with the same dependency problem as their patients will probably have difficulty being objective.

15. *Explain how the denial of health care has caused many misdiagnoses and the importance of the emergency and family doctor's role in recognizing AUD.*

16. *Discuss exposure to legal liability.*

An attorney who prosecutes and one who defends medical malpractice will discuss the importance of inquiring, screening, diagnosing, and referring an alcoholic for treatment. The attorneys will also explain the elements of medical malpractice and how doctors can avoid potential liability.

This session will clarify the rising community standards regarding AUD screening and diagnosis. For example, ignoring alcoholism, *choosing* not to treat the alcoholic, not screening the alcoholic, and not addressing alcoholism with an alcoholic patient are becoming substandard.

It's also helpful for the health care professional to understand the mechanics of a medical malpractice case.

Participants will learn that health care is largely self-regulating. Yet, like most groups, insiders tend to develop thinking unique to and in conformity with that group. So, to try and ensure balance and diversity, many groups rely on laypersons, to some extent, whose purpose is to provide unbiased feedback as part of the policy-making process.

Still, if anyone outside health care decides the existing policy is unfavorable to them, they can choose to litigate, and lay persons serving as jurors decide whether to maintain the current policy or change it. Unfortunately, it often takes litigation to change policy.

—

THE SOLUTION IS knowledge. As professor George E. Vaillant, MD, has said, health care's "lack of knowledge about alcoholism is astonishing." Yet it only takes a little knowledge, which isn't complex, to make a significant difference.

First, learning the symptoms, a small part of the neurobiology related to alcoholism, and how best to approach the alcoholic is critical. Second, awareness of alcoholic comorbidity is crucial. Finally, understanding the compulsive and insatiable characteristics of the alcoholic-craving is a must.

For health care to catch up, it must let go of its archaic stereotyping of the alcoholic and adopt the scientific, evidence-based view. Doctors can't treat a condition they don't recognize or understand. Yet, ignoring this 7,000-year-old problem hasn't made it go away.

Considering that *at least* 25% of patients, 16% of US residents, and 33% of medical students drink alcoholically, educators and accrediting bodies must make the long-awaited changes far past the expiration date that professional responsibility demands. Because of this prevalence, at *least* an alcoholism seminar should be mandatory during the first year in all medical schools and not merely a residency elective.

Researchers, universities, medical associations, and institutions like the NIAAA and CDC have done the heavy lifting. Health care practitioners only need to accept delivery. A wealth of easily accessible information is also available to assist practices in adjusting and integrating these solutions.

This information will enable primary and emergency doctors on the front lines, usually the first ones to see the alcoholic, to perform their responsibilities of screening and diagnosing, which means not merely placing a band-aid on the biological effects of alcoholism.

Still, it isn't only the responsibility of health care. The public can easily learn enough of the early signs to spot the alcoholic and intervene. Health care and the public should rely on each other and work together.

Doctors need to know that the alcoholic will not accurately self-report. So, training health care workers on how to identify probable alcoholism and interact with the alcoholic effectively is critical.

Additionally, recognizing this failure to self-report should also prompt updated and upgraded screenings and diagnostic tools, making them less transparent and more effective, resulting in many more alcoholics receiving the help they need.

Finally, health care must remain open to gaining valuable insights and perspectives about alcoholism from those outside the medical community.

Questions for Discussion

1. Do you believe health care should receive more training in alcoholism and diagnosing alcoholism?
2. Has this chapter altered your view about health care's treatment of AUD?
3. If you're a sober alcoholic, what experience have you had with alcohol screenings and diagnostic exams?
4. Do you strongly agree or disagree with anything in this chapter? If so, what? Why?
5. Have you learned anything from this chapter? If yes, please discuss.
6. Do you believe the AUD section of the DSM-5 should be updated and revised as suggested in this chapter?
7. Have you learned anything about alcoholic comorbidity from this chapter?
8. Has this chapter affected you? How?

THE AFFECTED
Caught in the Crossfire

CHAPTER 8

*You're probably an alcoholic if you
demand friends and family worried
about your drinking get counseling—now!*

MANY ARE CONVINCED the alcoholic lives a carefree life that is a continuous lifelong party. They don't know the real life of the alcoholic—it's unknowable to anyone other than those affected by the alcoholic and those afflicted with alcoholism. *It's not a party.*

Those of us affected by an alcoholic have not emerged unscathed. A drinking alcoholic affects *at least* 10 others, including former and current spouses, partners, in-laws, friends, coworkers, employees, and employers, as well as parents, children, siblings, aunts, uncles, nieces, nephews, cousins, and grandparents. Millions of men, women, and children have been affected in various ways.*

This chapter applies to everyone distressed by an alcoholic, but it focuses on the most affected—those who live or have lived with an alcoholic.° Still, this focus does not blur the alcoholic's effect on others.

---

*Seventy-six million Americans (about 45% of the U.S. population) have been *exposed* to alcoholism in the family, and an estimated 26.8 million of them are children.

°About 10.5 percent (7.5 million) of U.S. children ages 17 and younger *live* with a parent with AUD, according to a 2017 report by SAMHSA.

The emotional turmoil that parents of an alcoholic suffer is agonizing. The anguish of watching a loved one or close friend descend into alcoholism is tormenting. The frustration, anxiety, and resentment an alcoholic coworker or employee causes are also distressing.

However, a spouse, partner, and child living with an alcoholic are affected in ways rarely faced by others. The hardest hit is the child of an alcoholic. Adults have the tools to be resilient and cope with catastrophes, but children don't. The trauma endured by a child raised in an alcoholic home has been likened to the soldier's trauma on the battlefield.[1] They both suffer Post Traumatic Stress Disorder.[2]

Battle scars from a war they never fought mark these impressionable and silent bystanders. They're caught in the crossfire, unable to take cover without a say.

First Things First

RECOVERING FROM THE effects of living with an alcoholic is not an event but a process—*it takes time*. Still, the benefits of recovery begin the moment we exit the dead-end road we've been traveling.

In the world of physics, for every action, there is an opposite and equal reaction. But in the world of alcoholism, for every action, there is an opposite and *unequal overreaction*.

Alcoholics don't like change. With emotions running high in the alcoholic arena, when we change the road we've been traveling, there may be an abusive overreaction.

If physical or emotional domestic abuse is likely, you should take prompt action to protect yourself, especially if children are present. This may include escaping with the children to a safe place or calling the police.[1]* *You may also call the 24-hour National Domestic Violence Hotline at 1–800–799–SAFE*

---

*According to the Bureau of Justice Statistics, of those suffering violence by a current or former spouse or partner, three out of four incidents involved a drinking offender. This doesn't include the verbal and emotional abuse, often more damaging and ignored.

(7233), *which provides referrals to agencies in all 50 states.*

Many support services are available to help and encourage those affected by the alcoholic during this uncertain time while making necessary life changes. For example, we may seek guidance from a drug and alcohol counselor or anyone adequately trained. Once safe, we can pursue and receive soothing relief from *recovery.*

—

I have divided this chapter into three sections.

SECTION ONE — THE ENDLESS CYCLE discusses the cycle of alcoholism, the common characteristics of the alcoholic (dysfunctional) family with a focus on the children, how many children are affected, the signs exhibited by children more affected, ways to lessen the effect on children living in an alcoholic home, and the various support available for these children.

SECTION TWO — WHEN THE CHILDREN BECAME ADULTS discusses the adult children of alcoholics and the impact on their behavior, relationships, and self-esteem, the trauma they faced and how they faced it, and how many have recovered, including the sources for overcoming the effects of this trauma.

SECTION THREE — THE AFFECTED SPOUSE, PARTNER, OR PARENT discusses how the affected struggle with the issues affecting them, including making various life-changing decisions, common reactions to the drinking and sober alcoholic, how the denial of those affected supports enabling which supports the alcoholic's continued drinking, and the various support available.

Section One

The Endless Cycle

ALCOHOLISM IS A family disease affecting everyone. Studies consistently and convincingly show the adult child of an alcoholic will likely marry an alcoholic.[3] These studies also reveal that children of an alcoholic are more likely to develop alcoholism than the general population.[4] So, the children *affected* by an alcoholic often become *afflicted* with alcoholism, and *their* children and others become the *affected*.

If changes aren't made, this cycle continues and builds momentum with each generation. Either the afflicted or the affected must escape this darkness by walking into the light. Although this light may, at first, cloud our vision causing discomfort, as we acclimate, it will lighten our path to ending the cycle of alcoholism.

The Uncomfortable Truth

Some have suggested that contempt for the alcoholic is plenty and doesn't need a boost by writing about the difficulties our children have endured. But we can change nothing unless we see it. Although we know we can't change the past, we *can* prevent further harm and begin repairing the damage done.

To start this, we must reflect *reasonably* on the past without morbidly obsessing about it. This reflection is the gateway to recovery, allowing us to end the cycle. We must protect our children and ourselves.

Family Denial—Roadblock to Recovery

Of course, it's an abomination to *intentionally* harm our children. As parents, we instinctively love and protect them. Even if we *unintentionally* harm them, we agonize with guilt and remorse. Naturally, to avoid these dreadful feelings, we may easily conclude: "Luckily, my kids weren't *that* affected by my drinking."

Still, no parent is perfect. Upon further reflection, we may minimize the severity of any harm to cope with the emerging truth. Yet, that truth encourages us to move toward the solution. Whether we're an alcoholic, one affected by an alcoholic, or the adult child of an alcoholic who is now a parent, we must accept that our actions and reactions affect the ones we love. We *can* stop this endless cycle if we march forward, avoiding the landmines of useless guilt and sorrow as the light of truth brightens our path. Our children deserve it ... and so do we.

COMMON CHARACTERISTICS OF THE ALCOHOLIC (DYSFUNCTIONAL) FAMILY

UNDOUBTEDLY, THE ALCOHOLIC home is dysfunctional. The consensus is that children experience nearly the same trauma in a dysfunctional family absent alcohol as children raised in an alcoholic home. Both dysfunctional environments have common features.

These include a family member demanding, passively or aggressively, that other family members tolerate their behavior. For example, this could be a sober or drinking alcoholic or one with unresolved mental disorders (e.g., depression, narcissism, bipolar, anxiety, borderline personality). If the demanding one is a parent, the other parent is typically submissive. Yet, they come across as assertive and controlling with others. Submission is *only* to the demanding family member.

As a survival mechanism, alcoholic and dysfunctional parents usually become impulsive and self-absorbed, catering to their own needs, wants, and wishes. The submissive or affected parent spends so much time and energy satisfying the demanding one that they have less time for their children—there's simply not enough attention to go around. So, the children grow up without enough nurturing and guidance. It's a chaotic environment, although the chaos may manifest subtly.

Because family members usually receive unequal treatment, especially children, they have boundary issues and are in constant conflict. Children fear talking and expressing emotions, so they repress anger, as well as other feelings, as they slip deeper into denial.

They rarely do things as a family. Instead, there is often extended family disharmony—children seldom interact with grandparents, cousins, aunts, and uncles.

Everyone walks on eggshells to please one family member. Children quickly learn that 'cracking an eggshell' produces unpleasant and sometimes cruel consequences.

The Children

Children living in this dysfunctional environment are often disrespected, ridiculed, and held in contempt. Many alcoholic parents withhold love conditioned upon the children behaving according to their unreasonable expectations. These parents are often unforgiving, hypocritical, judgmental, and employ double standards. Gender disparity is common, where a sister may see her brother given unlimited freedom while she's strictly controlled.

Individuality is repressed. Parents are often too protective or neglectful, apathetic, and bitter with unpredictable emotions. They unfairly criticize and discipline their children.

When the child's behavior outside the home calls for discipline, the parent *randomly* defends or abandons them. This decision is not reasonable but based on the parent's temporary emotional condition. This teaches children that right and wrong are meaningless.

Siblings become caretakers, assuming too much authority over younger ones. Parents ignore their children's emotional expressions. Children must take part in extracurricular activities they dislike to please their parents.

Whether the family is physically intact or separated, children usually become the pawns—parents talk to the other parent through the children. For example, one parent may reward a child for snooping on the other parent and reporting their findings.

To cope, children assume roles. They may be the *perfect* one, the *scapegoat*, the *caretaker*, the *quiet and passive* child, the family *clown*, or the *opportunist*. They may adopt more than one role or alternate between them.

However, not all alcoholic families and relationships are similarly dysfunctional. Some are more severe and some more mild, but most fall between these extremes.

Many children need and will benefit from outside support, particularly victims of abuse.

Some grew up with a drinking alcoholic, and others with a sober alcoholic. Some never saw their alcoholic parent drink. Some alcoholic parents were merely abstinent, known as "dry drunks," one who displays all the behavior of a drinking alcoholic—sometimes worse—without drinking. They may have had a parent who relapsed often. Then, some grew up with both parents drinking.

Many children learn to communicate and cope in unhealthy ways. For example, children learn to distrust, keep quiet, repress feelings, and hide the few feelings remaining. The alcoholic family intuitively upholds this status quo to remain emotionally numb.

To cope with an alcoholic parent, children may isolate and cultivate denial, delusion, anxiety, shame, and confusion. Many feel chronic stress and fear, never knowing what to expect next yet always preparing for arguments, violence, and other destructive conduct, especially if they've been the victim of this conduct. Many feel abandoned because of a parent's inattention and neglectful permissiveness.

Their chaotic family environment deprives them of consistency, stability, and emotional support. Parents routinely act and interact with others in ways that embarrass them. They avoid inviting friends over or even making friends, fearing a shameful exposition of their secrets.

Children living in different alcoholic homes experience common feelings. Although they're struggling to cope, they act like they're doing fine. This facade escorts them into adulthood. They can't risk being real. They continue believing everything is their fault as their self-worth plunges. They feel separated and different from others. They assume an age-inappropriate responsibility and decide they're a failure when they can't make it better. Still, they keep trying, even when nothing is left to make better.

Children worry about their parent's health, expect unpredictable and inconsistent behavior, and feel increasingly unloved as they endure broken promises. Yet, they constantly and stubbornly defend their parents out of a strict sense of loyalty. This loyalty survives their childhood and strengthens in adulthood as it manifests in unhealthy ways.

Characteristics of Children Less Affected

Not all children of alcoholic parents experience the above. Some are resilient survivors who have similar characteristics. They are decision-makers and can identify and express feelings. They may inappropriately assume the role of a responsible parent. They have close relationships with adults they see as 'parental' figures. This is usually a relative, teacher, neighbor, parent's friend, or friend's parent.

They feel autonomous, sense a purpose at an early age, and enthusiastically look forward to the future. They appear in charge at home, school, and social events. They feel a need to control, especially when helping others. They earn high grades and are overachievers.

But the trauma remains, although they disguise it reasonably well. These traits carry over into adulthood as their emotional problems, ignored for years, begin surfacing.

Signs of Trouble

Although similarities exist, everyone is different and responds uniquely to specific events. So, living with alcoholism affects some children more than others, which their behaviors reveal. Although parents are often too preoccupied and self-absorbed to notice, teachers and relatives usually do.

Some of the similar signs exhibited by children struggling to cope include (1) doing poorly in school, (2) excessive unexplained absences, (3) frequent unexcused tardiness, (4) excessively isolating in their room, (5) avoiding social interaction and decreasing interaction with classmates, (6) a pattern of starting and explosively ending friendships, (7) distrusting others and having no close, intimate friendships, (8) feeling embarrassed so resists inviting friends over, (9) feeling lonely or expressing loneliness, (10) appearing depressed or expressing suicidal thoughts, (11) self-injury,* (12) playing online games or engaging in any activity obsessively and compulsively,° (13) often complaining about physical ailments, (14) engaging in risky activities, (15) increasing promiscuity, (16) repressing feelings,** (17) feeling unreasonable guilt (believing they're responsible for the alcoholic situation), (18) feeling or appearing anxious (always waiting for the other shoe to drop), (19) appearing or expressing confusion (caused by the alcoholic's moodiness), (20) acting aggressively (pushing a child in the lunch line), and (21) expressing anger about the alcoholic and the nonalcoholic parent, to their parent or others, for not protecting them.

Support for the Affected Child

When children belong to a support group, it benefits the entire family. Some of these benefits include reducing stigma and shame, which is life-changing. They do better in school and attendance improves. They learn to rebound from setbacks. The stress the entire family feels lessens.

Children in an alcoholic home need information to make

---

*While boys often cope with their distress aggressively, girls usually direct it inwardly. This could be burning, cutting, and causing other superficial injuries to their skin. (Although often hidden, a portion may be visible around their arms.)

°This activity may range from playing sports to abusing alcohol and drugs. Even if it's a healthy appearing activity such as sports, it's the *trauma* fueling the obsessive involvement that needs attention.

**The children of alcoholics experience many feelings they can't identify nor sort through so they repress them until they express them in hurtful ways.

sense of their lives. This includes information about (a) alcoholism, (b) treatment availability, (c) self-protection skills, (d) setting boundaries, (e) coping with their environment, (f) developing problem-solving strategies, and (g) asking for help. They must know it's alright to ask for help—that it's even expected.

They also need to know they're not alone and that many other children live in similar environments. They must understand that their parent's drinking is no one's fault. A support group can help with this and encourage them to share their feelings.

A support group will also connect children to others with similar difficulties. They will learn to separate their parent's behavior from their parents. They will discover healthy ways to express their anger as they build self-esteem. They will receive approval and learn about other healthy tools. Finally, they will feel safe sharing their thoughts and feelings.

Much can be done to help our children living in an alcoholic environment, whether sober or drinking. The old African proverb applies: "It takes a village to raise a child."

If one parent is drinking and the other isn't, both may be emotionally absent. With little attention devoted to the children, others outside the home can be essential. This may include relatives, teachers, friends, school counselors, and neighbors. A loving and nurturing adult almost always has a positive influence.

Minimizing the Trauma

Meanwhile, much can be done *now* to mitigate the adverse effects on our children.[5]

1. **Personal growth.** Children learn by copying role models, and we, as parents, are their role models. When the tension is thick, we can thin it with a positive attitude. Seeing us trying to improve our lives invites them to take similar steps. As we grow, we recognize that

nurturing our children is a priority.

2. **Communication**. Being only physically present is not being emotionally present. It's better than no presence, but we miss opportunities to emotionally connect with our children when we don't listen to them.

    Sometimes, we must listen to our children without criticizing, preaching, or even talking. This affirms that we value them. If we disagree with their thinking, this isn't the time to convince them they're wrong—we can address that later. We only need to open the lines of communication. Children must know their feelings matter. Being sensitive to subtle signs they need to talk and being available to listen fosters healthy interactions.

3. **Honesty**. Children must know that feelings aren't right or wrong, good or bad—it's how they express these feelings that matters. Still, they must feel free to express these feelings.

    If we feel anger toward the alcoholic, we can express it in healthy ways. Letting our children know it's normal to feel anger and suggesting productive ways to express it is healthy and honest. Telling them they shouldn't *feel* a certain way will cause them to repress feelings—feelings that will erupt later.

    We should avoid concealing evidence of the destruction the alcoholic caused. Children know when bad things happen, and hiding this causes them to *imagine* what happened, resulting in distrust, anxiety, and insecurity. We must not conceal or confuse reality.

4. **Information**. Children will have questions. Telling our children they needn't worry about something that causes them enough distress to want an answer is dismissive and not calming. Their questions deserve answers. If we don't know, we tell them we don't

know, but we will seek the answer. And when we have the answer, we tell them. This will increase their trust in us and others, increasing their sense of security and well-being.

5. ***Support***. Excellent support is available. Mental health professionals recommend Alateen as a companion to other support. Alateen is a support group and a safe place for children to express feelings. This results in improved self-esteem and gives them a sense of belonging. They will better understand that alcoholism is an illness. They will gain confidence and become more resilient to the potential damage caused by living with an alcoholic parent.

6. ***Fun.*** Children need and deserve to have fun. Since children rarely have fun while enduring the trauma of living in an alcoholic home, they may need encouragement to relax and enjoy. Plan fun times with them and watch them transform from sad and hopeless into smiling, laughing, bright-eyed, enthusiastic children.

7. ***Compassion*.** Children living in an alcoholic environment often act in ways seen as misbehavior. Yet, their behavior flows from feelings of sadness and hopelessness. Therefore, parents should address their children's misconduct suitably and with compassion.

8. ***Unconditional affection*.** Children benefit when told often, "No matter what, I love you and will always love you." But words aren't enough. Instead, they must see that our words match our actions. While telling our children how much we love them, we can also show it by hugging and holding them. We can also act in other loving ways, such as spending quality time and sharing appropriate feelings with them.

9. **Limits.** We should set reasonable limits, impose consequences when they ignore them, and praise them

when they abide by them.

10. ***Responsibility.*** If children are responsible for their conduct, they can make positive changes. Blaming others shackles us in chains, preventing us from changing. It gives those we blame the power over us. Being responsible improves self-worth and other character assets, giving us the freedom to make healthy choices.

—

Section Two

When the Children Became Adults

IN 1983, AS the children of alcoholics were becoming adults and sorting through the remnants of their childhood, Janet Geringer Woititz, Ed.D., wrote a book called *Adult Children of Alcoholics*.[6] Without promotion, it was slow-selling. Yet four years later, in 1987, based solely on word of mouth, it made the *New York Times Bestseller*'s list, where it hovered for a year, selling two million copies. The sheer volume of these sales revealed the large number of those affected by living in alcoholic homes.

The characteristics of the adult child outlined in her book interested these children, now adults, as they identified with them. These adult children felt apart and different for many years, knowing something wasn't right. Many believed they were the only ones feeling this way. But, for the first time, seeing an accurate description of themselves invited validation. They saw an escape hatch they could pass through, fleeing the solitary confinement their confusion fueled by alcoholism and other dysfunctions had self-imposed.

Spawned by Woititz's book, meetings called *Adult Children of Alcoholics* (ACOA)* began and mushroomed. These meetings were based on the 12 steps of Alcoholics Anonymous. Adult children were now healing and developing healthier relationships. With their self-image improving, their lives improved significantly. These improvements were filling their void and ending the cycle of alcoholism.

As the adult child in recovery began to understand alcoholism, this understanding freed them from the bondage of blaming their alcoholic parent. Many themselves had become alcoholic parents. They were no longer brooding in a morass of misery, reflecting on their childhood. They were no

---

*It is now called *Adult Children of Alcoholics & Dysfunctional Families*.

longer victims—they had become survivors striving to provide their children with a healthy environment.

Characteristics of Adult Children of Alcoholics

The adult child raised in an alcoholic home usually discounts how it affected them. It's even more challenging to accept when they have duplicated part or all of this imperfect childhood environment into *their* home, affecting their children similarly. For us to cope with this reality, some denial may be necessary.

It deserves repeating that those in an alcoholic home intuitively believe *what happens in the home stays in the home*. They see an inside and outside world. The boundaries separating the two worlds are embarrassment, shame, and an obscured sense of loyalty. It is this 'secret' that lives on and fuels the endless cycle.

Moreover, this trauma doesn't end when the alcoholic parent becomes sober, or the child reaches adulthood. Adult children often suffer social, emotional, and cognitive harm lasting a lifetime *if ignored and untreated*.[7] They engage in risky behaviors.[8] Ironically, although they have seen the damage alcohol causes, they're convinced they won't end up like their alcoholic parent ... until they do. They often drink or use other substances to cope with the darkness of their past, now blocking the light.[9] And so, the cycle continues.

These adult children are not only prone to alcoholism and substance abuse, but they have an increased risk of depression and anxiety.[10]

Certain features among adults raised in an alcoholic or other dysfunctional home are common. Although the general population may show some of these traits, they are much more prevalent in those who have lived in an alcoholic or dysfunctional home.[11]

Woititz was the first to outline the typical characteristics of Adult Children in her book.[12] Since then, research and observation have expanded and revised her list. Based on that research and anecdotal study, a combined list of these traits follows.

Identifying with one or more of these traits will often stimulate taking healthy action. Still, society views many of these traits as positive, and many successful people have them. Adult Children have most of these characteristics at various levels.[13]

1. *We take ourselves too seriously and have difficulty having fun.* We believe we don't deserve fun and feel guilty when having it. We appear rigid and too self-disciplined. We resist enjoyment, fearing we might look foolish or insist we don't have time to waste on such silliness.

2. *We are closed-minded, resist competing perspectives, and think in black and white.* Everything is right or wrong, and people are good or bad. We see compromise as a weakness.

3. *We disguise our low self-esteem and imperfections by being perfectionists and controlling.* We deny making mistakes. We evaluate everything we do, always hoping for a gold star. We're often obsessed with achieving high socioeconomic status. We gossip to solidify our contempt for others or discover new people to condemn. We appear and are selfrighteously judgmental, which artificially and briefly raises our self-esteem. We unfairly judge ourselves and others by rushing to judgment before we have the relevant facts. We're often self-centered, defiant, and seen as aloof and indifferent.

4. *Although we appear comfortable when socializing, we're not.* We feel like impostures and often isolate.

5. *Many obsessively and compulsively seek love and approval, although it's never enough.* Since we need everyone to like us, we can't be real, fearing that some-

one may not. We condemn and view anyone who dislikes us as an enemy. We believe everyone must see us as flawless, or they won't accept us. This causes us to view constructive criticism as rejection. Even though we may resent it, we remain loyal in situations and relationships that don't warrant it.

6. *We are uncomfortable around authority figures and misinterpret assertiveness as anger and control.* We are overly sensitive and feel immediate inadequacy when criticized. We sense criticism even when there isn't any. To avoid confrontation and criticism, we support but resent those in power while feeling inadequate. We are insecure and intimidated when in the presence of anyone we *sense* as angry, but we don't show it. And even when we're wrong, we overreact with anger or revenge.

7. *We will bend the truth even when not doing so would benefit us more.*

8. *We insist on being right, and we take everything personally.* We are competitive even when nothing warrants competition. We appear confident, even arrogant, to disguise our faults, low self-esteem, and incompetence. We fake self-deprecation to avoid rejecting those we might offend with our arrogance.

9. *We waver between being too responsible and too irresponsible.* We may assume others' problems or expect others to resolve ours.

10. *We are overly sensitive about others' feelings and needs to the point of ignoring our own.* We suffer unnecessary guilt when we take care of ourselves. We don't set defined limits and boundaries and become entangled in others' needs and emotions.

11. *We ignore our feelings by denying or repressing them.*

Since we can't identify our emotions, we can't accurately express them (e.g., we may express sadness as anger). We are unaware of the significant effect this has had on our lives.

12. *We fear rejection and abandonment, which prevents us from ending unhealthy relationships.*

13. *We experience denial, isolation, shame, and baseless guilt, which results in depressive feelings of hopelessness and helplessness.*

14. *We continually attract emotionally unavailable people with addictive personalities.*

15. *We often make excuses, blaming any mistake or flaw on stress, fatigue, or others.* Since we routinely blame others, we don't think we need to change. We feel victimized and attract friends and lovers who are self-victimizing. We feel 'love' for those we pity and rescue.

16. *We unknowingly and chronically fear the intimacy of committed relationships.* We engage in a "come here-go away" dance—a dance we know well, although we're unaware we're leading. And we withdraw sex to punish and seduce to manipulate, but we don't see it. We turn minor disagreements into battles and battles into wars.

17. *We are prone to extreme procrastination, nurturing our need to be perfect, which prevents us from completing projects on time or at all.*

18. *We must be in complete control.* When we're not, we become anxious and resist any change that isn't our idea.

19. *We are impulsive but not spontaneous.* We insist all events, even trivial ones, are planned. Some resist making plans, avoid commitments, and always demand instant satisfaction.

20. *We will abruptly volunteer without considering the nature or possible results of the commitment.* Then, we feel trapped and resentful while trying to escape our new 'burden.' We will spend excessive time and energy trying to wiggle out of our impulsive promises.

21. *We deny our feelings.* We are unaware of our obsessive-compulsive behavior and the shame, guilt, resentment, fear, rage, and other emotions that we repress.

Support for the Adult Child of an Alcoholic

Adult children respond well to recovery. Several excellent options include individual, family, and group therapy and psychopharmacology. Again, mental health professionals widely recommend a popular peer support program discussed above, Adult Children of Alcoholics & Dysfunctional Families. Many good books will benefit one seeking recovery. Four are 1) *Adult Children Of Alcoholics /Dysfunctional Families: Big Red Book* (ACA WSO Inc.); 2) *Adult Children of Alcoholics* by Janet G. Woititz, Ed.D. (Health Communications, Inc.); 3) The 12 Steps for Adult Children by Friends in Recovery (Recovery Publications, Inc.); and 4) *Bradshaw On: The Family* by John Bradshaw (Health Communications, Inc.).

Section Three

The Affected Spouse, Partner, or Parent

If we are the alcoholic's spouse, partner, or parent, we struggle with issues and making various decisions. Perhaps it's the difficult decision of deciding how much more we can tolerate. Or it's the anxiety of focusing on the alcoholic while blurring our own lives. It may be feeling ineffective or hopeless when thinking about failed efforts to get the alcoholic sober. It could be trying to stay afloat in our drowning sea of misery. If the alcoholic is our spouse or partner, it may include deciding whether we should divorce or separate. Ironically, the more we focus on resolving *our* issues, the more likely the alcoholic will recover, although that can't be *our* priority.

Denial: "But I'm Not the One With the Problem!"

Many of us will read this with tears in our eyes and fire in our hearts. We may assert, "I don't need any help. I'm not the one with the problem!" But we can admit we have one problem—the alcoholic.

Another problem is our confusion and indecisiveness when deciding what to do next. A third problem is finding the best way to protect ourselves and our children from further harm. A fourth problem is confronting the fear, anxiety, and resentment we suffer regularly. If the drinker is our spouse or partner, it could be the lack of intimacy and loneliness that shrouds us. Another problem is deciding the best way to start living *our* lives again.

We all have problems, but fortunately, we can take steps to change. Most never recognize much less resolve, the issues preventing them from fully living and enjoying life.

Our Reactions to the Drinking Alcoholic

Many of us obsessively try controlling the alcoholic's drinking by counting drinks, looking for hidden bottles, pouring out liquor, giving ultimatums, and so on.

We live in constant anxiety, worrying about the consequences of our loved one's drinking, which we try but fail to fix. We make excuses for the alcoholic's behavior. We are constantly stressed about the alcoholic's health and feel responsible for managing it.

As we helplessly watch alcoholism progress and the alcoholic's behavior spiral, our anger also progresses. The alcoholic is lying more about their drinking, claiming they only had "a couple." If they have become less responsible than we insist they should be, we feel used and abused. If the drinker is our spouse or partner, we have likely begun feeling lonely and unloved if intimacy has faded or has been redirected. We increasingly resent the alcoholic's drinking—and the alcoholic—feeling a constant desire to punish the alcoholic for the suffering we endure.

We often feel guilty believing we have contributed to the alcoholic's drinking. Then we're frustrated and feel inadequate when we can't stop or slow it down, insisting we haven't done enough and we are not enough.

Occasionally, we believe the alcoholic's promise to stop drinking. Perhaps the alcoholic is drinking less or has stopped drinking. We so badly want alcoholism to vanish that denial causes us to ignore the obvious signs and believe the drinking problem has disappeared. Yet, when it reappears, it's worse, and so are we.

Feeling *obsessive, anxious, angry, guilty,* and living in *denial* takes its toll. It leaves a mark that will remain even if the alcoholic stops drinking unless we remove it. But that's difficult and sometimes impossible unless we accept outside assistance.

Our Reaction to the Sober Alcoholic

We wait for the alcoholic to become sober so we can live 'normally' and be happy. Although alcoholism is incurable, it is treatable. And since drinking is only *one* symptom of alcoholism, although a significant one, the other symptoms remain.[14] Still, proper treatment can weaken and even end them.

Sobriety presents a new set of difficulties. For example, suppose the alcoholic is merely dry—exhibiting drunken behavior without drinking—and not actively in recovery. Then we'll feel guilty secretly wishing they drank again. However, if the alcoholic continues to treat the other symptoms, they may be more tolerable but not saintly. The changes the alcoholic experiences in early sobriety usually cause us to feel anxious and uncertain *if we allow them to.*

We may monitor sobriety with doubt, looking for clues of a relapse. If the alcoholic attends a 12-step program, we may count the number of meetings attended as we once counted the number of drinks. We may anxiously watch the clock for clues. We may wonder when the alcoholic will become the person we expect and perhaps demand.

If our spouse or partner is sober, we may question when they will contribute to the household responsibilities. We may resent their spending more time with sober friends than with us. We may ask ourselves why we now feel less intimacy when we've been expecting and perhaps demanding more. We may wonder why we don't feel the way we had hoped. We may be as lonely or lonelier than we were before sobriety.

If the alcoholic becomes more active, taking more control, we may feel less in control. *We* want to control those changes *we* feel powerless over. Although we wanted the alcoholic's involvement, we will not quickly accept that we are no longer the sole decision-maker. We may question whether we even know this newly sober person.

Hopefully, we will eventually accept that our feelings need not depend on the feelings of another, nor do we need to live our lives according to the dictates of someone else.

Often, we find that our problems remain even when we separate from the alcoholic through divorce or death. Some worsen. To our surprise, we remain affected. The feelings of anger, anxiety, loneliness, obsession, and guilt remain until we accept that *our* thinking has become distorted, focus on *ourselves,* and improve *our* lives. We no longer have the alcoholic's drinking to blame. Instead, we must treat our issues with caring support and help.

Enabling

INVOLVEMENT WITH AN alcoholic for any period impacts us. We will naturally try to help the alcoholic we love. This 'help' often transforms into *enabling,* which can and usually does go on forever. It allows the alcoholic to continue a destructive course of conduct with impunity. I define enabling in this context as:

> When one is close to and affected by the alcoholic encourages continued drinking with action or inaction that shields the alcoholic and the enabler from suffering consequences that might have persuaded the alcoholic to seek sobriety.

The Ways We Enable

The enabler is unaware that their enabling is delaying the alcoholic's sobriety by interrupting the flow of natural consequences that the alcoholic would endure, which would motivate seeking sobriety.

For instance, we may call the alcoholic's employer and explain tardiness or an absence with a lie. We may perform many of the drinker's typical responsibilities as a parent, spouse, or partner and complete the alcoholic's daily tasks, further obstructing the flow of consequences. We do this besides handling our duties. We make excuses to others to reduce our humiliation. We feel increasingly overwhelmed while our anger toward the alcoholic swells.

The Reasons We Enable

We enable for several reasons. One may be to prevent the

alcoholic from losing a job and income, which would affect us.

Or we minimize the severity of the alcoholic's condition to friends and relatives, sparing us shame and embarrassment as we try to avoid stigmatization. We feel chronic confusion and less control, causing us anxiety. We live in the fictional future where we project disasters. We're continually fearful. If we don't enable, we feel guilty for not 'helping.'

We want everything to look 'normal' so we can pretend everything is normal. Coping this way feels normal. And we're frustrated that we can't help the one we love while watching them dig a hole so deep we're convinced they can never crawl out.

We become obsessed with everything looking flawless. We display a facade as if we're living on Main Street in the Norman Rockwell Christmas painting, surrounded by a white picket fence. Yet we live anxiously, knowing the pickets are rotting just below the surface and waiting for a gust of wind to topple them and expose the damage. We are as fragile as the pickets, yet we insist on appearing as strong as the fence posts.

Enabling and Denial

As I describe in Chapter 5, "The Darkness and Lightness of Denial," the power of denial can be so robust and compelling that it's often contagious, and the alcoholic's entourage is usually more in denial than the alcoholic. We tend to believe that everything and everyone else unrelated to drinking causes the consequences suffered by the alcoholic—the alcoholic drinks *because* of these problems. Alcohol doesn't *cause* these problems, or so we tell ourselves repeatedly . . . for a time.

Support for the Enabler

The enabler will need help recognizing their obsessive, compulsive, and ineffective conduct and taking healthy action. These changes often 'encourage' the alcoholic to seek sobriety.

Many programs provide support and comfort for those

affected by an alcoholic's drinking. Al-Anon is the best-known and most recommended by mental health professionals. (See a list of contact information after this chapter.)

Al-Anon is for friends and relatives affected by an alcoholic—sober or drinking.* It provides a community for those enduring a common problem to exchange ideas and experiences, giving hope to the hopeless.

Al-Anon and most mental health professionals believe alcoholism is a family disease. The one closest to the alcoholic is in a unique position to 'motivate' sobriety. Learning about alcoholism and effective intervention methods will help those affected by another's drinking. (See Chapter 10, "The Alcoholic Intervention.")

Learning more about its symptoms will allow us to identify alcoholism, especially in the early stages when it's typically missed. The path we blaze while recovering is often trailed by the path the alcoholic staggers when considering sobriety.

When we realize the behaviors we despise are the symptoms of alcoholism, not the person, we can avoid reacting. For instance, the alcoholic prefers to drink when resentful and may provocatively address us, prompting our defensive posture. Any argument will do. Still, no one likes to be the target of another's wrongful and abusive accusations or condemnations. But when we understand the alcoholic's verbal abuse flows from an illness, we don't take it so personally or excuse it.

It takes two to engage in a tug-of-war. When we grasp that our engagement with the alcoholic is optional, we can release our end of the rope. Soon, the alcoholic, while tugging on a loose rope, will drop their end, allowing us to release and detach with love, freeing us to take healthy action. It takes practice before these become routine, but the journey toward

---

*Al-Anon is based on Alcoholics Anonymous and practices the same twelve steps. Still, it remains independent and autonomous and is not controlled or influenced by any entity, including Alcoholics Anonymous. It never engages in outside controversies or causes. It doesn't accept any funds from anyone other than members who may voluntarily contribute.

this solution doesn't start until we take our first step. And when we do, change begins instantly.

The Victorious Surrender

Eventually, the experience of trying desperately to hold everything together and mend the destructive trail of debris littering the alcoholic's path takes its toll. Often, the emotional harm we suffer is more severe than the alcoholic endures. Although we once believed it's only the alcoholic who needs support, we've learned otherwise.

Typically, loved ones and close friends finally recognize the alcoholic needs help long after they wish they would have. This is when many interventions happen.

If you surrender to the victory of recovery through counseling, a support group, or both, your life will improve. You will receive new tools to reshape your life. You will wish you had done this sooner. You will feel freedom, unlike you've ever felt before. Confidence will improve your decision-making and actions. You will meet people and make friends who have walked your path and who lovingly and non-judgmentally understand you. You will walk with dignity. You will touch the lives of those who care about you and who you have come to genuinely care about. The light you radiate will brighten the darkness surrounding those near you. Your life will become better than you could have ever imagined, regardless of whether the alcoholic seeks sobriety.

Questions for Discussion

1. Do you believe someone's drinking has affected you? Who? How?

2. Has this chapter changed your thinking about how another's drinking may have affected you?

3. Are you or someone close to you the adult child of an alcoholic? If so, which characteristic do you recognize?

4. Have you taken any steps toward recovery? If so, discuss.

5. Have you ever enabled an alcoholic? If so, who benefited from your enabling?

6. Has this chapter affected you? Explain.

7. Do you strongly agree or disagree with anything in this chapter? If so, what? Why?

8. If any sober alcoholic has *affected* you when drinking, how did you feel about them in sobriety?

9. Have you ever attended an AA or ACOA meeting? If so, was it helpful?

THE RELAPSE
Returning to the Darkness

CHAPTER 9

> *You're probably an alcoholic if you've ever said, "I don't know why everyone thinks I relapsed. I'm simply curious to see if I can control my drinking after ten years sober."*

—

THE ALCOHOLIC RELAPSE is little talked about, little thought about, and little sung about. Perhaps the relapse has the same dark cloud hovering over it as suicide since many see it as 'choosing' a slow, agonizing death. The prevailing notion is that a relapse is harmful to long-term sobriety, but that's not *always* so.

WHAT IS AN ALCOHOLIC RELAPSE

IN ITS SIMPLEST form, a relapse occurs when one stops and then resumes drinking. Yet, it's much more than that.

Not All Relapses are the Same

Relapses are not black and white, success or failure, or defined by their duration. A relapse can be a valuable part of recovery. Some need a relapse to convince themselves that they can't control their drinking and to remove any doubt about their alcoholism.

For example, suppose the relapser is one of the fortunate few who regains sobriety. They often treasure their new sobriety and insist, "It's different this time." They now value sobriety as a gift, not an everlasting curse to endure. They usually commit to sobriety with a resolve they never knew.

Others stop making the changes needed to remain sober. They quit a recovery program, relapse, and never regain sobriety. Some endure multiple relapses yet eventually become and stay sober. Others briefly relapse during early sobriety, then return to a sober life. Still, a few who have been sober for years, have a one-time relapse yet quickly return to a sober life. However, before relapsing, alcoholics never know into which category they will fall.

Relapsing isn't unique to alcoholism or other substance abuse disorders. It's also a problem with all conditions where one needs to change behavior to treat it.[1]

THE RELAPSE: A CASUALTY OF DENIAL

DENIAL IS THE reason most alcoholics relapse. When sober alcoholics drink, including those sober for years, most observers believe they did so abruptly, without warning. The truth is they questioned their alcoholism long before they lost their defense to that seductive drink.

Denial is a chief component of alcoholism, and the level of denial increases as alcoholism progresses. That's why it's so difficult for early-stage alcoholics to quit drinking. Why would they when no one sees a problem?

Periodic alcoholics and those who escaped before their alcoholism progressed to the latter stages with irreparable consequences are especially susceptible to relapsing into denial. They never quit thinking, "I didn't have to drink every day." They never *fully* accepted their admission of alcoholism. They never stopped asking, "Am I *truly* an alcoholic?" They resumed comparisons: "I never did that when I drank" or "I never had a DUI, so I'm probably not an alcoholic."

Denial causes one to forget the relevant past. Many alcoholics, including those sober for years, tiptoe in and out of denial, silently debating their alcoholism. Risking relapse, the realities of their past fade away. "Now that I've been sober for years, and everything is going well, I wonder if I could drink normally?" They feel so good they're convinced they can control their drinking. Yet it's universally accepted that alcoholism is progressive, never regressive. So, when alcoholics relapse, their drinking almost always resumes at the same severity as when they quit, often worse.

If any sober alcoholics question if they're truly alcoholic, that's a grave sign of a probable relapse. So, not keeping this doubt a secret and discussing it is vital. Of those continually struggling with denial's appeal, many drink, but some don't. Even if this doubt doesn't lead to drinking, this constant uncertainty lessens the enjoyment of sober living.

Not all Sobriety is the Same

FOR MOST ALCOHOLICS, quitting drinking is much easier than staying quit. Although relapsing is a choice, choosing to drink is easier for some than others.

Many confuse "abstinence" with "sobriety," but they differ. Abstinence is not drinking any alcohol. Sobriety includes abstinence *and* not craving alcohol to change their feelings—to change their mood. Chapter 12, "The Happily Sober Alcoholic," discusses the difference between simple abstinence and quality sobriety.

For example, some suspend drinking only to avoid legal, marital, employment, academic, or health problems. They want to drink but don't—for now. They struggle to make it through each day without a drink. They believe that once their marriage, health, and other drinking-related problems improve, they can drink again, and most do. Still, some decide they enjoy sober living and remain sober. They do so because *they* want sobriety, not because others want them sober.

Those with quality sobriety would not drink even if they could. Why would they want to drink if they preferred sobriety? Also, why would sober alcoholics want to drink if they could control it? Drinking only one or two drinks doesn't appeal to most alcoholics.

An emotional relapse, also known as a "dry drunk," is when dry alcoholics act the way they did when drinking. An emotional relapse usually precedes a physical relapse.

So, the quality of sobriety is relevant.* Low-quality sobriety invites a relapse.

Relapsed Again?

A relapse is not always the opposite of recovery. If a relapse occurs and recovery continues, it's helpful to realize that relapsing can be a part of recovery, like other illnesses with relapses and remissions. Many seeking sobriety after relapsing are closer to lasting sobriety, while others will never have it.

Also, the length of sobriety is relevant. *The longer alcoholics stay sober, the better their chance of remaining sober.* According to the Journal of the American Medical Association (JAMA), two-thirds of alcoholics who receive treatment will relapse within the first year, and 90% will relapse during the first four years of sobriety.[2]

Only 15% of those sober for five years will relapse. For each following year, the likelihood of relapsing declines by half (six years sober: 7.5%; seven years sober: 3.75%; and those sober 10 years or more are at less than a one-percent risk of relapsing).[3]

So, for each day alcoholics remain sober, they not only get another sober day, but they get a statistically improved probability of staying sober.

Because relatively few long-term sober alcoholics relapse, research on the severity of relapses in this group is scarce. However, I have repeatedly seen the few who relapse after long-term sobriety have more difficulty regaining sobriety

---

*Recovery statistics reflect quantity (percentage who became sober and length of sobriety), not quality (enjoyment of sobriety).

than those with short-term sobriety.

Avoiding Relapses

Avoiding a relapse requires a commitment to sobriety by making *persistent* efforts to remain sober. And this is more than a mere commitment to abstain. It includes learning coping skills, having the confidence to stay sober, and taking the necessary action.

Finding adequate support is helpful and often essential to avoid a relapse. For example, this might include 12-step or other peer support meetings, inpatient or outpatient treatment, aftercare, individual talk therapy, or a combination thereof.

Finally, avoiding a relapse includes building a new life with new behavior.

Triggers

Drinking alcoholics are more likely to drink during times of overwhelming stress, depression, anger, self-pity, loneliness, anxiety, guilt, and hopelessness. Even when sober, these feelings can trigger a relapse. Although recovery doesn't abolish these feelings, it can lessen their triggering effect. A recovery program does this by showing how changed behavior can diminish these feelings. It also prepares the alcoholic to cope with these feelings when they arise. Unfortunately, the alcoholic outside recovery is rarely aware of these tools.

Healthy triggers also exist, which one learns in recovery. For example, the thought of drinking triggers calling a supportive person and avoiding people, places, and things in early sobriety, which once prompted their drinking. Also, when alcoholics romanticize the good times when drinking, it triggers recalling the associated consequences they suffered. Loneliness triggers contacting another recovering alcoholic. Anger triggers meditation and other relaxation techniques. So, these positive triggers promote coping with dangerous triggers without drinking.

Some Warnings of a Relapse

FOR THOSE WHO relapse, it's essential to know why they relapsed. Unfortunately, many relapsers were unaware they had been edging toward a relapse because they didn't see what others saw.

Perhaps it was one of the warning signs outlined below. Relapsers must know what to look out for. Recognizing the behavior preceding the last relapse will prepare them to see it the next time it's present.

Warning signs of a pending relapse often include:

1. *The alcoholic-craving.* The alcoholic-craving prompts a relapse. As discussed in Chapter 3, the alcoholic-craving isn't a desire to drink—it is a need to feel differently. So, the alcoholic must be ready to deal with triggers that create an abrupt thought of a drink—a thought that can quickly become an obsession and then a compulsion to drink.

2. *Announcing they will never drink again—drinking is no longer an issue.* The alcoholics announcing this suggest they have their alcoholism under control. It also reveals they haven't surrendered to alcoholism as an involuntary, incurable, chronic, progressive, metabolic, biochemical, central nervous system disease needing continued care. So, they don't need recovery, nor do they need to follow the path other alcoholics with long-term sobriety have traveled.

3. *Ego inflation when life is going well.* When alcoholics first become sober, feeling hopeless and helpless, their ego deflates. They will do anything to change. But in time, while their life is going better than they ever dreamed possible, many experience ego inflation.

    This is the reason recovery stresses humility.

Without it, sober alcoholics forget the problems that caused them to seek sobriety. And with this memory 'lapse,' they take, and some demand, credit for their good life. Recovery is no longer a top priority. They decide they have done such an excellent job managing their lives they can now control their drinking. This thinking often prompts a relapse.

4. *Defensive about their recovery or sobriety.* If anyone mentions any concern about their recovery or sobriety, they are defensive and ignore these concerns as overreactions. They've often decided that they're not as alcoholic as they once thought.

5. *Negative attitude or behavior change.* They aren't enjoying life as much as they once did. They may quit or reduce activities that once pleased them. Sobriety feels dry and is losing its appeal. Drinking seems reasonable.

6. *Complacency.* Some may believe they have conquered alcoholism. This belief denies reality and ignores the risks of relapse. They are in a dangerous comfort zone without realizing it.

   Since they have figured it out better than others, they no longer need to exert effort to remain sober. Instead, they become close-minded to the suggestions of others. While they may continue to seek the safety, comfort, and security of attending a support group, they no longer contribute. They no longer feel gratitude for their good fortune of sobriety.

7. *Relationship issues (lying, arguing, and resenting those helping).* Relationships are becoming more difficult. For example, alcoholics might nurture old resentments and develop new ones toward loved ones. Rather than accepting responsibility for their actions, they casually blame others. Without even reviewing their conduct, they quickly decide they are faultless.

They may lie and argue more since they must always be right. While tolerant of their own mistakes, they are intolerant of others. They treat others worse than they expect and demand others treat them. They become more judgmental and trust the motives of others less and less.

8. ***Lessening attendance and problem behaviors during support meetings or therapy.*** Perhaps one is going to five support meetings weekly. A month later, their attendance drops to four. The following month, they attend one meeting. Then, weeks pass with no meetings.

When they do attend, they may focus on their cell phone with their attention sliding in and out. When it's time to share, they have nothing to say or confiscate time discussing everything except their alcoholism. Or they may share detailed facts of their drinking days ("war stories") in a tone reminiscent of the 'good times.' They may talk about another's experience or recount their day in tormenting detail. Some only focus on their problems to dump them on their captive audience in the hopes of provoking sympathy. Unfortunately, they don't hear the solution.

When those with shaky sobriety are in meetings, they usually don't hear others because they're so deep in their world, preoccupied with preparing their speech for when it's their turn to ramble.

When some with wavering sobriety attend meetings, they become teachers pontificating about some esoteric concept irrelevant to recovery. They define terms, explain the irrelevant, and intellectualize to remain emotionally sterile and emotionally anonymous. They can't be real.

Others may preach at meetings, insisting that their understanding of God is the only path to recovery from alcoholism. After sharing, they may leave since they can't see any benefit from listening to others. They may mock recovery slogans or sobriety talk.

Some are court-ordered to attend and consider mandatory meeting attendance a punishment. Convinced they're at a meeting because they were merely at the wrong place at the wrong time—just bad luck—they count the days until they discharge their 'sentence.'

A few consider meetings a dating site and prey on the vulnerable. Others are always late to meetings, while some habitually leave early as if walking on a fashion show runway, hoping to get the attention they can't ever seem to get enough of.

Some flirting with a relapse may focus on the differences more than the similarities between themselves and others during meetings. For example, they think, "I never did that" or "That never happened to me." Instead, they focus on one immaterial difference rather than the whole healing message to support their denial. They compare themselves to those they believe were worse alcoholics, making the same comparisons they made when drinking.

Research shows members of Alcoholics Anonymous who are more engaged in the fellowship are less likely to relapse because of their social connection with other recovering alcoholics. This connection reduces the alcoholic-craving. They usually enjoy better and longer sobriety than those remaining anonymous within the anonymity. A predictor of relapse is distancing from other members and isolating more.

9. *Other interests are taking priority over recovery.* This may include a job, a relationship, the casino, yard care, or other activities that substitute for alcohol dependence. One repeatedly hears and sees alcoholics losing anything they have placed between themselves and

sobriety.

10. *Avoiding sponsorship by not selecting or keeping in regular contact with a sponsor and not sponsoring others.*

11. *Not contacting or helping others in recovery.* They may try to sidestep accountability by isolating more to avoid hearing the concerns of others. Their self-absorption results in them dominating conversations without listening. They disbelieve the paradoxical axiom: One must give it away to keep it.

12. *Glamorizing past alcohol use.* A familiar hint of a likely relapse is selectively recalling the 'good' times spent drinking and discussing these times with old friends while ignoring the bad. They may contact past drinking companions and reduce the time they spend with sober friends.

    Some may minimize their drinking or blame it on someone else, deciding if that person were out of their lives, they could drink normally. They often feel they're missing out when they see others drinking with impunity.

13. *Failing to treat co-occurring (comorbid) disorders such as depression and anxiety.* Studies show that about 40-60% of recovering alcoholics have another mental disorder besides alcoholism, which also needs treatment. This is especially so if the comorbid disorder existed before their alcoholism and contributed to it. The most common comorbid disorders affecting alcoholics are depression and anxiety.

    If it's alcohol-induced, it will usually disappear within 30 days of sobriety. But if the disorder prompted their drinking, then sobriety may remain elusive. So, alcoholics with co-occurring conditions may relapse without a proper diagnosis and treatment or if they fail to follow their treatment plan.

14. *Not following suggestions from trustworthy sources.* A trustworthy source may be one who helped the alcoholic achieve sobriety, a health care provider, or a sponsor. These suggestions may include regularly attending support meetings, outpatient care, psychiatric care, individual therapy, group therapy, and taking prescribed medication, which is a part of the treatment plan. It also includes helping others by sharing what they have been so fortunate to receive. Failing to take this action often ends in a relapse.

15. *Using a mouthwash with alcohol or other drugs containing alcohol (Nyquil®) or drinking nonalcoholic beer (near beer).**

16. *Keeping a secret while violating one's trust.* Hiding activities from a loved one, a business partner, or a friend that causes guilt or resentment is dangerous. It can easily provoke a relapse since drinking dilutes guilt, and resentments fuel drinking.

17. *Not ready for sobriety.* Some are only dry to avoid problems, please a loved one, or not worsen a medical condition. Unfortunately, they haven't yet drunk the value out of drinking.

—

NOT EVERYONE SHOWING one or more of these warning signs will relapse. I've seen alcoholics display similar behavior and stay sober. This reveals probabilities, not certainties. And the more warning signs alcoholics show, the higher their likelihood of relapsing. Although not all-inclusive, it describes the most common actions and thoughts typically seen before relapsing.

Like the movement of the hour hand, many of these warnings appear so slowly they go unnoticed. Those on the bluff

---

*There is a trace of alcohol in "nonalcoholic" beer. About six "nonalcoholic" beers equals the alcohol contained in one regular beer.

often see sober alcoholics treading dangerous waters better than those caught in a crosscurrent dragging them out to the sea. Despite this, before relapsing, many convinced themselves they would never drink again—until they did.

The road to relapse can be dark and silent. The alcoholics who relapsed were often unaware of their destination. Still, many won't see it even if pointed out to them. However, if they feel part of a recovery community, are aware of triggers, and don't want to drink, they are more likely to remain sober.

The quickest way to lose sobriety is not to appreciate how fortunate one is to be sober and taking sobriety for granted.

Questions for Discussion

1. Has this chapter affected you? How?
2. Has this chapter changed your thinking about how you understood the alcoholic relapse?
3. If you're an alcoholic, have you ever relapsed?
4. Do you identify with any of the listed warning signs of a pending relapse? If so, which ones?
5. Do you believe that not all relapses are the same?
6. Did the discussion about "Triggers" help? If so, discuss.
7. Do you believe the neuroscience discussion was helpful? If so, in what way? Discuss.
8. Before reading this chapter, did you believe there was an emotional relapse before a drinking relapse?
9. How has this chapter helped you?
10. Do you strongly agree or disagree with anything in this chapter? If so, what? Why?
11. Have you learned anything from this chapter? If yes, please discuss.

Contact Information

Suicide & Crisis Lifeline:
Call or text **988** or chat at **988lifeline.org**

Suicide Prevention Lifeline:
1-800-273-TALK (8255)

For confidential information about help for alcohol dependence, contact one or more of the following:

NIAAA ALCOHOL TREATMENT NAVIGATOR
"Pointing the way to evidence-based care"

A service of the U.S. federal government providing unbiased information for finding quality alcohol treatment through mutual support groups, therapists, doctors, and outpatient & inpatient care.

www.alcoholtreatment.niaaa.nih.gov

Mutual-Support Groups

(AA) Alcoholics Anonymous
www.aa.org | 212–870–3400
(or local phone directory)

Al-Anon Family Services/Alateen
For Those Affected by Another's Drinking
www.al-anon.org | 888-425-2666 for meetings

Adult Children of Alcoholics & Dysfunctional Families
www.adultchildren.org | 310–534–1815

AA Agnostica
A space for AA agnostics, atheists and freethinkers worldwide
www.aaagnostica.org | admin@aaagnostica.org.

Celebrate Recovery
A Christ-Centered Recovery Program
www.celebraterecovery.com | 800-723-3532

LifeRing
Secular (nonreligious) Recovery
www.LifeRing.org | 800-811-4142

Moderation Management
www.moderation.org | 212–871–0974

Secular Organizations for Sobriety
www.sossobriety.org | 314-353–3532

Secular Alcoholics Anonymous
AA meetings for agnostics, atheists and freethinkers
www.secularaa.org

SMART Recovery
An Alternative to AA, Al-Anon, and other 12-Step Programs
www.smartrecovery.org | 440-951-5357

Women for Sobriety
www.womenforsobriety.org | 215–536–8026

INFORMATION RESOURCES

The Alcohol and Drug Addiction Resource Center
(800) 390-4056

Alcohol and Drug Helpline
www.alcoholanddrughelpline.com | (800) 821-4357

Alcohol Hotline Support & Information
(800) 331-2900

American Council on Alcoholism (ACA)
www.recoverymonth.gov | (800) 527-5344

National Child Abuse Hotline
1-800-25-ABUSE

National Clearinghouse for Alcohol and Drug Information
www.ncadi.samhsa.gov | (800) 729–6686

National Council on Alcoholism & Drug Dependence, Inc.
www.ncadd.org | *HOPE LINE*: 800/NCA-CALL (24-hour)

National Domestic Abuse Hotline
1-800-799-SAFE

National Helpline
Treatment referral and information 24-7
www.samhsa.gov | 1-800-662-HELP (4357)

National Institute on Alcohol Abuse and Alcoholism
www.niaaa.nih.gov | (301) 443–3860

National Institute on Drug Abuse
www.nida.nih.gov | (301) 443–1124

National Institute of Mental Health
www.nimh.nih.gov | (866) 615–6464

THE INTERVENTION
Shining the Light of Truth

CHAPTER 10

*You're probably an alcoholic if
you've attended a seminar entitled
"How to Convince Those Involved in an
Intervention to Apologize and Never Return."*

—

SHINING THE LIGHT of truth into the darkness of denial* is often a life-saving event. Although this chapter isn't a manual on conducting an intervention, it describes various interventions, perspectives, offers suggestions, and presents options for those considering one.

If you're undecided about whether to intervene, this has likely been a difficult time filled with frustration, confusion, and uncertainty. Your frustration may come from trying 'everything' but failing to convince the alcoholic to see what others clearly see. Perhaps you're confused about your future course of action, if any, and uncertain if you can do anything to help the alcoholic. Most see the intervention as their final effort.

Understandably, if you've suffered stress and invested significant time, effort, and money into 'getting the alcoholic sober' unsuccessfully, you may be questioning whether to

---

*Denial in this context means more than the alcoholic just denying a drinking problem. It includes denying the severity of the problem, denying drinking is causing problems, denying treatment will help, and denying now is the time to stop drinking.

reduce your involvement in the alcoholic's recovery, which you might now see as a probable waste of time. If that is so, less involvement might be healthier.

However, if you have decided to intervene, this chapter will ease your confusion and uncertainty, reduce frustration, and improve your effectiveness. If you're undecided, it will help you make a reasoned decision.

What is an Intervention?

An intervention occurs anytime anyone questions, addresses, prevents, restricts, or interferes with the alcoholic's drinking or prompts them to consider that they may have a drinking problem that needs treatment. It includes any action that softens the alcoholic's denial or "raises their bottom."*

Interventions can be informal, formal, or both.

The Informal Intervention

Informal interventions include pouring the alcoholic's liquor down the drain, a bartender refusing to serve "just one more," or announcing "last call." They occur when anyone tells the alcoholic if they don't stop drinking, there will be consequences. They happen when one is charged with DUI and the court orders an alcohol evaluation, AA attendance, treatment, installation of a vehicle alcohol interlock device, wearing an alcohol monitor, or sentences the alcoholic to incarceration.

The Formal Intervention

A formal intervention is when family, friends, coworkers, employers, and others affected by the alcoholic's drinking join in planning and structuring a meeting to persuade the alcoholic to consider sobriety and treatment.

One obstacle is that by the time most interventions finally

---

*"Raising the bottom" is when alcoholics realize they have a problem with alcohol, have not yet suffered irreparable consequences, know the consequences they *and others* have and will suffer if they continue drinking, and decides to stop drinking.

occur, most alcoholics know, and many admit they have a drinking problem but insist, "I like drinking—I don't want to stop!" Yet how can that be without anything to compare it with? How can they know they like drinking and don't want to stop unless they know what life would be like if they did? Aren't they really saying, "I'm afraid I can't stop, and if I stopped, I'm afraid I would feel worse than I feel now?" Wouldn't they want to stop if they believed they would enjoy a sober life more?

It's widely recognized that alcoholics don't quit drinking until they're ready—until they have drunk the value out of drinking—until they realize that the harm their drinking causes far outweighs the benefits.

So, one goal of an intervention is to open their minds enough to see that they are ready, that they have drunk the value out of drinking, that their drinking has been harmful, and that they do want to stop.

The intervention includes helping them see their drinking is destructive to them and others by each participant gently and firmly explaining how the drinker has harmed each one.

This also includes helping them realize that if they don't stop drinking, the consequences they have suffered will worsen. This may be done by the participants calmly and firmly giving ultimatums, which they are prepared to follow through with, such as a spouse promising to divorce or a boss committing to fire the alcoholic if they continue drinking or refuse treatment.

So, the intervention strongly encourages the alcoholic to explore sobriety by explaining they have nothing to lose—they can always return to drinking. Still, if they at least explore sobriety, they will be able to compare their current drinking life to a sober one before rejecting it. Hopefully, the intervention will persuade them to enter treatment.

These interventions may be invitational—inviting the alcoholic's participation, or confrontational—surprising the alcoholic with a meeting. (The common types of interventions are outlined later in this chapter.)

The following illustrates an intervention that includes several intervention methods.

The Bleeding Heart

HE AWAKENS TO light, intensifying the throbbing behind his eyes. Scattered events from hours ago sprinkle his memory, but his memory lapses prevent any useful recall.* He tries filling the gaps . . . it's no use.

His intensifying anxiety, self-hatred, and hopelessness are unbearable. He quietly and slowly scans to his left so he doesn't disturb anyone he may have 'fallen in love with' last night. Relief. No one is there.

He's heard a drink or two can help with a hangover, but he's reluctant to do that because that's what alcoholics do. To convince himself he's not an alcoholic, he only drinks on weekends and never before sunset.° And he knows it's Sunday morning because this is how he feels every Sunday morning.

He feels like he's been crawling in the desert with sand blowing through his parched lips.

In keeping with his Sunday morning ritual, he staggers to the kitchen, chases aspirin with orange juice, checks to see if his car is damaged, and then returns to bed to convalesce.

An hour later, he sits up while groaning, "Why? Never again." The throbbing is now pounding.

He walks out of his bedroom and sees his parents forcing contrived half-smiles. He then sees his brother, sister, ex-wife, 8-year-old son, boss, girlfriend, best friend, and an empty, isolated, gray metal folding chair facing everyone.

"Great. A surprise party. Aren't you supposed to scream, 'Surprise!' although I'm not sure what we're celebrating?" No

---

*The blackout isn't an inability to remember; it's the brain's failure to record information, so no memory exists to refresh.

°The alcoholic self imposes rules to support denial. So long as they adhere to these rules, they believe they haven't crossed the line into alcoholism. These rules are made to fit their misconception of an alcoholic. Examples are in Chapter 2, "A Description of the Alcoholic," which discusses this rulemaking in more detail.

one says a word. The silence expands the explosions in his head. "You all know this is illegal—breaking and entering." Still nothing.

"Do you know why we're here?" asks his Dad.

Everyone pulls out pieces of paper.

"What are those? Notes with your threats? Look, I just don't have time for this. I'm not feeling too good, and I'd like everyone to leave so I can take a shower. And I mean now—please."

His Mom gestures toward the chair. "Why don't you sit down, dear? You don't look so good!"

Again, he glares at the lonely chair. "I'm good."

"We're here to discuss your drinking," his friend announces.

"Oh, yeah . . . my drinking. What a relief. I thought it was something serious. No problem there. I can take it or leave it. But, I could take you to a place where your services could be useful, where drunks are homeless and drink every day. Look, . . . I agree . . . I agree that I drink a little too much every so often. But I enjoy drinking; I could stop if I wanted to, but I don't want to. I don't drink during the week and never before sunset. Hey, open your eyes—things are good. I've got a car, a home, and a good job. In fact, I'm doing better than most of you. I appreciate what you're trying to do. I'm not saying it's none of your business, but I've got a busy day, and I haven't had a drink in . . . a week or two."

"You were with me last night and so drunk that—" his girlfriend says before he interrupts her.

"I meant a week or two before last night."

"I love and care about you very much, but if you continue drinking, I can't see you anymore."

His boss interjects, "You may have a good job, but you've missed several Mondays during the past few months. And on the Mondays you did show up, you were late, sluggish, and unproductive."

"Well, that's going to change. I know I've said that before, but this time is different. I plan—"

His boss interrupts, "I'm going to be straight with you. If you continue drinking, I'm going to have to let you go, and I'm serious about this."

His son says, "Dad, I haven't seen you for a long time. Lots of times when I'm sad, I think about seeing you, and it makes me happy. Sometimes, I wait for you to pick me up all weekend, and I run to the window when I think I hear your car. But it's not you. Then I feel sad again."

"I love you very much, son, and that will change, too. I'm sorry we've had a scheduling problem. We're going to have fun together. I've got lots of ideas, okay?"

"Okay, Dad."

His ex-wife remarks, "If it doesn't change now, I will be making a call first thing tomorrow to change the paperwork. It's no longer acceptable."

"Hey, here's the deal. I know you've all invested a lot of time into this, and I'll give you what you want. But I have some commitments I need to attend to, so let's get back together at a better time. So you win, okay? I'll do whatever you want if everyone leaves right now. I promise. Please leave."

"That's great to hear because three of us are ready to leave right now and take you with us to a place with a room waiting for you," his brother calmly but firmly states.

"Now? No way. I'm sorry, but I can't go right now. I've got too many irons in the fire, but—"

"We've taken care of everything. We've got you covered, and there's nothing to worry about," promises his best friend.

"And don't worry about work; you're covered there, too. We all want to see you healthy and feeling better. You're worth it to us," his boss says. "But if you don't go with them now, you no longer have a job. I'm sorry."

He glances at his son, who has a teardrop staggering down his right cheek, which splatters on the crumpled heart he drew on his frayed note. While they watch the heart bleed, his son stammers, "Please, Dad, please go with them. I miss you."

With tear-filled eyes, he walks over to his son, hugs and kisses him, looks at his brother, and says, "Let's go."

—

Although this is not how every intervention unfolds, it is similar. However, as later described, most effective interventions are no longer surprise meetings with aggressive attacks shaming the alcoholic into treatment.

So, what do you do if you're considering an intervention?

THE PARTICIPANTS AND EXPECTATIONS

IF YOU'RE ONLY intervening because you're convinced the alcoholic will agree to treatment and never drink again, you're setting yourself up for a possible letdown. Projections about the alcoholic's recovery are unproductive and reduce the chances of success. Moreover, science tells us that such predictions are nothing more than chance—only a crystal ball can tell us if an intervention will work.

Compassion and Empathy

Shining the light of truth without empathy or compassion is like someone shining a flashlight into our eyes. It causes discomfort and defensiveness and darkens the darkness even more.

Again, to increase the chances of a successful intervention, the participants must know that recovery from alcoholism is a process, not an event. They must know that this process requires open-mindedness, patience, compassion, and honesty, which includes learning to express their concerns gently and lovingly while firmly prepared to follow through with their requirements. Still, a well-deliberated plan is often best when it is flexible. The symptoms of alcoholism didn't appear overnight, and its chief symptom, denial, has been strengthening for years. Therefore, compassion requires us first to view the intervention from the drinker's perspective.

One way to gain this perspective is to attend a few Alanon

and *open* AA meetings. In these meetings, you will find others who have walked similar paths. Hearing their experience, strength, and hope will reduce your anxiety by revealing a new perspective, fostering a better understanding of the intervention, and helping to manage expectations. (Chapter 8, "The Affected," provides suggestions for coping with the issues created by alcoholism.) These meetings will also help you understand recovery from the alcoholic's perspective.

You may see the intervention as an honest and loving method of inspiring abstinence by helping the alcoholic see the problems their drinking is causing, which will encourage them to "want to stop." But the alcoholic doesn't see it that way.

The alcoholic sees the intervention as an attempted deprivation of something needed to cope with and endure life —it doesn't feel loving. The alcoholic, feeling ganged up on and attacked and sensing this risk to survival, feels threatened and frightened by the intervention. The alcoholic is convinced the participants don't realize how essential drinking is.

Although less common now, if the intervention is a surprise to ensure the alcoholic's participation, the alcoholic will feel deceived. No one enjoys others questioning their behavior, especially an alcoholic who feels tricked into a confrontation about their drinking.

Expectations

Having expectations about a potential intervention is natural. Still, these expectations must be realistic to prevent more harm to everyone and must not fuel your participation. The goal here is to help you have reasonable expectations.

Recovery comes in many forms. And since the future isn't ours to see, it's a mistake to decide to intervene based on predicting the chances of recovery. Still, a *cautiously* optimistic attitude is more productive than a pessimistic one.

It's also helpful to know what a 'successful' intervention is.

The Successful Alcoholic Intervention

Assessing an alcoholic intervention is challenging, especially when the term "successful intervention" is ambiguous.

Our impatience requires immediate results. Still, if one is patient and remembers the intervention is a process, not an event, any softening of denial is a success. If the intervention didn't increase the alcoholic's drinking but increased the alcoholic's thinking about their drinking and how hurtful their drinking has been, it's a success.

For example, the alcoholic may storm out in a rage only to seek treatment the next day. Or, they may enter treatment immediately, then leave early or drink the day they're released.

Sure, it would be wonderful if the alcoholic agreed to treatment within the first two minutes of an intervention and lived a sober life. And that could happen, but it probably won't. However, as discussed later, using an interventionist increases the odds of the alcoholic at least agreeing to treatment above 90%.

According to the *Journal of the American Medical Association* (*JAMA*), more than half of all alcoholics receiving inpatient treatment will relapse* within weeks of discharge.[1] Still, half will remain sober beyond the first year—a significant success. Either way, it's not a predictor of sustained sobriety.

If a relapse occurs, it's helpful to know that it's often a part of recovery, like other illnesses with relapses and remissions. As mentioned in Chapter 9, "The Relapse," it often takes a relapse to prove to themselves that they can't control their drinking and are alcoholics. Many who stop drinking after a relapse are closer to lasting quality sobriety than some who haven't relapsed—yet. Still, the intervention planted the seed, and in time, many who relapse eventually recover. They usually do this with a new resolve and a firmer commitment to sobriety, becoming and remaining sober, and *enjoying* stable

---

*A relapse is drinking alcohol after a period of abstinence, as described in Chapter 9.

and lifelong sobriety.

Some firmly grasp sobriety at first but then lose their grip and struggle with it for a lifetime. Yet, many others embrace sobriety and live a life never dreamed possible.

It's essential to understand that the intervention, treatment, and recovery are a process—a series of events. Only time will tell if the intervention succeeded. For those that need the certainty of numbers, give it two years. For those that don't, disregard the last sentence.

Since alcoholism is progressive, the alcoholic's drinking, thinking, feeling, and living worsens if drinking remains uninterrupted. Still, one thing is for sure: *An intervention can never succeed if it never occurs.*

Denial and the Intervention

THE LIGHT OF truth can be too bright, like an interrogation, or too dim, like a casual visit—both illuminate nothing. Those living in the darkness of denial will do better with the light of truth gradually shining brighter so their eyes can adapt enough to see the truth, just as our eyes need time to adjust to light when leaving a dark room. Eventually, the shadows will disappear and reveal the consequences of the alcoholic's drinking. Patience is a must.

An alcoholic often views a genuine concern as an accusation, which excites defensiveness. A poorly done intervention, which is nothing more than judgmental and accusatory ramblings, can reinforce the alcoholic's denial.

Just as there are different levels of denial, there's a clear contrast between the denial of the periodic alcoholic who drinks occasionally and the chronic alcoholic who drinks daily. Although the intervention approach is similar, it's not the same.

The Periodic Alcoholic's Denial

The periodic drinker is usually more in denial than the daily drinker. They preserve their denial by focusing on the 'real' alcoholic—the stereotypical alcoholic who drinks daily and drinks upon awakening. They are unaware or ignore that whether one drinks daily does not determine alcoholism.

They don't see all the problems their drinking has caused and disregard their inability to predict, with reasonable certainty, how much they will drink once they start—a symptom that does determine alcoholism.

The periodic alcoholic usually experiences more alcohol-related consequences and challenges than the daily drinker. Despite this, most periodics believe they don't have a drinking problem. And if they do, they're sure it hasn't reached the level of alcoholism. Instead, they view anyone's concern as an overreaction, which means the intervention must address the periodic's denial. To do this, the intervenor must see what the periodic sees.

The Chronic Alcoholic's Denial

The reaction to an intervention by alcoholics who drink daily will depend on the type of denial they are in. Regardless, they will probably be less resistant than periodic alcoholics and those who insist they "enjoy drinking and don't want to stop."

Those who don't think they have a problem will find the intervention absurd. They may be even more defensive if they know they have a drinking problem but think they've hidden it. Feeling exposed and betrayed, they could become angry and run for the exit. Or, realizing their secret is out, they may be reasonably open-minded and accept treatment. Again, there's no way to know for sure.

The Timing of an Intervention

The timing of an intervention is crucial since alcoholics are more in denial at various times. The alcoholic should be as sober as possible. It's best to wait until they feel their worst, are remorseful, and are suffering the consequences caused by their excesses. Those close to the alcoholic have seen a pattern develop and usually know the best time to intervene, such as the Sunday morning hangover.

The Addiction Specialist

Addiction specialists are physicians who have continued their study and training beyond the primary medical curriculum, focusing on the prevention and treatment of alcoholism and other addictions.*

According to the American Society of Addiction Medicine (ASAM), the nation's largest professional society of addiction specialists, alcoholism is a chronic brain disease that can be treated. It is not bad behavior or poor choices related to excessive drinking.

The addiction specialist has extensive training in all aspects of alcoholism and other addictions. This includes interventions, detoxification, rehabilitation, treatment, therapy, withdrawal-related symptoms, and much more. They can competently assess if one will require medically managed detoxification, determine the appropriate treatment, and suggest an effective intervention.

The ASAM website (asam.org) provides a search locator for addiction specialists in all cities and includes information about each doctor.

Although not always practical, I recommend that anyone considering an intervention consult an addiction specialist.

THE INTERVENTIONIST

ALTHOUGH NO ONE knows how an intervention will go, it almost always goes much better with an intervention specialist, known as an *interventionist*. This is one trained, experienced, and skilled in conducting interventions.

---

*According to ASAM, 40% of addiction specialists are psychiatrists.

The Benefits of an Interventionist

Although many 'successful' interventions occur without an interventionist, they have proven more effective with one, and I encourage using one if feasible. The National Council on Alcoholism and Drug Dependence (NCADD) found that in over 90% of interventions with an interventionist, the alcoholic agreed to treatment.

For example, an interventionist can study the proposed intervention, decide the best approach, and select helpful participants. They can also describe problems that may arise, prevent or lessen surprises, choose the best time for the intervention, and suggest a treatment plan.

During the intervention, the alcoholic will likely claim it's unnecessary and try deflecting the focus away from them. Also, those most affected by the alcoholic usually harbor justified resentments that have been bottled up for years and can explode without warning. In the likely event those resentments are triggered, an interventionist can prevent the event from turning into an unproductive and angry shouting match.

Finding an Interventionist

When searching for an interventionist, I recommend reviewing the website of the Association of Intervention Specialists (AIS), a network of interventionists located throughout the country and abroad. This website provides information about credentialed interventionists who are part of the network and is easy to navigate. It states: "All full members are Certified Intervention Professionals, thereby meeting or exceeding educational and performance standards. All members adhere to the AIS Code of Ethics."

A professional familiar with alcoholism is also an excellent source for finding the right interventionist.

Interventionists can include physicians (e.g., addiction specialists, psychiatrists), mental health professionals (e.g., psychologists, psychotherapists, alcohol and drug counselors, social workers), nurse practitioners, or physician's assistants. Or they may be trained informally with no formal credentials* but with extensive intervention experience, often with an impressive record.

Consultation with or participation by a sober alcoholic may prove invaluable if the interventionist is not in recovery.

Intervention Types

Before interviewing potential interventionists, it's helpful to understand the most common intervention methods. Depending on the personality and severity of the alcoholic, the interventionist will likely use one or more of these models:

1) **Confrontational Model of Intervention:** This was the first method of intervention used, although it's rarely used today. It is harsh. Without warning, participants confront the alcoholic with ultimatums that are carried out if the alcoholic doesn't immediately agree to treatment. It laid the groundwork for interventions that are much gentler today.

2) **Johnson Model of Intervention:** Vernon E. Johnson, the pioneer of interventionism, created this model. It flowed from the Confrontational Model, the most familiar form, in which an interventionist confronts the alcoholic without notice. The aim is to "raise the bottom" by explaining the disease's progressive nature and describing how it affects loved ones. The interventionist guides the family and moderates the meeting.

   The participants prepare by meeting with the interventionist to create a workable plan. They also learn techniques for interacting with the alcoholic during the intervention. Finally, the interventionist encourages family members also to seek treatment and discover how alcoholism has affected them and how they've contributed to the condition. According to the American Psychological

---

*Credentials for interventionists include Certified Intervention Professional (CIP), and Board Registered Interventionist (BRI-I or II).

Association, this method is gentle and efficient.

3) ***Invitational Model of Intervention:*** This model focuses on the entire family, including the alcoholic, in a workshop-type atmosphere and discusses the roles each has played related to the alcoholic. This intervention doesn't surprise the alcoholic since the drinker is invited to attend with their family. It reduces hostility and defensiveness. It encourages the alcoholic *and* the family to seek treatment. It is less threatening, and the interventionist may stay involved for over a year, helping the family adjust.

4) ***Systemic Family Intervention Model:*** This model is like the Invitational Model but has some differences. One chief difference is that it may continue for months, with several meetings each week until the family and the alcoholic accept a proposed treatment plan. This method is more than one brief workshop.

5) ***The Field Model of Intervention:*** This is like the Johnson Model but has added benefits when dealing with an alcoholic who has an emotional disorder in addition to alcoholism (e.g., bipolar, depressive, and anxiety disorders). It allows the interventionist experienced with this model to assess the alcoholic's chances of becoming violent, suicidal, or self-harmful.

6) ***The ARISE Intervention:*** This combines the benefits of various models. The interventionist refers the alcoholic and the family for treatment. When family members accept treatment with the alcoholic, the chances of the alcoholic entering treatment exceed 80%.

7) ***The Brief Intervention:***[2] This differs from the above models in that the brief intervention is usually not considered when planning a traditional intervention. It is used in a wide range of settings,* including online, and encourages one who isn't seeking treatment to change unhealthy or

---

*Settings include health care, criminal justice, workplace, education, and more.

risky alcohol abuse. In health care, it's typically incidental to a patient seeking treatment for a related medical issue. A brief intervention occurs when a screening indicates a drinking problem, and the doctor advises the patient to reduce or stop drinking based on health concerns. It could be as brief as a mere mention or more involved, including up to four counseling sessions. It is efficient and effective.[3]

Selecting an Interventionist

After you've found one or more prospective interventionists, the following provides suggestions for selecting the right one for your situation.

Choosing an interventionist is a decision most feel uneasy making, but it's not as difficult as it first seems. You should feel comfortable with the interventionist during the first interview. If not, move to the next one on your list. When interviewing prospective interventionists, inquire about the following:

- *Education, certifications, experience, and association memberships.*[*] Although credentialed interventionists aren't *necessarily* more effective than uncredentialed, their certification shows they have the necessary skills, training, and experience to assure you they likely know what they're doing. Also, certified intervention professionals follow an ethical code. If they don't disclose this information or are evasive, you should consider moving on to the next candidate.
- *Experience and the number and types of interventions conducted.*
- *Success rate with an explanation of their definition of success.*
- *Fees, payment methods, services performed, and refund policy for unused services.* If hired, all these terms should be in writing. If the interventionist doesn't charge or

---

[*]The associations are private and unregulated.

charges a low fee, confirm the information in the following inquiry.

- *Full disclosure about any connection to, preference for, or interest in any treatment centers or treatment plans they recommend.* You have a right to know if they are a salesperson posing as an interventionist and if they receive any referral benefit such as a commission, gift, or rebate. While this is ethically frowned upon, especially if undisclosed, it happens, and the alcoholic will likely sense this, supporting their protests about treatment.

  Although having a connection, interest, or preference may not be a deal-breaker, their full disclosure will help you identify conflicting interests. If their employer's interest motivates them more than the alcoholic's interest, it could be a serious problem.

- *A description of the intervention models they prefer and the reasons for this preference.* They should also discuss the ones they've had the most experience and '*success*' using.
- *An explanation of what happens in the intervention.*
- *The usual number of meetings they have with the participants to prepare for the intervention.*
- *If they conduct video conferencing.*
- *The percentage of their initial consultations that resulted in a recommendation for intervention.*
- *A description of the aftercare plans they usually recommend after release from treatment and for the long term.*
- *If the intervention involves a periodic alcoholic, find out their experience with periodic alcoholic interventions.*
- *The extent of their experience with an alcoholic who is also a drug addict.*
- *Their experience and training in identifying dual disorders (e.g., depressive, bipolar, alcohol-induced psychosis, and other alcohol-related disorders).*

- *If their services end or continue after the intervention.* If it continues, you should know the details of the services provided.
- *Description of treatment recommendations typically made for those affected by the alcoholic's drinking.*
- *A disclosure of what prompted the candidate to become an interventionist.*
- *The likelihood of any other obligations preventing the interventionist from providing the services as scheduled.*

Always use and tell an interventionist if the alcoholic has:
- a history of suicide attempts or thoughts,
- been using other mood-altering substances,
- a history of mental illness, or
- a propensity to harm others.

COSTS AND COVERAGE

IT'S UNDISPUTED THAT drinking alcoholics incur more medical costs than sober alcoholics. Since it makes financial sense, more policies cover interventions, and all carriers will likely cover them in time.

A carrier may cover the intervention under "outpatient counseling" or another description that doesn't mention the word "intervention." Additionally, a policy may cover a credentialed interventionist differently than one without the same qualifications.

It's essential to read the policy carefully since many different ones exist. However, if it excludes coverage, the insured can appeal by following the simple instructions in the policy.

So, before any interviews, discover if intervention coverage exists. If it does, seek preauthorization from the insurance carrier.

Remember, interventionist fees vary substantially. For example, the fee charged by an addiction specialist is usually much higher than the fee charged by an uncredentialed interventionist.

THE INTERVENTION TRIES to soften the alcoholic's denial and 'raise the bottom.' If it does, this may allow the alcoholic to exit the downward spiral, hopefully before irreparable harm has occurred.

Ideally, an interventionist will facilitate the intervention. Still, although the success rate is higher with an interventionist, the benefits of intervening without one outweigh the harm of doing nothing. This is especially true when considering that most alcoholics, left alone, endure misery and strike bottom long before they ever recognize they have reached their bottom.

In other words, doing something is better than doing nothing.

QUESTIONS FOR DISCUSSION

1. Has this chapter changed your understanding of the intervention?
2. Have you been involved as a participant or subject in an intervention?
3. Were you aware of interventionists before reading this chapter?
4. Were the questions for the interventionist helpful?
5. How has this chapter helped you?
6. Do you strongly agree or disagree with anything in this chapter? If so, what? Why?
7. Have you learned anything from this chapter? If yes, please discuss.

"God"?

CHAPTER 11

*You're probably an alcoholic if
you've ever been cut off during
communion and asked never to return.*

―

WHY IS THIS chapter in this book? What does "God" have to do with the denial of alcoholism? How relevant is a concept commonly called God to the atheist or agnostic alcoholic? Must the alcoholic believe in this Concept to escape denial and breathe a sober breath?

Preaching to the atheist or agnostic alcoholic that they must believe in God to become and remain sober could be a death sentence. They could easily view it as insisting they believe in Tinker Bell and have faith that she will use her magic wand to sprinkle pixie dust and shower them with magical feelings, removing the compulsion to drink. And if they believe this, their lives will be better than ever.

Those comfortably believing in a power greater than themselves that they call God may find this reminds them of what they already know. This chapter focuses on those who struggle with the God notion and have resisted receiving the benefits of sobriety because, as they claim, "For God's sake, all they do is shove God down my throat."

SECTION ONE

BELIEFS IN GOD

I'VE SEEN MANY alcoholics repelled by well-meaning sober alcoholics in recovery preaching that *their* belief in God is the only salvation from alcoholism. Although they meant well, it was harmful.

One purpose of this chapter is to reduce this harm. It offers uncommon ways, rarely talked about in recovery circles, of viewing the God idea. This chapter does not promote religion or seek to convert or convince anyone of anything. Such intent would defeat this chapter's purpose: To offer alternative views to the open-minded seeking recovery.

Einstein said, "We cannot solve our problems with the same thinking we used that created them." Instead, we must open our minds to think differently before finding a solution to a problem created by our thinking.

For example, our mind contemporaneously *orders* us to drink while *demanding* we not drink. We often need Something to intervene that we trust and is powerful enough to ignore the brain's *order* to drink. It must be more potent than the alcoholic-craving. This power exists for the theist, atheist, and agnostic. Most of us look outside ourselves for the power to value sobriety before finding it within.

THE GIG IS UP

WE BECOME DESPERATELY open-minded while flopping around like a fish out of water, trapped on the sun-parched sand, suffering unbearable desolation, and seeking any solution.

Now, as we approach our final curtain, we realize that drinking is no longer a solution while we grasp in terror for some obscure lifeline in the darkness and tell ourselves the big lie: *Drinking will work for us again—someday.*

The window of opportunity is short. We don't consider not drinking as a solution. Yet millions who are free from their alcohol obsession and compulsion to drink experience a life they never dreamed possible. Still, we believe our condition is as unique as the millions now free once thought and the millions more in misery still think.

Nevertheless, escaping the darkness and accepting that we have a drinking problem, unable to see any solution, is hopelessly terrorizing. If we do nothing, we're doomed. Not only doomed to drink but also doomed to despair and suffering when not drinking. So, where do we go from here?

We must trust in Something more influential than the influence of alcohol. Nor does it matter what this Something is or how we get this trust. It could come from others telling their experience, displaying their strength, and sharing their hope. Wherever it's from, whatever its form, and whatever it is, reliance on anything more potent than the grip of alcohol will nurture sobriety. And it's not as difficult as the atheistic or agnostic alcoholic may think.

We trust many things we can't see will cause an effect we seek and may need. We trust gravity will ground us. We trust that the air we breathe will keep us alive. We trust that the signals we receive and send with our devices will become voices or images. We even trusted a bottle would relieve us even when it no longer could.

Whether it's trusting a group of people, principles, a traditional religious concept, the rising sun, the universe, or a spiritless object symbolizing a higher power, it doesn't matter. We must grasp and cling to our trust—whatever it is—as if it were a life preserver cast our way while gasping for our last breath.

By surrendering to the victory of trusting in *Something* more powerful than we are, we will gain trust in sobriety and ourselves. At last, we will know a new power—a new freedom. But if we don't, we will sink to the indifferent bottom, melding with the millions who miscalculated and had faith they had more drinking time.

The Final Miscalculation

An open mind is essential. The suffering many alcoholics endured opened their minds. They're ready to do whatever it takes to change their feelings. This open mind includes a willingness to believe in something more compelling than the compulsion to drink.

Those alcoholics who aren't ready haven't suffered enough. While floating in the sea of misery, they keep a close eye on the shoreline, calculating a safe distance. They calculate, recalculate, and miscalculate their remaining drinking time. They will quit tomorrow and believe it every day they say it. But the drowning thinks only about their next breath—not the shore. The darkness of denial blinds them from the tidal wave approaching. It strikes. Entombed within this mass and plunged to an unrecoverable depth, all they struggle for is their next breath—even though they've already had it.

An openness to consider that a power greater than alcohol and us might exist only comes when we're ready. The theological web is tangled. No one understands it enough to disentangle much of it. All that is necessary is a mind open enough to consider a unique or alternative perspective. The mere process of *seeking* a higher power opens our minds and floods us with benefits. The benefits of this open mind encourage us to consider a different way of living—of living sober.

The Meaning of the Term "God"

Those who stumble on the word God mostly stumble on semantics—we think the word means what someone else says it means.

Yet the term "God" means something different to each of

us, whether we believe in God. How can we discuss God if everyone's conception of God is unique and indescribable? What causes the open-minded to reflexively close their minds when hearing the word God? We must have some idea of God causing this reaction—an idea we adopted from others and has never been ours. We think we understand the term as it's used, but we don't—we can't.

Our conception of that Abstract Being is the thoughts, feelings, and images that emerge when we hear the word God. The *term* God, which alone has no meaning, is the name for *Something* that does have meaning.

—

WHAT IDEA OF God does the witness imagine when sworn in and reciting, "I solemnly swear ... nothing but the truth, *so help me God*?"* By custom, the United States Presidential Oath ends with "So help me God." From what belief of God is the President asking for help? When U.S. currency reminds us, "In God We Trust," what idea of God do we Trust?

When we exclaim: "Oh my God!" "For God's sake!" or "Honest to God!" what belief in God do we have? We speak the word often—regardless of our beliefs.

So, what does the term "God" mean? For this chapter, God means *our* idea of *anything* we believe is more powerful and persuasive than alcohol, more knowing than we are individually, and that may comfort and support us in sobriety. It doesn't matter if anyone else believes it; all that matters is that we believe it.

What Does a Belief in God Mean?

Where is the line separating the believer from the nonbeliever? What does "I believe in God" or "I don't believe in God" mean? And who decides?

When we use labels to describe beliefs, we risk

---

*In most jurisdictions, the oath has changed from "swear" to "swear or *affirm*," and "So help me God" has been removed.

stereotyping. Many kinds of theists, atheists, and agnostics exist. The following is a broad definition of these terms as used here. The *theist* believes in some higher power, the *atheist* believes no higher power exists, and the *agnostic* believes that since a higher power can't be proven, we can't know if it exists.

What if our higher power is the infinite universe, or the sun, moon, and stars, or the collective wisdom of a group, or a soothing feeling within, or a powerful energy that is everywhere? Are we believers?

What if we believe God is a man in the heavens, waiting to grant all our prayer requests, so long as we register green/good on the 'faithometer?'

Doesn't our reaction to the word "God" depend on what we think God is?

What if we believe something exists that is omnipotent but doesn't care about the details of our lives? Are we believers? Can we partially believe in God?

What if we have times of doubt? Are we atheists or agnostics during these doubtful periods?

Consider self-described atheists who believe in a force for good that drives away evil. Aren't these 'atheists' believers in their conception of God?

What belief does it take to cross the line from a believer to a nonbeliever . . . and who says?

These rhetorical questions merely invite us to reflect upon our views. Since none of this is black and white and we know so little, theological differences are the rule.

Herbert Spencer* said, "Contempt prior to investigation leaves a man in everlasting ignorance." And I would add to that, "Contempt after a *biased* investigation could leave an alcoholic in everlasting misery or worse." So, to avoid everlasting ignorance, misery, or worse, we must be willing to hear different perspectives.

---

*Herbert Spencer was a famous English philosopher, biologist, anthropologist, and sociologist. He coined "survival of the fittest."

A Description of the Power

SO, WHAT IS this elusive Higher Power? It's a power that can alter and raise our awareness. It creates a passion for celebrating life and cherishing the present. It provides us with a purpose—a higher purpose. It opens our minds.

It encourages humor—we can laugh and stop taking ourselves and others too seriously. It promotes connecting with others and resisting isolation. It removes our compulsion to change who we are and how we feel artificially. It replaces despair with hope. It blazes a trail we can walk on with dignity, confidence, and self-respect. It adjusts our ego and dissolves arrogance, allowing us to walk with humility, not thinking too little or too much of ourselves.

It opens our hearts. It provokes contributing to others. It helps us recognize our past as valuable for helping others and ourselves. What went before is no longer a destructive memory fueling our excessive guilt, regret, and remorse.

It dissolves our unproductive fear of our forecasted fictional future. It strengthens our emotional elasticity, providing us the resilience to recover from setbacks reasonably. It invites us to mature suitably.

It nurtures a feeling of gratitude, shrinking our greed, so we want what we have rather than frantically searching for what we *think* we want. It creates a desire to give, occasionally anonymously, expecting nothing in return.

It provides us with fearless freedom to look in the mirror of introspection. It excites our compassion and empathy while softening our distorted envy. It allows us to see our imperfections, traits, and motives, making us less judgmental and accepting of those who think, act, and believe differently.

It removes our need to blame, giving us the freedom to accept responsibility for our actions. It allows us to replace resentment with contentment and recognize the benefit of forgiveness. We no longer expect others to be perfect; we expect them to be human and imperfect. We no longer expect more of others than we expect of ourselves. Others no longer continually let us down.

Finally, it cultivates a neutral feeling toward alcohol. It enlightens our vision, empowering us to see and welcome the wonders surrounding us. We realize we find true joy, meaning, contentment, and happiness when we shift our focus to the greater good—the higher purpose. We no longer desperately search for the good life from a bottle.

How Atheistic or Agnostic Alcoholics Find This Power

Endless ways exist to benefit from a power greater than ourselves without getting bogged down by what we see as the constraints of religious dogma. An effective way to do this is to congregate with other alcoholics in recovery.

Those with long-term sobriety usually enjoy life more than the constant relapser. And those enjoying sobriety more have searched for and believe in *Something* more potent than they are, which helps them value sobriety.

Our Comprehension of the Incomprehensible

IF GOD IS all-knowing, then we can't understand God. But we can imagine something even though we can't understand it— an imagination undoubtedly flawed. Our imagination of God reveals more about who we are than what God is.

Various Conceptions of God

The number and uniqueness of conceptions of God equal all the fingerprints in the world. Many are similar, but no two are identical.

Describing our imagination of God would be more difficult than describing blue in a monochrome world, which is only possible with a blue sky to compare it with. But we may describe the Conception we created, limited by our imaginations.

Most conceive God as a power greater than us—or even an

Omni-God: a God who is omnipresent (everywhere), omniscient (has infinite knowledge), omnipotent (has unlimited power), and omnibenevolent (is all good and all-loving).

Many believe the God most spoken about is like humans. God has feelings, like a loving parent—available to protect, teach, and nudge us, allowing us to exercise our free will. They believe God thinks and feels sad, happy, mad, and glad. Some insist that God is aware of and cares about every thought we have and action we take.

Some see God as a concept by which we measure our pain.* Others see God as a feeling, and some sense God as love. Many insist God lives in the heavens, and others believe God lives in our hearts. Some define God as anything science can't explain.

Some reject the masculine reference, while others imagine God is a woman, man, or genderless.

Countless others believe everyone worships the same God, though their understanding of that God differs.

Although many mainstream religions believe in one God, not all religions are monotheistic. Some are polytheistic, and although these faiths believe in more than one God, many are henotheistic—worshiping one supreme God but believing assistant gods could exist. Then there are atheistic religions, such as Buddhism, whose followers believe that no God exists and don't worship anyone or anything.° And it becomes more complicated as the exploration continues. Fortunately, alcoholics can find 'salvation' in any conception they choose.

The Genesis of Our Conception of God

The branding iron of indoctrination seared an idea of God in our memory during childhood. This branding molds and may

---

*Lyrics from a song called "God" from John Lennon's first post-Beatles solo album, *John Lennon/Plastic Ono Band*, released December 11, 1970.

°Buddhism is the world's fourth-largest religion. Contrary to popular belief, Buddhists do not worship Buddha, but during prayer, they may focus on a painting or statue of the enlightened and spiritually influential Buddha.

scar our spiritual beliefs.

Transcending religious indoctrination is difficult. Occasionally, we must discard childhood remnants. When our theological baggage forbids us to imagine any acceptable religious or spiritual concept, it may be time to overcome it. An effective way to overcome indoctrination is open-mindedness. If we feel uneasy hearing the word God, perhaps it's time to rise above our thinking by opening our minds a little more.

Imagine two children discussing God. One pictures God as a gray-haired, bearded, angry, scowling man with clenched teeth and a knitted brow, hovering above, leaning over storm clouds, blowing damaging gusts of wind, warning us with frightening thunder, and ready to hurl a lightning bolt at the first sinner walking by.

The other sees a loving, smiling, curly and silky silver-haired bearded man hovering above, leaning over white fluffy clouds, breathing a gentle, soothing breeze like a guardian angel.

One child fears God, and the other loves God. Neither understands nor believes in the other's God. Their discussion goes nowhere.

I've heard of two people attending the same church and listening to the same sermons for years. One heard of a loving God, and the other learned of a vengeful God. As children, one believed God would punish him if he misbehaved or sinned, and the other understood that God would unconditionally love him despite any wrongdoing.

Most of us received our understanding of God from our parents. Others from religion, media, friends, neighbors, and relatives. We learned about God from those who led us to believe that Santa Claus,* the Easter Bunny, and the Tooth Fairy are real, and a pot of gold glitters at the end of every

---

*This belief flowed from Saint Nicholas, who was a generous gift giver to the poor. It transformed into good and nice children are given the best toys—the naughty and bad don't fare as well, sending the message that wealthy children are good, and the poor are bad.

rainbow and two at the ends of double rainbows.

Despite this, alcoholics seeking sobriety will do well to develop their own understanding of a higher power, not the understanding they've been spoon-fed, which will ignite a new appreciation for sobriety.

THE ALCOHOLIC SKEPTIC AND LOGIC

IF WE ASSERT that no higher intelligence or greater or higher power exists, we'd be claiming we have *all* knowledge. And wouldn't that be the most blatant display of ignorance? As we acquire more knowledge, the more we discover how little we know.

How can we know something doesn't exist when we don't know what is beyond our knowledge? So how can we claim that no God exists when we can't know what we don't know?

Still, if we say God doesn't exist, we must conceptualize the God that doesn't exist. Once we do, our conception of God exists. So, even skeptics have their unique concept of God and may have a better-defined concept than some believers.

Moreover, if we say, "I don't believe God exists," then aren't we saying we don't believe *our* conception, or anyone's conception, exists? But we can't know everyone's conception, and even if we did, how can we say their conception doesn't exist? For example, if some believe God is a calming presence, how can we disbelieve they experience this presence? Conversely, if we say we believe in God, aren't we saying we believe in *our* unique idea of God?"

To further illustrate, when one answers "Yes" to the question, "Do you believe in God?" the answer heard is, "Yes, I believe in the same God you do." But this answer means nothing unless followed with: "What is your understanding of God?"

The Power of Words

Certain words cause some alcoholics to recoil from sobriety

because these words relate to a Concept they don't believe in. These include God, Deity, Devine, Him, Father, Lord, Thy, Worship, Bless, Prayer, Sin, Heaven, Miracle, Grace, Hell, and Amen. Historically, these words have been connected to a traditional religious God.

Millions of alcoholics have missed *quality* sobriety because of the *word* "God." But we can't let a misunderstood word hinder survival. If it's a problem, why not substitute the words Collective Wisdom, Collective Energy, Creator of the Universe, Good, Loving Force, Higher Consciousness, or Good Orderly Direction for the term "God" or any other word that works?

Regardless, they are only words. Nothing changes its character and properties based on what it's called. Still, words alone must not dissuade the alcoholic from seeking help. We can easily translate thick religious jargon into more comfortable language.

Although believers and nonbelievers may view the world in different terms, both view it from a human perspective, and the effect is the same.

For example, the theist may follow scripture: "Love thy neighbor, as thyself." The agnostic may follow the golden rule: "Treat others how I want to be treated." Yet both are acting equally good.

Both may be philanthropists, making large gifts to charities and those in need. One may consider philanthropy God's work, and the other may view it as a good deed. Both experience a pleasant sensation when doing for others.

Perhaps the believer sees walking on water and the parting sea as miraculous, while the skeptic sees one walking on a sandbar that divides the sea during low tide.

The theist sees a burning bush, and the atheist recognizes

the *Dictamnus* plant.* Both are in awe.

One may see a series of events resulting in a mysterious experience as Godly. The other sees luck and coincidence, which is easily explained by the theory of probability. Both are in wonder.

Both may feel a soothing presence—one by praying and the other by meditating and quietly contemplating, sensing oneness with nature and the universe.

Still, sobriety is available to both, regardless of their views.

An "Act of God"

An "Act of God" is a legal doctrine. It doesn't define God; it only ascribes acts to God.[1]

An "Act of God" means an unforeseeable, intervening force so potent we can't prevent or affect it.° Most know this force is usually a natural disaster.

Nonbelievers pay insurance premiums to reimburse them for any loss arising from an Act of God. For example, one never hears of an insured refusing to accept an insurance payment for damage caused by an Act of God because they didn't believe in God. Instead, they sign contracts that excuse them from performing their contractual duties if prevented by an "Act of God."

Therefore, someone else's conception of God in an "Act of God" is unimportant when seeking to minimize the loss caused by a flood, tornado, earthquake, or another natural disaster. They know the word God reflects no precise idea of God other than a power greater than any human power. This doctrine doesn't suggest that the God of any religion causes this harm, and we know that. So, using the God in an "Act of

---

*The *Dictamnus* plant releases volatiles near the flowers and seedpods that can easily ignite, enveloping the plant with flames. After the flame extinguishes, the plant remains uninjured. It is marketed under its common name, "The Burning Bush."

°Insurance companies use it to exclude coverage for natural disasters. Supplemental policies covering acts of God are available. A common one is flood insurance.

God" will avoid preconceived notions that prevent us from seeking protection from the disaster of alcoholism.

Devine Providence is an act of God that results in good—a miracle. We've heard, "Nothing short of an act of God will help him now." People who usually shut down when hearing one discuss God are neutral about the God 'acting' in an Act of God.

For an alcoholic to become and stay sober takes something that science can't explain; it takes an Act of God. So, how does the sobriety-seeking alcoholic, with no belief in a God, benefit from an Act of God?

We must get past our preconceived and rigid belief of the word God—our lives depend on it. The rest of the answer follows.

WHEN ATHEISTS AND AGNOSTICS PRAY AND MEDITATE

THOSE WHO DON'T believe in God won't pray to something they don't believe in, will they?

Well, according to the Pew Research Center, eight percent of adults who claim not to believe in God pray to Something several times a year, and some pray daily.[2] Ten percent read scripture, and 41% occasionally attend religious services, some bi-weekly. Four percent participate in prayer groups, scripture study, or religious education groups. Over half describe seeking and feeling spiritual peace and well-being. One-third think it's essential for religion to be a part of their lives, and they meditate regularly. Eighty-five percent sense a wonder about the universe, while two percent believe in heaven and hell. So, belief in traditional notions of God is unnecessary to explore and benefit from prayer and meditation.

Neuroscientists have discovered that repeated prayer and meditation can cause favorable changes in the brain that can become permanent.[3]

Neuroimages show that prayer and meditation strengthen the brain's frontal lobes. The more vital this part of our brain, the better our focus, concentration, movement, coordination, problem-solving, memory, language, actions, judgment, impulse control, reasoning, and social and sexual behavior.[4] Also, it can stabilize our mood, breathing, blood pressure, and sleep. These positive changes have a significant healing effect.[5]

And we need not pray to Something outside us as many traditional religions routinely dictate. We can direct it within, wherever that place may be.[6]

It is well known that meditation is so practical and powerful that significant world leaders, including U.S. presidents and CEOs, have regularly practiced it before making challenging decisions.

ONE OF THE most effective prayers I know of is the agnostic or atheist prayer. Praying to Something we don't believe in takes an extraordinary willingness, often by those who are desperate and have been crawling in an endless circle on the damp, cold, indifferent ground, shivering while dodging fireballs of truth and surrounded by walls of distorted reflections and horrifying sounds, repeating and reverberating endlessly. They feel hopelessness, frustration, and self-hatred. They have reached their bottom and see no way out.

Their desperation gives them the willingness to try anything to escape their misery, including surrendering by praying to a God they don't believe in. These desperate prayers typically start with a demand: "God, if you exist, show yourself and help me stop drinking!"

As mentioned in Chapter 3, "The Alcoholic-craving," although rare, some have experienced a life-changing, incredible event when simply asking God for help. Many call this a "spiritual experience." Suddenly, a diffused and soothing bright white light partially clouds their vision. They sense an unusual feeling and an indescribable presence. This results in an immediate psychic change—their thinking radically changes. The alcoholic-craving disappears and rarely returns. The abstinent alcoholic feels no dysphoria. Instead, they often feel a sudden euphoria embrace them. This event reportedly lasts from a few seconds to a few minutes.

This astonishing incident occurs when certain emotions mix with the alcoholic's complete surrender. Although they may need medical stabilization during physical withdrawal, no emotional withdrawal occurs.

This is even more inspiring when described as a "spiritual experience of sorts" by the self-proclaimed atheist or agnostic chronic alcoholic.

But this sudden spiritual experience, followed by an abrupt psychic change, is the exception—the transformation is usually gradual. Still, it occurs in all who want it enough to seek it.[7]

Although the Radiance bestowed is likely the same at all levels of the alcoholic descent, we're most receptive when hopelessly crawling in an endless circle, dodging the fireballs of truth—the consequences of alcoholism. Perhaps that is why we never hear of the high-bottom* alcoholic having a sudden spiritual experience—they're not desperate enough.

ONE BENEFICIARY OF this experience explained that hearing the word "God" would spark an unpleasant feeling. He didn't believe in a Supreme Being that cared enough to manage the details of his life. Instead, he substituted Creative Intelligence, Universal Mind, and Spirit of Nature for the word *God*. He said:

> When they talked of a God personal to me, who was love, superhuman strength and direction, I became irritated and my mind snapped shut against such a theory. To Christ I conceded the certainty of a great man, not too closely followed by those who claimed Him.[8]

---

*The term "high-bottom" refers to the alcoholic who became sober before losing everything.

But there he was, once again, detoxing in a hospital or, as they called it, drying out. He was considered hopeless, considered himself hopeless, and he appeared hopeless. But as he lay in the hospital bed, desperate and defeated, he finally earned enough humility to ask that Supreme Being for help. He then had the "spiritual experience" described above.

He surrendered and gave himself to what he now called God to use him for any purpose. This self-described agnostic had simply asked God for help. Flowing from this millisecond decision to surrender was the birth of Alcoholics Anonymous (AA).

His name was Bill Wilson, co-founder of AA. The year was 1934. He never drank again. This birth resulted in millions of helpless and desperate alcoholics—considered hopeless—becoming sober, transforming their lives and the lives of loved ones. The events leading to this world-progressing phenomenon flowed sequentially perfectly.

The Perfect Sequence

It's Saturday afternoon. Bill Wilson is now six months sober. Devastated by a failed business opportunity, he paces the hotel lobby with the thoughts and feelings that often prompt an alcoholic to drink. No one is watching him for the first time since he quit drinking.*

At one end of the lobby is a bar where music, laughter, light, and fun radiate. At the other end is a lonely darkness, with a telephone and a directory dangling above, listing local churches and ministers.

He panics while deciding which direction to walk and feels drawn to the bar. This surprised him because he's never panicked when thinking of drinking—only when he couldn't get a drink. He then feels a sliver of sanity.

He realizes the reason he's sober is that he's been trying to help other alcoholics quit drinking. He's then drawn to and

---

*Bill Wilson's last drink of alcohol was on December 11, 1934.

walks toward the silent darkness. He scans the church directory, hoping to find a minister who might know of a hopeless drunk he can try helping. So, he 'randomly' selects Reverend Walter Tunks, who 'fortunately' understands and provides Bill with 10 names.

Bill calls everyone on the list except the last one. Discouraged, he returns to his room. But soon, compelled to make the final call, he returns to the lobby, paces, and then calls the last name on the list, Henrietta Seiberling.*

As luck—or *Something*—has it, a friendly and kind woman answers. She invites Bill to meet her at once because she knows of a severe alcoholic who might be receptive.

After Bill arrives, she calls the hopeless alcoholic, whose wife answers. The wife is receptive but explains that her husband isn't in any condition to talk. So, Henrietta invites the wife and her husband to dinner the following day. The wife accepts, provided her husband isn't too drunk to attend.

The next day arrives. It's Mother's Day, 1935, and the alcoholic and his wife appear for dinner. After dinner, the alcoholic and Bill visit in the library for hours. The alcoholic's name is Robert Smith, M.D. (fondly known as Dr. Bob), who becomes and eventually stays sober as the co-founder of AA. On June 10, 1935, the day Dr. Bob had his last drink, AA was born. Soon, they both visit another hopeless, hospitalized alcoholic who becomes sober and the third AA member.[9]

Undoubtedly, Bill's motive for his decisions was not selfless. He could not have known his 'arbitrary' selection of the Reverend or making the final call—*that he almost didn't make*—would result in millions of alcoholics recovering. Nor did he know that avoiding the bar or attending Mother's Day dinner would have a global impact. But he knew it was *his* only

---

*The final name on the list was Henrietta Seiberling, according to *Alcoholics Anonymous Comes of Age*, and Bill thought she was the wife of the Goodyear founder, which intimidated him (this was Bill's account). According to *Pass it On*, the last name on the list was Norman Sheppard, who referred Bill to Henrietta Seiberling.

chance of staying sober. Still, nothing could've happened without him acting.

A perfect sequence of events also occurred for the millions who came later and sought, received, and cherished sobriety. Merely focusing on this perfect sequence could propel many past doubtful thoughts about Something beneficial outside themselves.

Prayer and Meditation, and Sobriety

TO ENJOY AND deepen our relationships with anyone, we must first connect with them. We connect through verbal and nonverbal communication. Every relationship needs communication to thrive. This connection is just as essential when relating to a higher power. Communicating with a power greater than ourselves is often called prayer.

As a relationship matures and deepens, communication often becomes nonverbal and occurs when merely with each other. Talking is unnecessary to sense contact with each other. Sometimes, simply being with another is connecting. This person may be outside our view, in another room, or far away. Still, we sense we're together, like the presence of a higher power, which many sense through meditation.

Prayer and meditation allow us to feel universally connected. It inspires us to rise above the nonsense that provokes drinking. It encourages raising our consciousness to where we embrace life rather than reject it by saturating and hoping to drown our lives with alcohol. It gets us through the rough spots when giving in to the alcoholic-craving would be disastrous.

There's no right or wrong way to connect or pray for this to be effective. This connection doesn't require us to be in any position or place, provided we're not distracted, nor does it require wearing unique clothing, so long as we're comfortable. Still, without a connection, there's no benefit.

Prayer is a method of centering ourselves to soothe our thoughts and feelings. It allows us to recognize our self-will and question whether it's helpful or hurtful to us or others. During this time, we can express gratitude and appreciation, which causes us to feel grateful and appreciative. We can mention our regrets and reflect on possible remedies for our misdeeds. During difficult times, prayer is often comforting.

Prayer can give suffering alcoholics the strength to walk out of the valley of hopelessness and climb to the mountaintop of sobriety, which turns out to be much closer and easier to climb than we ever imagined.

A Soothing Concept to Consider

Imagine something radiating equally on the believer and the nonbeliever, much like the sun radiates light and heat.

Whether we're aware of this Illuminated Warmth doesn't reduce its radiance. We can avoid the light and warmth we receive by burrowing in the ground and escaping some or all this radiance. Or we can remain surfaced and open enough to prosper from it. This Power is continuously present and working in our lives without praying or paying for it. We benefit the most when we pause to notice this Power.

We don't pray to please this Power—we pray to feel connected. Prayer and meditation allow us to know and *feel* this presence. So, we tune in for our benefit to soothe and comfort us. It helps *us* become more centered and in tune with others and the universe.

We are mostly theologically unaware and bewildered. That is the apparent design. This Power *expects* nothing from us and exists infinitely beyond us.

So, many accept and feel the Illuminated Warmth with gratitude and open, loving arms, while others ignore it and some reject it. Many with long-term quality sobriety accept and *feel* this Warmth.

PRAYER AND SELF-WILL

I'VE NOTED TWO primary types of prayer discussed in

recovery forums: One seeks the knowledge of and the ability to do God's will, and the other seeks something for us or others *with specificity*.

The General Prayer

The first prayer is other-centered. This prayer doesn't seek sainthood but often enables the alcoholic to recognize self-will. This recognition is essential because many alcoholics experience an abundance of adverse results from exercising self-will. Self-absorption guarantees this, and these undesirable results often prompt drinking.

The difference between God's will and self-will is often blurry, but not always. We know it's likely not self-will if we're doing something we don't want to do, which helps others.

Conversely, uneasiness usually identifies self-will. We can't put our finger on it, but we know it when we feel it. This uneasy feeling includes our conscience creating discomfort when we resist doing what we sense is right. It's typically characterized by planning to act in a way that we don't want to tell anyone, including those we trust enough to tell everything else. We may also become closed-minded and resist feedback about our proposed self-centered action, from which only *we* can benefit.

An exception is the alcoholic praying for the common good and discovering their role in working for the common interest.

This prayer helps the alcoholic to feel connected to a purpose—a higher purpose.

The Specific Prayer

The other prayer is praying for something we or someone else wants. It's questionable and often prompted by our or another's self-will.

For example, aren't we hindered by shortsightedness if we pray that Jane does well at the casino or John gets the pay raise he demands? It might be catastrophic if Jane won the jackpot.

She may suffer the rest of her life repeatedly and compulsively, pursuing elusive jackpots and enduring endless consequences, much like the alcoholic chasing the murky euphoria once enjoyed when drinking.

And how do we know whether a pay raise for John is best? What if he declines another position because he receives a pay raise? The job he rejected may have been best for him and others.

Or consider this. Julia is an alcoholic with her fifth DUI charge. She's fearfully asking everyone pray that she avoids prison. Yet perhaps imprisonment could enhance or save her or someone else's life. Prison programs have produced positive and significant life changes for many alcoholics.

If we agree to pray for Julia, how could we resolve that with what we believe is God's will? Would our prayer seek God's will or Julia's will? Who knows? Regardless, is it our call to make, and wouldn't any omniscient being ignore such a prayer?

On the other hand, if we see that her fear has prematurely imprisoned her emotionally and we connect her with a sober alcoholic who has benefited from prison, perhaps that might be God's will or perhaps not.

Then there's Mark, who is distraught because his drinking finally caused his wife to end their 15-year marriage. Still, he continues to drink despite the breakup of his marriage, an intervention, and his chronic misery. Feeling hopeless, he asks everyone to pray that his marriage doesn't dissolve.

Wouldn't it be presumptuous to request that God salvage his marriage and abruptly end his suffering? If prayers reduced his suffering, this could extend his drinking and inhibit recovery. Or, if he becomes sober before he's ready, he might repeatedly relapse, never enjoying continuous sobriety. In retrospect, the times I walked through the most difficulty were the times I grew the most spiritually, intellectually, and emotionally, and that growth has given me a passion for helping others, including writing this.

If we pray for specifics, aren't we trying to use prayer to support our manipulation and control of those around us to get what we want or think others need? Doesn't this prayer presume we know what's best, even more than God? Can we trust and believe in a God needing our suggestions to make the right decision?

Dangers of Self-Will for the Alcoholic

Some believe they have a direct line to God. Their way is the only way. Whatever they do, God tells them to do it. They populate our psychiatric hospitals and prisons. If we pray for a decisive answer and act on it without talking with someone we trust to be objective—how can we trust our biased perception of the answer?

We've heard sober alcoholics talk about making major life decisions like changing jobs, ending a marriage, or moving to a distant city. They present their decision-making directly to God through prayer. Then we hear, "I prayed about it, and God answered my prayers. I've decided to end my marriage, accept the job transfer, leave my children, and move across the country."

Their rationalization affected their decisions, and their strong will to take the action they prayed about distorted the answer they heard. Many would love our significant choices rubber-stamped with "APPROVED BY GOD." This would reduce any guilt, especially if it turns out to be the wrong decision. It would allow us to briefly escape responsibility for our choices, which *we* believe would soften others' contempt for us.

But this fantasy doesn't last forever. Eventually, they may wonder why their disabling guilt remains and why they're unable to stay sober. If they ever escape denial, they must cope with the devastating realities—the consequences of "God's" decision. They will then understand why their children want nothing to do with them. Their explanation that God approved of them abandoning their children will not diminish their children's disdain for them.

Had they gone to their God via their therapist, sponsor, unbiased friend, or trusted spiritual adviser, they may have seen that their decision was self-will and not God's will. Had they foreseen the likely result, they may have decided differently. Others, who aren't influenced by our self-will and ego, can often see the next right move for us better than we can.

Even religious leaders, including the Pope, consult with others without relying solely on their direct contact with God for answers.

Faith

IT IS COMMON to hear "the God of our understanding" in 12-step recovery meetings.* What does it mean? Isn't it an oxymoron? If I could understand God, God would not be knowledgeable or powerful enough to be my higher power. A more accurate reference is "the God of our misunderstanding." Still, we often need to understand and identify whatever we believe.

Most have had a passion for learning since birth. Our innate curiosity is compelling. We want, and sometimes think we need, immediate answers to our questions—and if not at once, sooner than later, and better later than never. Unanswered questions nag for answers. But we finally realize, and at times accept, that some spiritual knowledge exists that isn't for us ever to know. I call it our "mandated ignorance," which includes our ignorance about God.

Faith and Doubt

If we never knew doubt, faith would never be an issue. Although we speak of faith in absolute terms, it's seldom all or nothing. Faith and doubt are companions and dynamic, much

---

*The phrase "God of our understanding" originated in Alcoholics Anonymous, but developed a wider use, and people unrelated to AA it has been adopted by.

like a teeter-totter with faith and doubt at opposite ends. When doubt strikes the ground, faith often soars and then plummets at other times, causing doubt to rise. But they usually swing pendulously.

Many prefer to root our beliefs and conclusions in evidence, and since we can't prove faith, we believe it can't exist.

Yet many truths are incapable of proof. We call these truths axioms. Something is axiomatic if it's self-evident—a universal truth that needs no proof—its truth is obvious. An axiom is a foundation for deductive reasoning, and science accepts axioms.

An example is Euclid's axiom: things equal to the same thing are equal to each other. It is self-evident and needs no proof. Thomas Jefferson wrote in the U.S. Declaration of Independence, "We hold these truths to be *self-evident*, that all men are created equal ..." Although it can't be proven, it's an accepted truth—an axiom. We have faith that axioms are true.

To illustrate, if I ask a believer to prove God exists, they may have difficulty obliging. They have all the evidence *they* need to prove it to themselves because they feel it. So, faith senses *Something* that moves and comforts us that we can't understand, identify, explain, or demonstrate. It is self-evident.

It's like traveling down the road in a blinding rainstorm. Though we can't see the road ahead, we continue traveling because we have faith that the road continues.

The Power of Faith

Faith is powerful. Even the placebo effect shows this. In the scientific testing of the effectiveness and safety of a drug, many participants, with faith that a drug would cause an expected effect, experienced that effect even though they took a sugar pill.

For instance, giving what one believes is aspirin for a

headache will often relieve the headache even though the tablet contains no aspirin. Additionally, of those given a tablet with inactive ingredients and told to report any side effects, many reported side effects.

These findings prompted further research, which revealed that the placebo effect applies to many areas of our lives. It proves the power of suggestion—a self-fulfilling prophecy—the power of faith.

"Why?" is Not a Spiritual Question

We ask "why" when we lack faith. It isn't a question but a complaint disguised as a question oozing from our self-absorbed attempts to justify our self-pity.

Examples of the "why" question are: "If a God exists that is all kind, loving, present, and powerful, *why* do I see malice, hatred, evil, and suffering everywhere I look? *Why* do bad things happen to good people? *Why? Why* me? Poor me! Pour me another drink!" But we choose where to look. We could look elsewhere and see all the good that abounds and all the good that happens to good people. We could focus on the good in our lives and feel gratitude. We could conclude, "I am fortunate," "I am blessed," or "I am lucky."

I'm not suggesting we ignore all wrongs. Still, we didn't create this universe, and the world we see as flawed may be more flawless than we understand. Without being all-knowing, who are we to say? Accepting our limits and realizing how little we know invites faith.

I've often heard, "I think something is out there; I just don't know what it is." Yet, shouldn't the highest power be unknowable? To imagine and believe something may exist that we don't understand provides the humility of open-mindedness.

Our beliefs can't change the truth, can they? Although they can't change objective reality, our beliefs can and do change our subjective reality. Whether God exists depends on the beholder. Although we know other conceptions of God exist, we believe our conception must be the right one, or we would adopt a different one.

The consensus is that we benefit from faith. Whether it's the placebo effect when benefiting from faith is irrelevant.

So, it's axiomatic that God exists for those who believe God exists or have felt God's presence. Though it can't be proven to one who has never felt the Presence, it's been proven to one who has. It's self-evident. Again, God wouldn't be God if we could understand God.

To re-emphasize, we can't comprehend the incomprehensible. Although we're driven to search for answers, faith relieves our spiritual anxiety, allowing us to accept our *mandated ignorance.*

What's It Going To Be: Sobriety or Not?

THE DILEMMA OF whether to seek sobriety haunts alcoholics for life or until we finally make a decision. Selecting sobriety requires courage, trust, faith, and balance. It's like learning to ride a bicycle. The following story illustrates recovering from alcoholism with a support group.

I'M CLIMBING on my bike for the first time since my training wheels were removed. My father had gradually raised them over the past month until neither wheel touched the ground the faster I pedaled. So, even though the bike balanced the same with or without the training wheels, I believed they were helping, which gave me faith and confidence they would protect me from falling. Now I knew they were gone.

My father balances me while we're still. "Okay, you ready?" he asks.

"Yeah ... no ... no ... not yet, Dad."

His massive hand covers most of my back as he holds the handlebars straight with his other hand.

"Okay, here goes!" he warns.

We move but not much because I have slight pressure on the brakes. To balance, I must courageously pedal and move forward.

"Let off the brakes—start pedaling." He's running beside me, his left hand pushing my back. Your bike will stay up if you go faster, but you'll fall if you go too slow."

"Don't let go, Dad!"

"You've got it. You're doing great. Keep pedaling!" He continues running by my side, but now his hand barely touches my back. He thrusts me forward—I can no longer feel his hand. He sounds distant—and confident.

"Don't brake. You're doing great!"

I tell myself that so long as I pedal, I'll remain balanced and won't fall. Then I realize I must stop . . . eventually.

"Okay, don't brake, but don't pedal as fast, and when you're ready, start turning slowly! Don't brake!"

I complete the turn.

"Good. Start pedaling again, but not too fast, and ride toward me."

"I'm coming; you going to catch me, Dad?" I panickily plead.

"You bet I am ... you're fine. Okay, don't break, but stop pedaling . . . now you can break just a little bit . . . a little more . . . good . . . just a bit more . . . perfect! I've got you!" he says with a wide smile. "You did it!"

"That was fun. Can we do it again, Dad?"

—

I NEVER FORGOT how to ride a bike and passed it on when teaching my children. Nor did I forget that courage is not acting fearlessly—but acting fearfully. My child learning the quickest had the most courage to act in the face of fear. At the moment, their courage paralleled their trust and confidence in me, a power they thought to be greater than themselves.

It's like seeking sobriety. Those alcoholics with the most courage to change will gain sobriety the quickest. As they pass it on, they realize that some will grasp it more quickly than others.

Those who give without wanting, expecting, or accepting anything in return except our well-being are trustworthy. Those achieving sobriety trusted those worthy of trust, which seeing it work for others made possible.

They eventually realize that many have no veiled agenda. Trusting the trustworthy supplies them with courage and a faith they never knew. When they are ready to pedal without being held and knowing the caring hand of others is always within reach, those who helped them will smile and watch them pedal on to help another alcoholic prepare for the ride.

To keep balance and prevent a fall or relapse, they continue pedaling. They don't rely on their past pedaling to move forward and avoid falling . . . for long.

It works this way. This is recovery—the Power—a higher power for many new in recovery.

Many Paths to Recovery

MANY AVOID SEEKING recovery, claiming those offering it promote religious views incompatible with their comfort. This conclusion seldom follows open-minded, durable, and personal observation but often comes from an abbreviated experience or another's experience—usually one not ready for sobriety.

Yet, this view doesn't flow from a vacuum. Many sober alcoholics insist their path to recovery is the only one because it's all they know. Still, we can find many paths to sobriety, and we should choose the most comfortable one.

The misunderstanding that 12-step support groups *require* a belief in a religious doctrine is the view some have of Alcoholics Anonymous. A pamphlet published by Alcoholics Anonymous entitled *Many Paths to Spirituality* discusses this.[10]

Also, Bill Wilson, co-founder of AA, in 1965 said:

> Newcomers ... approaching AA ... represent almost every belief and attitude imaginable. We have atheists and agnostics. We have people of nearly every race, culture and religion. The full individual liberty to practice any creed or principle or therapy whatever should be a first consideration for us all. Let us not, therefore, pressure anyone with our individual or even our collective views. Let us instead accord each other the respect and love that is due to every human being as he tries to make his way. Let us always try to be inclusive rather than exclusive; Let us remember that each alcoholic among us is a member of AA, so long as he or she so declares.[11]

So, attending AA doesn't require a belief in God. No one pressures members to believe anything. Instead, members may discuss their religious or spiritual beliefs or disbeliefs, but no member speaks for AA.

Alcoholics Anonymous is not a religion or religious. Half the new members are atheists or agnostics.[12] Some AA groups meet in churches (where they pay rent), and some close meetings with a universal prayer (that some skip and others change), which bolsters the misperception of a religious connection.

Many consider the power of AA, the principles, or the group to be their Collective Wisdom or Higher Power. Some believe their Higher Power is the special feeling one has when "one alcoholic shares their experience, strength, and hope with another alcoholic." Members practice whatever faith works best for them, or they practice none. They conceive of a higher power as they wish, or they don't.[13]

Some have cited the 468 times the "Big Book" of Alcoholics Anonymous mentions God as proof that AA promotes a religious connection. But this chapter alone mentions God 209 times and encourages only theological freedom.

Nevertheless, many alcohol recovery organizations exist. Some publicize a religious base, as does Celebrate Recovery, and others promote a secular view, including primarily atheists and agnostics, although many of them believe in *some* higher power. These groups include Secular Alcoholics Anonymous, Agnostics AA, AA for Atheists, Agnostics, and Freethinkers; AA Agnostica; and AA Beyond Belief. Still, based on many experiences, some connection with *Something* more persuasive than alcohol and ourselves is necessary to reach *content* sobriety, whatever that *Something* is.

So, whatever one's belief, programs exist to accommodate those beliefs with sobriety as its primary purpose.

Section Two
Spirituality and Religion: A Comparison

Writing this section has changed my views. I started searching for evidence to support my preconceived notions years ago. But when I opened my mind enough, I saw where I was closed-minded.

Bias toward spirituality and against mainstream commercial religion plagued me. When I compared spirituality and religion, committed to suppressing any prejudice, I invited and considered opposing views.

I paused and wondered whether I would want a world where religion never existed.

I searched for and found the advantages and disadvantages of both. The more I considered it, the more I realized my views were myopic and judgmental. That realization further opened my mind. After comparing spirituality and religion, I decided that one is no better than the other—they're different with similarities. And what some consider a negative trait, others see as positive. So, I realized religion benefits billions with all its imperfections, and I wouldn't want a world where religion never existed.

The Differences Between Spirituality and Religion

Many in recovery express confusion about the differences between spirituality and religion, with some claiming there is no difference.

Although no scholarly consensus exists concerning the definition of religion, most consider it a formal organization that usually, but not always, promotes belief in a defined God and dictates behaviors and practices. It typically offers unique ritualistic worship where attendance is *strongly* encouraged.

However, spirituality glistens with many meanings and is often confused with spiritualism (mortals communicating with the departed using clairvoyance, Tarot cards, Ouija boards, mediums, and other paranormal paraphernalia).

Spirituality means walking an alternative path to connecting with a power greater than ourselves instead of following the trail blazed by organized, traditional religion. Others can't control or interpret one's spirituality. It is understanding oneself in relation to one's conception of the Highest Power.

Personalities are unique—what works for some doesn't work for others. For example, if one concept of God fit everyone, only one religion would exist rather than the estimated 10,000 religions worldwide.[14] Even organized religions haven't even reached a consensus on what God is.

Twenty-five percent of the U.S. population describes themselves as "spiritual* but not religious," and nine percent identify as "religious but not spiritual."[15]

Sixty-eight percent of us believe in our childhood faith.[16] Eighty-four percent of us have the same faith as our spouse or partner.[17]

Many spiritualists don't reject religion; they reject what they see as religious limits. Instead, they value their freedom to explore their spiritual curiosity and conceive their own God. This exploration often focuses on God *within* more than "God above."

Many established religions claim to believe in the same or a similar conception of God, although their methods of worship and ideas of this God distinguish them. Further, religious denominations are subgroups comprising those with the closest beliefs.

Spiritualists seek higher levels of consciousness, where they put everyday life in perspective, and base instincts don't blindly drive them. Instead, they strive to increase awareness of their unawareness or unconsciousness.

Living in the present is paramount instead of wasting

---

*I noticed the word "spiritual" includes the word "ritual," but found no etymological connection.

energy, regretting the past, and fearing the imagined future. Still, this doesn't mean ignoring the past or the future; it means not emotionally focusing on it needlessly. It means recognizing and disallowing those instinctual demands, which are no longer helpful in a civilized society, to control our every move and sensing a more significant, higher purpose.

The spiritualist searching for and finding their conception of God is like building a custom house. One can make changes while building it. It allows one to be free of spiritual blueprints and boundaries drafted and imposed by others.

Religion provides tract housing with move-in-ready homes by describing the God in which to believe. It removes discovering God on our own.

Spiritualists don't have volumes of revered writings describing their beliefs. Instead, they may have books by individual authors that support their views. For example, many include *A Course in Miracles* in their library.

Religion provides sacred writings, including the best-seller, the *Holy Bible*. Others are the *Qur'an, The Book of Mormon,* the *Torah,* and *The Sutras*. These writings explain the differences and similarities between various religions.

Spiritual people may have adopted all or part of a religious code or created their own values and principles they strive to follow.

Each religion has a set of laws, codes, doctrines, principles, commandments, or other names for rules designed to dictate a member's thinking and behavior. These rules have many interpretations. And it's common for different interpretations to exist within a religion or denomination. These rules and rituals provide values to live by and simplify one's connection with the God of that faith. Religion also offers traditional prayers.

Many spiritualists create their prayers and affirmations instead of using established ones. This includes unique and unconventional meditation and prayer, which many spiritualists consider a private event. Although they have no consistent place to congregate and worship with others, some attend a traditional place of worship periodically, such as on religious holidays. The spiritually minded can experience their beliefs anywhere. They contend their God doesn't care where or how they seek a connection with God.

Religion reduces the struggle some experience during their spiritual journey of seeking a higher power. For example, it may exempt the entire voyage by spoon-feeding one with a packaged conception of God.

The spiritual journeys traveled are diverse. Though some beliefs have destinations, for others, it's an endless lifelong journey, believing they find God when they start the voyage and improve their connection with God throughout the journey.

Spiritual thinking believes it's essential to transcend the material world and connect to something higher. This connection is comforting.

Accountability and gentle confrontation encourage self-honesty. The less contact with others, the more the spiritualist may avoid accurate introspection. Others see us more clearly than we see ourselves. If they notice one adrift, they can gently nudge the drifter back on course. Organized religion provides this, as do recovery programs.

Religions often provide many services to their members, including weddings, sermons, funerals, worship services, prayer and meditation, mission opportunities, ministries, education, tutoring, bible study, alcohol and drug recovery services (celebrate recovery), workshops, support groups, public services, childcare, and other services.

Spirituality involves the mind, body, and spirit. Although religion is becoming more inclusive of this, its primary focus is worshiping God.

We instinctively need one another to prevent extinction. Those facing a threat to our survival will often benefit from another's help. Empathy encourages this. Those in the middle of the herd are more protected than the stragglers.

Isolation stimulates emotional disorders and is a high-risk indicator of suicide. The profile of those committing aberrational acts is often: "He was a loner—quiet, never saw him." Isolation is also a symptom of late-stage alcoholism and other disorders.

Feeling lonely prods us back to the herd when we stray too far. Like other instincts, some of us feel an *excess* of loneliness and dread being alone. Conversely, the loner feels little loneliness. Then, others often feel lonely when they're mingling in a crowd. These deviations are considered disorders.

Religion provides a flock for those who wouldn't have one—providing community—a feeling of belonging. Mutual support groups work similarly.

I'm not suggesting that all loners are dangerous to themselves or others. We need our alone time, but most don't need it continuously and pathologically. Religion provides a relief valve for loneliness.

Although further distinctions exist, this presents a general comparative summary of religion and spirituality. As shown, the alcoholic trying to find a higher power has many ways to find a comfortable one.

Religious and Spiritualist Views

ALTHOUGH SIMILARITIES EXIST, the religious and the spiritualists have many contrasting views.

Both the religious and the spiritualist see inequities and human suffering saturating our world. Yet the religious are often more active, conducting global missions that help those in distress. Spiritualists usually passively talk about it.

Many spiritualists see the religious avoiding accountability by projecting false appearances while hiding behind a façade of righteousness.

They see the religious as hypocritical, fake, closed-minded, and judgmental. Spiritualists say the religious portray a saintly persona on Sunday morning, but the rest of the week, they act godlessly.

Yet the religious suggests that opinion is as hypocritical, fake, closed-minded, and judgmental as the views that formed it. Sunday morning worship *should* bring out the best in those attending. And falling short of their goals during the rest of the week is not hypocritical—it's human. It's doubtful that spiritualists consistently adhere to their self-imposed principles around the clock. If they attend a public event, they presumably act their best.

Many spiritualists view ritualistic worship as nonsense, rigid, and without benefit. Yet, others contend formal worship allows their members to feel connected. And as a bonus, attending worship congregates like-minded people, fostering a sense of well-being—a connection to a higher *purpose*.

Many spiritualists see the religious as self-seeking and not as other-centered as they portray. Yet others say spiritual practices seeking merely self-knowledge are casual self-improvements without theological meaning. They consider seeking an understanding of self is unrelated to seeking an understanding of God. Some claim it's self-absorption.

Many spiritualists see organized religion as big bureaucratic businesses competing for new customers to increase revenue by spreading the word and promoting conversion. They view organized religion as seeking strength in numbers. The more members, the more income.

Some view spiritualists as ignoring practical realities while seeking to transcend the material world—a world in which they live, receive a benefit, and denounce without contributing. Spiritualists avoid donating a part of their labor to support the business of religion, while the religious often tithe a part of their income.

Spiritualists see the religious as having an intellectual relationship with God in contrast to their emotional connection.

Spiritualists suggest that the religious are intolerant of different views. The religious contend that any of their thinking or behavior perceived as intolerant flows from love and goodness.

The anti-religious suggests religion breeds catastrophic wars. Still, others argue that those conflicts are more political, ethnic, or geographical. They say that only extremists proclaim these conflicts are religion-driven and publish false information, provoking hostilities between faiths.

I'm not suggesting these views are correct or incorrect. Still, general awareness of them illustrates the differences between them.

Many alcoholics *struggling* to find a higher power will prefer a spiritual path rather than a belief spoon-fed to them from another. So much depends on one's personality, indoctrination, environment, and desperation. While some like the stability and convenience of established religion, others select a mixture of both or none.

The Spiritual and Religious Blend

More than half describe their theological path as a religious and spiritual blend.[18] This provides a communal spiritual journey rather than traveling alone as a spiritual tourist. This blending takes what it likes from the religion most resembling their spiritual beliefs. Some religious doctrines are more tolerant of this method, inviting theological variety.

THE PERFECT PRAYER (OR AFFIRMATION)

ONE OF MY favorite prayers is known as the St. Francis of Assisi prayer. Most believe St. Francis of Assisi wrote it in the 13th century, but scholars have disproved this, discovering that an unknown author wrote it in the early 1900s, and the Vatican agrees.[19] Still, it remains attributed to St. Francis since it vividly reflects his life and teachings.[20]

Numerous versions of the prayer exist. It became widely popular during World War I and II.[21] Modified versions have been set to music, sung at prominent funerals and weddings, quoted by world leaders, and recited in movies and series.* A popular version appears in the *Twelve Steps and Twelve Traditions* (*12 & 12*), published by Alcoholics Anonymous,[22] and is often referenced by AA members as the "Eleventh Step Prayer."

The version thought to be the original is in French, and this is the English translation of the original:

> Lord, make me an instrument of your peace.
> Where there is hatred, let me bring love.
> Where there is offence, let me bring pardon.
> Where there is discord, let me bring union.
> Where there is error, let me bring truth.
> Where there is doubt, let me bring faith.
> Where there is despair, let me bring hope.
> Where there is darkness, let me bring your light.
> Where there is sadness, let me bring joy.
> O Lord, grant that I may not so much seek
> to be consoled as to console,
> to be understood as to understand,
> to be loved as to love,
> for it is in giving that one receives,
> it is in self-forgetting that one finds,
> it is in forgiving that one is forgiven,
> it is in dying that one awakens to eternal life.

I changed it to make it more contemporary and inviting for those of various beliefs and those without a belief. It shows how simple it is to transform almost any prayer into a secular affirmation and keep the beneficial effect, which could help many seeking recovery.

---

*It was part Princess Diana's funeral, Mother Teresa prayed it daily, quoted by Presidents Bill Clinton and Joe Biden, and Speaker Nancy Pelosi.

This prayer or affirmation is unique because it doesn't ask for anything except for us to recognize and help satisfy the needs of others. It shifts our thinking away from us and our problems. It prevents us from forgetting the difficulties millions face, which minimizes focusing on our troubles. It reminds us:

- We can improve nothing unless *we* act.
- Hoarding a surplus of money manifests fear.
- Our achievement of true happiness is proportional to how much we give to others.*
- Many, including children, are suffering from hunger because most of us, out of fear, collect an excess of food that we eventually discard since we can't ever consume it.
- Before we condemn the deeds of others, we ought to focus on *our* blemishes and misdeeds.
- It feels better to love than to be loved.
- To understand someone, we must listen to *them* and resist our desire to interrupt and talk about ourselves. When speaking, we may ask, "What am I trying to achieve with my words?"
- Most of our envy comes from delusions: comparing our hidden world, thoughts, and feelings to the imaginary world of others.
- One person *can* change the world—let it begin with me.
- To treat others as we treat ourselves.
- To rise above ourselves and consider what we can do for others.
- To make positive changes that radiate goodness, caring, faith, hope, love, courage, and truth.

---

*Harvard Business School research supports this.

- To feel grateful and express this gratitude when we are with others.

—

My version of the prayer or affirmation follows:

> Let me seek to be an instrument
> of love, peace, and inspiration.
> Let me try to be of service to others.
> Where doubt, let me cast faith;
> where injury, let me help heal;
> where hatred, let me show love;
> where I see fault, let me forgive;
> where hunger, let me share food;
> where despair, let me offer hope;
> where sadness, let me radiate joy;
> where fear, let me display courage;
> where poverty, let me shed wealth;
> where delusion, let me reveal truth;
> where darkness, let me reflect light;
> where conflict, let me create harmony.
> Let me seek to comfort rather than be comforted;
> to understand rather than to be understood;
> to love rather than be loved.
> For it is by giving that we receive;
> it is by forgiving that we are forgiven;
> it is by self-forgetting that we are found.
> It is by surrendering to a Higher Purpose that gives us
> the passion to be of service to others,
> which awakens us to eternal Truth.

—

Questions For Discussion

1. Has this chapter affected you? How?
2. Do you consider yourself religious or spiritual?
3. Are you now, or have you been, an atheist or agnostic, or have you thought you might be? Has this chapter altered your thinking about your religious or spiritual past? If so, how?
4. What are your thoughts about prayer?
5. Do you pray? How often? Do you pray for specifics?
6. Have you asked "Why" questions? What are your thoughts about "Why" questions compared to having faith?
7. What are your thoughts about faith?
8. Were you surprised that those who don't believe in any God could benefit from prayer?
9. Were you ever confused about the differences between the spiritualist and the religious? Where do you fit in?

THE HAPPILY SOBER ALCOHOLIC

CHAPTER 12

*You're possibly an alcoholic if
you refuse to pay your bar tab because
you just weren't that happy at happy hour.*

—

THE PHRASE "HAPPILY SOBER ALCOHOLIC" in this title refers to alcoholics who enjoy life more without alcohol than with it. Here, "happiness" includes feelings of serenity, contentment, pleasure, joy, cheerfulness, optimism, hopefulness, enthusiasm, delight, fun, humor, confidence, and gratitude for sobriety. "Sober alcoholic" refers to an alcoholic in recovery who doesn't drink and is thoughtful, calm, clear-minded, moderate, honest, reliable, mindful, and emotionally balanced.

Still, always feeling happy is neither realistic, natural, necessary, or healthy. Many emotions we perceive as negative or distressing, such as fear and anxiety, protect us. Humans would have perished long ago if we never feared. Life also includes times of sorrow and sadness, often caused by events we can't control. Only when these protective feelings are dysfunctional or unbalanced do we feel unhappy. So, being happy includes times of unpleasant emotions.

THE HAPPILY SOBER ALCOHOLIC

ALL REFERENCES TO the "happily sober alcoholic" are to the

fictional character in these pages. Not every alcoholic must have the same traits, behavior, thinking, and feelings to be happy and content. However, many alcoholics enjoying high-quality sobriety have many of these characteristics at varying degrees.

This description of the happily sober alcoholic doesn't suggest or seek to impose any standards of morality, and it has no moral or immoral implications.

For alcoholics to choose a life without alcohol, they *must* know they will enjoy a sober life more. They must know they will have more self-respect, self-confidence, gratitude, trust, courage, contentment, social support, and other similar feelings produced by alcohol in their early drinking days.

For the alcoholic to know this requires continuous and frequent reminders to act and think differently. These reminders are the purpose of treatment and ongoing recovery support.

Alcoholics, like all people, have different values. While certain conduct might threaten the sobriety of some, it may have little or no effect on others. Still, many principles are naturally universal. For example, most agree that living with intense resentment and remorse leads to a less enjoyable life than living without them. Another principle is the age-old paradoxical axiom: *To keep it, one must give it away.*

Through self-examination, the happily sober alcoholic has discovered these principles, seeking to change the behavior that caused him difficulties. Some principles have been time-tested. Adhering to these principles has allowed many alcoholics to remain sober rather than unhappily abstinent.

Although the happily sober alcoholic may seem spiritually perfect, he's not. Still, he tries living by *self-imposed* principles—a prerequisite to enjoying a sober life—to being happily sober. Many of these principles follow.

Happiness

HAPPINESS IS HARD to describe, although we know when we

feel it and when we don't.

We would never know happiness had we never known sadness. Each of us conceives happiness differently. Our view of happiness typically relates to when we were the happiest. For some, their happiest time may be contentment or euphoria, yet for most, it's somewhere in between.

According to the longest-running Harvard happiness study, now 86 years old, the secret to happiness is close connections with others and focusing on the greater good, which keeps people happier than money, high IQ, fame, or genes.

Although we think of happiness differently, most agree it's the absence of unpleasant emotions flooded with pleasant ones.

THE PURSUIT OF HAPPINESS

THE FOUNDERS OF the United States believed the pursuit of happiness was so vital that they declared it inalienable—a birthright that one could never take or give away. This right is so fundamental that they proclaimed it one reason for declaring independence: "The right to life, liberty, and *the pursuit of happiness.*"

Some have a natural inclination for happiness, while others struggle with unhappiness.* Most fall somewhere in the middle.

As infants, we demand happiness. We smile and coo when happy and cry and scowl when unhappy, endlessly swinging between these extremes within seconds. Our unhappiness, expressed with a shrill scream, can't be ignored.

Over time, we learn we can't always be happy, but we keep trying. We soon enter the "Terrible Twos" and discover an effective technique—the temper tantrum.

We chant, "No, no, no!" while jumping, wildly swinging our arms, and thrashing about. As we see those panicking to

---

*This may include those who are diagnosed with clinical depression requiring medical treatment.

pacify our tantrums, we learn we can control the people around us. Those who quickly satisfy us teach us that we can quickly manage our emotions to get what we want on demand.

As we mature, most of us learn restraint. The lows aren't as low, the highs aren't as high, and they don't change as quickly. The older, wise ones display only minor mood variations—it's almost unnoticed. They don't act like babies when not getting their way. They adapt 'their way' to the way it is.

Then some throw adult temper tantrums. Perhaps they rush out without saying goodbye when their demands aren't met or pout when affection is withheld. Some might stray because they don't get the attention they 'deserve' and 'need.' Others toss a wrench across the floor when provoked by a stubborn bolt or abruptly end a call, ignoring future calls because another isn't acting as they think they should.

Many pursue happiness by getting things their way and getting what they think they want.

Alcoholics, from the first swallow of happiness, obsessively and compulsively insist on getting everything their way and living happily ever after—like an infant.

Many alcoholics abuse alcohol to fulfill their demands and expectations for continuous happiness. They continue using a version of the temper tantrum to get what they want, preferably handed to them on a silver platter. Alcoholics often mimic a two-year-old when not instantly gratified. It could be grumbling, "What's it take to get a drink around here?"

Since drinking reduces inhibitions and self-restraint, the roads that drinkers travel while seeking happiness are often endless and treacherous. Drinking can lead to dangerous adult temper tantrums, causing harsh emotional and physical harm to people and property.

Although alcoholics drink to be happy, in time, alcohol no longer produces the happiness it once did, and as alcoholism progresses, they drink to avoid unhappiness.

So, although many pursue happiness, many others have

learned that happiness does not come from pursuing it but arrives when we take the action that causes it.

To be happy, our lives must feel meaningful—significant—with a sense of community, belonging, and purpose—a *higher purpose*. Thinking of and trying to increase others' happiness is the surest way for the happily sober alcoholic to achieve this.

Recognizing and Sharing Happiness

Abraham Lincoln said, "Folks are usually about as happy as they make their minds up to be." I've seen happiness in those who simply believed they were happy. We must recognize our happiness to feel it, and we must enthusiastically share our happiness—hoarded happiness ceases to be happiness.

Those who are miserly with their happiness feel it evaporate. When we share happiness with others, we deepen and nurture it. For example, if we dine out, we usually prefer to enjoy that pleasure with another. We prefer a companion when enjoying most activities.

Happiness is contagious. There are many ways to share happiness. We might share happiness through community with a support group, with friends and family, by volunteering, or at our place of worship. Perhaps we connect with loved ones to express our happiness. However we do this, there is power in sharing and verbalizing our happiness, which is often contagious. For most, the happiness we feel when we share it is more than when we don't.

So, people strive to be happy differently. Many seek it by seeking pleasure.

SEEKING PLEASURE

PLEASURE IS IN the mind of the beholder. Everyone's notion of pleasure is unique, and it was different yesterday and will likely be different tomorrow. Some sources of pleasure are more popular than others. Once we choose our source of pleasure, our methods of seeking it flow mostly from our experiences and values.

I see two kinds of pleasure: real and artificial. Real pleasure naturally comes from within us, and artificial pleasure unnaturally comes from outside us. Real pleasure is innate—we're born with it. We derive artificial pleasure from something we have learned is pleasurable. Money is an example of something we've learned is pleasant. We weren't born with an appreciation of money. We learned that we can turn money into something that pleases us. Still, both artificial and real pleasure are useful.

A pleasure that soon evaporates signals an artificial pleasure. A real pleasure is timeless and often deepens with time.

Seeking Real Pleasure

PEOPLE SEEK REAL pleasure in various ways. These include practicing moderation, the golden rule, altruism, introspection, creativity, gratitude, forgiveness, or restitution. They could also involve developing genuine connections with others, contributing to the greater good, loving, connecting with a higher power, or recognizing and living for a higher purpose.

When enjoying real pleasure, one often feels confident, hopeful, grateful, forgiving, self-restraint, empathetic, loving, understanding, humorous, content, optimistic, humble, unenvious, introspective, nonjudgmental, patient, honest, and open-minded.

Seeking Real Pleasure Through Moderation

Living moderately is more rewarding than living excessively. Immoderation leads to suffering. Too much of anything is harmful, and examples of this surround us. We suffer when we overeat, drink too much, overspend, or do anything obsessively, compulsively, and excessively.

Overindulgence takes more time, effort, and money than moderation. The sacrifices we make for overindulging detract from and often exceed the pleasure we receive from our excesses. For example, one may buy their dream house, which they can only afford by working so much that they have no time to enjoy it. So, they enjoy it less than the home they replaced.

The happily sober alcoholic avoids self-indulgence and tries living moderately.

According to the Greek philosopher Epicurus (341-270 BC): "The good lies in happiness and happiness is gained in the prudent pursuit of pleasure."

Although Epicurus concluded pleasure was the only goal in life, his meaning of pleasure differed from our common understanding. According to Epicurus, pleasure is not the result of a continuous party of orgies, excessive drinking, eating, and other excesses. Instead, he believed we gain pleasure from self-restraint, sober and moderate thinking, reasoning, seeking knowledge, avoiding drama, and not trampling upon others. He believed one earns it by living a well-respected, unselfish, modest life. That's an example of real happiness, according to Epicurus and others, including the happily sober alcoholic.

Seeking Real Pleasure by Connecting with Others

The paradox is that the more pleasure costs, the less valuable it often is. We don't always get what we pay for. Those with friends are usually happier than those without friends. Who we eat with is more important than what we eat. Sitting alone in our new car will not produce as much pleasure as sitting in it with another. Going to the theatre will often wait until we find the right person to enjoy it with. So it is with most events.

No one disputes that we need each other. We feel lonely when we're alone and want to be with others. Whenever we ignore our need for companionship, we feel discomfort or worse. Ignored loneliness often turns into distressing feelings of sadness, depression, fear, and anxiety and can breed suicidal thoughts.

Still, loneliness isn't a bad feeling—it only feels bad. In earlier times, when alone, we were susceptible to attacks. Like a herd of animals, the one in the middle of the pack is the most protected. So loneliness is a helpful reminder for the happily sober alcoholic to "get with the herd" and socialize.

For example, using solitary confinement as punishment has proven our need for others. Forcing one to be alone is the most severe punishment in prisons. Some have described solitary confinement as "death before dying." Social isolation deprives us of the stimulation our brain needs. Isolation causes psychosis, suicidal ideation, hypersensitivity, problems with reasoning and concentration, paranoia, and hallucinations, even in those with no former mental disorders.

Those enduring this cruelty have said extended isolation is more painful than physical torture. Recently, the courts have also found isolation is "cruel and unusual punishment." So, today, it is only used briefly for temporary protection under strict conditions and can no longer be used as punishment.

The alcoholic's increasing time drinking alone often identifies the final stage of alcoholism. The alcoholic, who has progressed to drinking mostly in isolation, is typically more severe than one drinking socially in crowded bars.

We can't feel happy if we're lonely, and we can't feel lonely if we're happy and feel a sense of belonging.

Not that alone time is always unpleasant. Being alone when we choose to be alone, without isolating or feeling lonely, is healthy, pleasurable, and essential. It creates a suitable atmosphere for effective meditation, contemplation, and self-reflection, which provides us with the strength, insight, and energy we need to serve others. Some need more aloneness than others.

On the other hand, pathological attention seekers try to avoid loneliness by always being the life of the party—the center of attention—dominating conversations.

The spread of social media also reveals our need to socialize. Those who are introverted and uncomfortable mingling find this method more compatible with their personality.

For many today, online gaming (not gambling) fulfills this need to socialize. Having an opponent, even an anonymous one, allows many to feel a part of a larger community. Yet it has become so popular and is so potentially addictive that the American Psychiatric Association is considering including it as a mental disorder in a future edition of the DSM.[1]*

People satisfy their need to socialize in various ways. For example, the consensus is that most join terrorist or other hostile groups out of a compelling need to feel a sense of belonging.

Moreover, many worthwhile organizations thrive because of our social needs. One benefit of Alcoholics Anonymous is the community it offers. Those AA members most involved typically enjoy a quality of sobriety exceeding and outlasting those loitering on the fringes. One predictor of relapse is the alcoholic isolating from others in recovery.

Seeking Real Pleasure with Thoughts

Thoughts produce feelings. Negative thoughts create unpleasant feelings, and positive thoughts fuel pleasant feelings. And even though we know this, we often forget it when feeling down. Some of us are prone to pleasant thoughts, while others lean toward unpleasant ones. The happily sober alcoholic is mindful of this and strives to think positively.

For example, thoughts of someone we blame for harming us could cause resentment, anger, hatred, hostility, anxiety, self-righteousness, and condemnation.

Thoughts of pleasurable times with friends, anticipating a fun event, or appreciating what we have rather than focusing on what we don't have will produce pleasurable feelings. These feelings include affection, well-being, trust, gratitude, confidence, self-esteem, tranquility, and contentment.

---

*China has treatment centers for the treatment of online gaming addicts.

Seeking Artificial Pleasure

SEEKING ARTIFICIAL PLEASURE to achieve happiness may temporarily make us happy if the cost of the pleasure doesn't exceed the value it produces. Still, some methods of achieving happiness are healthier than others.

For example, some people seek pleasure in hobbies. This is healthy unless it becomes obsessive and compulsive, causing problems such as missing work, important events, family time, or other essential obligations.

There are many common ways people pursue fleeting artificial pleasure, such as acquiring money and property, controlling others, getting what they think they want, chasing fame, involvement in a new love relationship, enjoying a pleasant physical sensation, self-righteously judging others (seeing others as inferior to falsely inflate self-esteem), and using drugs and alcohol.

Seeking Artificial Pleasure by Avoiding Displeasure

Most of everyone's actions and inactions, including alcoholics, are primarily motivated by seeking pleasure and avoiding displeasure. The alcoholic's tolerance for displeasure is exceptionally low. Alcoholics can't recapture the euphoria enjoyed during their early drinking days as drinking becomes less pleasurable. This is caused by the alcoholic's brain constantly adjusting to the pleasure produced by drinking, known as tolerance. But the alcoholic's brain often demands nothing less than the most pleasure ever felt. The more pleasure alcoholics feel, the more they want and think they need.

The primary method the drinking alcoholic uses to achieve this pleasure is by drinking, and drugs often assist. However, the alcoholic often obsessively seeks this elusive pleasure even after it's lost forever, which usually results in displeasure or worse.

In recovery, the happily sober alcoholic has learned many ways to feel pleasure other than by drinking. He avoids destructive methods, which produce brief pleasure trailed by displeasure and unhappiness. Recovery has provided him with healthy ways to feel pleasure.

Seeking Artificial Pleasure with Money

Not all money is the same. For example, money has no value if it can't be spent. How we get and spend money determines how much we enjoy it. What we do with a surplus of money regulates our happiness. Those who hoard large sums seem less happy than those who create foundations to help others.

If one believes pleasure is amassing wealth, there are several ways to do this. Some will pursue a higher education only to earn more. Whether they're happy or unhappy in their career is less important than their salary.

Some steal. Some manipulate others by pretending to love them so they can live a life they believe will bring them happiness. They do this with little effort, blindly sacrificing the real pleasures of a genuine relationship. They ignore the harm they cause because they see their victims as merely objects to acquire pleasure from.

Others seek money through manipulation, fraud, fear, extortion, terror, force, or other self-centered and destructive methods, further disregarding others.

However, the wealthy know that a surplus of money will not buy happiness, and the not-so-wealthy would like enough wealth to reach their own conclusion.

Many try accumulating much more than they need. They soon discover that a surplus of possessions brings little pleasure. Instead, it produces displeasure as the fear of losing possessions lingers, requiring effort to defeat this useless fear. Wealth also demands accountability, which requires time and effort and distracts from pleasure. The wealthy endure other money-related difficulties proportionately related to their net worth.

For example, many lottery winners endure these difficulties. It can be unsettling when former and current friends, unknown distant relatives, acquaintances, and strangers repeatedly ask for money. Relationships often become strained, rarely returning to normal if one refuses or gives less than requested.

Those who believe having more will make them happier often sacrifice real pleasure to accumulate more and more for fleeting moments of security and pleasure. But it's never enough, and feeling one never has enough is unpleasant, especially when it's never enough of what one has plenty of and doesn't truly want or need.

A Harvard Business School study found that "spending money on others makes us happier than spending it on ourselves."[2] This study reveals that if one can afford shelter, food, and clothing, one has most of the happiness money can buy.[3*] Beyond this, more money, from a small amount to billions, may produce slightly more or less happiness—yet it's hardly noticed.

The happily sober alcoholic knows one way to have enough is to realize he has enough. He knows that no financial fortune alone will bring long-term or real happiness. His self-worth is unrelated to his net worth.

Seeking Artificial Pleasure with Things

Artificial pleasure doesn't last as long as natural pleasure, which the familiar phrase, "The newness wore off," supports. An example of fleeting artificial pleasure is the new car experience.

We're happy with our new car until the novelty and pleasure soon fade. We make each payment less eagerly than the last one. Some try reviving this pleasure by tricking their minds into thinking it's a new car again with popular air fresheners described as "new car scent." We ignore that the

---

*Enough money is considered a $64,000 annual salary in Mississippi, $67,000 in Oklahoma, and $104,300 in New York. The happiness benchmark for the national average is $75,000.

fragrance we're trying to recreate is toxic fumes off-gassing from plastics, adhesives, paints, sealers, and compounds used to create the car's interior. It's not the scent we desire; it's the pleasure we once associated with that scent we seek to 're-sense.' If it were the "new car scent" we sought and not the brief pleasure of owning a new car, it would be a cologne fragrance.

Seeking Artificial Pleasure with Romance

Although rarely acknowledged, the 'in love' feeling is often a fleeting artificial pleasure, usually lasting a few months to a few years. The 'symptoms' of being in love are like the symptoms of various emotional disorders, which foster the misbelief that passionate love could and should last forever.

Those seeking but failing to preserve this vanishing 'in love' high will soon decide the bond isn't real and move on to the next one, discarding it as if it were a spent disposable item. They repeat this pattern of finally finding the right one only to discover, once again, that they erred, insisting they were deceived. Yet, they remain motivated to continue searching for a fairy-tale relationship.

Their craving for the intoxicating effects of the pleasure they seek will tumble with unpleasant emotions, sometimes suicide-provoking, until death they do part. Many sober alcoholics fall into this addictive trap.

Despite this, for many, a commitment survives this 'honeymoon period' and evolves into genuine love and companionship, lasting forever and enhancing real happiness. It becomes a real pleasure. (This is discussed further under "Romantic Relationships In Sobriety.")

Seeking Artificial Pleasure Selfishly

Those who focus only on themselves are emotionally isolated and usually unhappy. Within this isolation emerges a conviction that no one understands them or their 'unique' situation. They feel no gratitude, only lingering self-pity while forecasting doom and gloom.

When we're down, it's a struggle to be other-centered. But I have repeatedly seen unhappiness, sadness, and self-pity instantly vanish when helping another, and I've often seen the opposite when one is self-absorbed.

The happily sober alcoholic asks himself at the end of each day, "Who did I reach out to today? Did I call or text someone wishing to brighten their day?" He accepts that to be happy and content, he must be *reasonably* other-centered.

Higher Purpose, Meaning, And Connection

ALTHOUGH TO SOME, pursuing a purpose, meaning, and connection may sound too esoteric and intangible to pursue, the happily sober alcoholic and others know, "Of course, you can't be happy without this pursuit!"

We're unhappy if we feel in an isolated rut and our lives are mundane, insignificant, and unimportant. We may feel we're nothing more than a cluster of cells the world neither recognizes nor cares to recognize nor is worthy of recognition.

Perhaps we endure chronic dissatisfaction—a feeling that things just aren't right. Some feeling this way often believe they're the only ones feeling this, while others believe everyone feels this emptiness. The truth is, the happily sober alcoholic and many others don't feel this way but feel fulfilled.

We may endure a nagging, persistent feeling that there must be more to life and that we're missing out. We should trust our feelings. If we feel there's more to life and we're missing out, there *is* more to life, and we *are* missing out! The good news is this situation is a choice we can change.

So, if we're missing out, what are we missing? Of course, to find what we're missing, we must know what to look for. Yet that becomes difficult when we vaguely sense we're missing something but don't know what it is. We will begin to discover the answer simply by starting the search.

The happily sober alcoholic has found the answer. He doesn't ask what he can get from others but asks what he can give. His transparency attracts, and he's often joyful and optimistic. He feels recognized and significant. He feels good and is good. He awakes eager to start the unpredictable day because he has a higher purpose.

The Higher Purpose

Having a higher purpose and meaning in life is essential to happiness. No research disputes this, and here is more good news: Those who strive to improve the lives of others are happier than those who think only of themselves.

To live a life with a higher purpose starts with asking ourselves, "How?" Asking this one-word question begins a new life with a higher purpose, a better life than ever imagined. It is a purpose that convinces us we are significant yet reminds us we're not too significant. The higher purpose causes us to focus on the significance of others.

The principles of the higher purpose help us realize that we receive by giving and are understood by understanding. The happily sober alcoholic strives to provide love, faith, hope, light, and joy where he sees hatred, doubt, despair, darkness, and sadness. His life has meaning, and he experiences real, timeless contentment.

These principles are not new. They have existed since humans have. Still, it's not as unselfish as one might think. When we *strive* to help others, we benefit. If no one ever helped another, we wouldn't exist. It's natural law or, if you will, higher law. Noncompliance ensures less pleasure.

Striving *only* for personal success is not a goal of a higher purpose and will fail. Nothing I'm saying implies personal success is wrong or unpleasant. Whether it feels right and pleasant depends on how we get it and our motives.

If we pursue happiness by only thinking of ourselves, happiness will remain elusive. Yet, striving to improve the world will inevitably shower us with happiness and satisfaction. Also, as we build character through our service to others, our meaning of happiness will change.

Some discount those who have made a widespread, valuable impact, claiming they were merely at the right place and time to exploit it. And while that may be true, it ignores that many who were similarly situated could have acted but didn't.

Often, those who acted assumed enormous risks without expecting any return. They endured sacrifices that they didn't view as sacrificial. Others failed to act because they didn't choose to assume the risk or make the sacrifice. Also, many others who took similar action yet received no external credit still reaped countless benefits.

That's because they had a higher purpose for acting. Their life had meaning. They felt significant. They didn't feel they were missing out. They believed that struggling to realize a goal and missing it is better than never trying. Great intentions, shackled by self-distraction, stop us from taking action and yield nothing. The higher purpose is free from the distractions of focusing on self.

Feeling Connected to the Higher Purpose

We must *feel* connected with others to fulfill a higher purpose, which will lead us on the right path. The happily sober alcoholic feels passionately connected. He helps others gain and maintain sobriety through a peer support program or other similar society. If another's drinking has affected us, we can help others similarly affected by becoming involved in a program like Al-Anon or another organization.

If we have religious or spiritual beliefs, we can visit our place of worship or engage with other like-minded people. Additionally, involvement in compatible organizations will give us the gift of community as we connect with others.

The happily sober alcoholic has gained a new perspective

and a more profound sense of meaning and hope by taking the right action. He makes the center of his attention something other than only himself. He doesn't allow the trivial incidents that, at the time, seem much more significant than they are to dissuade him from his higher purpose.

He has formed meaningful friendships. He may pray and meditate and enjoy quiet and calm contemplation, which allows him to help others and support his community. He feels contently connected.

NAVIGATING LIFE FOR THE HAPPILY SOBER ALCOHOLIC

THE HAPPILY SOBER alcoholic does not drink nor endure the alcoholic-craving. He no longer feels shackled by active alcoholism, and this freedom supports his happiness and contentment. He doesn't want to drink. He feels neutral about alcohol. He doesn't silently wish that someday he can drink; the thought of a drink doesn't move him. He accepts his alcoholism with gratitude and doesn't question it. He appreciates his sober life, made possible by his affliction, and it shows. His enlightenment has altered his vision.

He knows his sobriety must come first or be threatened. He realizes if he loses his sobriety, he will lose whatever he placed before it, including work, family, loved ones, and anything or anyone else. So, he prioritizes effectively.

He has no desire to engage in other unhealthy, self-seeking, pleasure-producing, addictive activities.

He is helpful and contributes to society. He doesn't feel overwhelming guilt, remorse, anger, or resentment. He is other-centered, not thinking too much or too little of himself.

He's proactive, not reactive. He lives modestly. He accepts responsibility for his actions, allowing him to manage his behavior. He's fearlessly introspective. He engages in meditation, self-reflection, and contemplation. He's physically and emotionally healthy. He seeks knowledge. Instead of seeking love, he seeks to love and give more than he receives.

He has inner strength and is appropriately self-confident. He resists seeming arrogant since that could separate him and prevent him from being helpful to others. He believes in himself, his goals, and his wisdom. His self-confidence prevents him from feeling threatened when his belief system is challenged. He appreciates challenges as an opportunity to see where he may be wrong and invites opposing views for growth. This identification of his wrongs allows him to walk on the right path.

Humor

Many say that genuine laughter can't occur when one is feeling sad. Yet I've seen humor rescue many from sadness, parting the way for laughter, which heals and is an essential tool for healthy, long-term sobriety.

Most of us have acted in ways when drinking that caused harm to ourselves and others. However, the happily sober alcoholic can laugh at his past behavior without insensitivity to those affected by it. He knows that without this humorous perspective, he may remain so chained to the past that guilt and self-loathing may reach a crescendo so painful and debilitating that it prompts a relapse.

So, he has a good sense of humor and doesn't take himself, others, or anything too seriously. He can easily laugh, even at himself.

Gratitude

The happily sober alcoholic is grateful for what he has and doesn't focus on what he doesn't have. If nothing else, at the moment, he's sober. This mindfulness of sobriety creates immediate contentment and pleasure. His gratitude usually crushes displeasure and includes the desire to give away what he has been so fortunate to receive.

Often, throughout the day, he focuses on his appreciation for sobriety and life. He briefly concentrates on his breathing—slowly inhaling and exhaling—feeling gratitude, focusing on the abundance of good in his life. This attitude edges out self-pity triggered by self-deception. His optimism is contagious. He knows that his happiness is his responsibility, not anyone else's. This knowledge gives him a positive attitude, enriching his happiness and sobriety.

He connects with a Power he doesn't understand, allowing him to experience the many benefits of unselfishness. This connection is uniquely his.

He sees others discouraged who believe they're missing out on the make-believe, glamorous life presented as reality by much of commercial entertainment. He doesn't pursue negative entertainment or information and is cautious when seeking superficial pleasure. He has reminders that trigger positive thinking while resisting negativity.

Relations With Others

The happily sober alcoholic's relations with others result in real pleasure more than artificial pleasure. He strives to live by the Golden Rule, treating others how he likes to be treated. Regularly attending a support group reminds him to practice positive principles.

Whether a lawyer, refuse worker, doctor, painter, CPA, plumber, teacher, published author, or Indian chief, he doesn't define himself by his occupation. Instead, he knows his status is situational. He doesn't look up to or down on anyone based on their socioeconomic standing, nor compare it to his.

He's comfortable socializing with the poor or wealthy, the dropout or the professor, the intellectually challenged or brilliant, the inmate or warden, the accused or judge, the atheist or preacher, the old or young, and the alcoholic or nonalcoholic.

He does not demand respect—his actions invite it. Rather than complain about something, he acts to change it. He knows his actions, not his intentions, make a difference. He often does for others anonymously and resists revealing his good deeds to anyone. He appreciates compliments but does not solicit nor need them. He doesn't boast about his accomplishments.

He learns and benefits most when listening, so he's often silent. He doesn't monopolize nor compete to talk during conversations. He doesn't believe what he says is more important than what others say. He knows everyone has a story worth hearing.

He is gentle with himself and others. He avoids loud, thoughtless, self-centered, and aggressive people. Although he sees injustices globally, this view doesn't stop him from focusing on the good that abounds. He's realistic yet not cynical. Rather than grumbling about the thorns on a rosebush, he appreciates the roses on a bush of thorns.

He's unenvious. He knows envy is comparing a distorted view of what he has with a distorted view of what another has, yielding an illusion. Since envy is the product of this illusionary thinking, it's meaningless, whether he's the envied or the envier. He doesn't invite envy from others by boasting about his good fortune. So, he can't measure if he has it better or worse than the target of his comparisons and believes it doesn't matter.

Open-Mindedness

The happily sober alcoholic is emotionally, intellectually, and spiritually flexible. He reminds himself to be open-minded and realizes his way is not always the only or the best way. He is open to suggestions and opposing views. The more knowledge he receives, the more he recognizes how little he knows. He continuously seeks alternative views and isn't intellectually lazy.

Counseling With Others

The happily sober alcoholic is aware that his self-perception differs from how others see him. He knows the perceptions of others are likely more accurate than his self-reflection. He considers and respects feedback from others.

He doesn't see constructive criticism as condemnation. He appreciates those who care enough to confront him about his conduct rather than those who tell him what they *think* he wants to hear. He invites enlightening criticism, enabling him to grow, expose areas of denial, and strengthen his sobriety.

Likewise, he offers no advice unless it's invited and from an earnest desire to help. He's cautious and refrains from advising about a problem he has neither had nor knows enough about. He knows he can be helpful by sharing his experience, strength, and hope rather than his irrelevant opinion, weakness, and despair. As a result, the time he spends improving his character leaves little time to focus on the flaws of others.

He follows through with his commitments. He doesn't accept unacceptable behavior nor try to control another's conduct to make it acceptable—he knows that would be futile. He respects the boundaries of others and avoids those who disrespect his.

Right or Wrong: Does it Matter?

The happily sober alcoholic realizes that it's unrealistic to think he can or should avoid *all* disputes. Still, he selects his battles carefully. The emotional expense of a conflict must be worth the potential benefits. Not every wrong is his to make right. Not every battle is his to fight. And what he perceives as wrong today, he may see as right tomorrow.

He doesn't need to control others. He responds rather than reacts. He doesn't feel compelled to debate issues with anyone holding a different opinion. Before trying to persuade one to agree with him, he asks himself, "Why?"

He understands that specific subjects provoke heated debate. So, he's cautious about discussing politics, religion, or any sensitive topic with those holding different views. Before he does, he asks himself, "What useful purpose will it serve if I persuade this person to agree with me?" Usually, the answer is none.

He realizes that convincing a stranger he's right is often meaningless, and even with those he's close to, not every disagreement can or needs to be resolved. He's aware that when trying to solve one problem, several others often arise. Although unintentional, they can become so unmanageable, unproductive, and hurtful that it's usually best to agree to disagree and move on.

He knows that when emotions are involved, logical resolutions are scarce, and a cooling-off period usually proves beneficial, increasing the probability of a productive discussion and identifying a solution.

Therefore, before deciding whether to discuss an issue or try to persuade one to see it his way, he asks himself:

1. Why? What is my purpose and motive? What am I trying to accomplish?
2. How important is the issue?
3. How meaningful is the relationship?
4. Can the issue or disagreement be resolved?
5. How helpful will any discussion be?
6. What could be the benefit if I persuade someone to believe as I do about a topic?
7. What could be the outcome if no resolution is reached?

This self-inquiry allows him to prevent trivial issues from becoming wars, causing resentment. He's also keenly aware that resentments once fueled his drinking, and they never support quality sobriety.

Secrets

He's aware that secrets can hinder his openness and connections with others, resulting in feelings that don't support sobriety. So he has those he trusts and confides in to share any secrets. Likewise, others trust him, and he protects their trust.

Expectations

He believes any demand or expectation he has that others adhere to his prescribed standards of conduct is destructive. He neither places people on pedestals nor invites others to elevate him, knowing that those glorified can't sustain the image cast upon them and will ultimately fail those glorifying them. Although occasionally disappointed by people's actions, they don't let him down because he expects people to be human and imperfect.

Friendships

He doesn't avoid people. Instead, he makes friends and avoids creating enemies. He values his friendships and doesn't judge his friends' thinking and behavior in terms of black or white, good or bad. He is flexible. He realizes that a true friendship is a commitment, and he doesn't casually end a friendship because his friend made a mistake and didn't live up to his rigid expectations.

He knows that as friendships develop, imperfections are revealed and that real friendships are unconditional—real friends befriend the whole rather than a part of the person. Real friendships are rare and aren't constrained by inflexible conditions and contingencies. Instead, friends work through issues that arise.

His friendships are mutually supportive, and he gives without keeping score.

If the end of a friendship is inevitable, he strives to close it amicably and with dignity without casting blame or talking badly about the other.

In short, he knows his friends are a valuable part of his sobriety, and he cherishes his friendships.

Dealing with Guilt and Remorse

Although guilt and remorse are closely aligned, there is a difference. Guilt is a distressing emotion that we feel when our wrong behavior harms others. This distress from guilt can include anxiety, low self-esteem, embarrassment, sleep disruption, and other conditions that alcoholics tend to treat with alcohol.

Remorse is regretting past actions that harmed others and wanting to make it right.

The happily sober alcoholic knows happiness doesn't coexist with guilt and remorse—emotions that call for a drink. Still, he has tools to lighten or abolish guilt and remorse. One of these tools is righting his wrongs by admitting and expressing remorse for the wrong, keeping his promise not to repeat it, and *trying* to repair the damage he caused, *if* reparable.

When he has wronged another, he quickly tries to make it right. He knows it becomes more difficult to admit his wrongs as time passes, so he tries doing it as soon as appropriate and practical. The longer he delays, the more time he has to justify his actions and falsely shift blame onto another.

He realizes that repairing the harm he caused usually requires more than a simple apology. He aims to restore the damage to where it was before his transgression. If appropriate, he will ask the person harmed if they have any suggestions for him to make it right.

He must be sure that any proposed reparations won't hurt anyone. He can't see the ripple effect of his actions as clearly as others can. So he doesn't undertake significant repairs without talking with someone he trusts. He is open-minded to various viewpoints.

He understands that forgotten mistakes are often repeated, and without identifying or *only* focusing on the problem, a solution can't be found.

He sees and accepts the role he plays in all events. When wrong, he admits it and doesn't blame others to avoid responsibility. When right, he doesn't need to convince others of this.

He has removed or reduced guilt to tolerable levels and acts to avoid future guilt and remorse.

Romantic Relationships in Sobriety

AS DISCUSSED EARLIER, romance can be the source of real or fleeting artificial pleasure or both and can also be a source of misery. The happily sober alcoholic approaches romance with cautious optimism, understanding it can be deceptively inviting and pervasively destructive.

Sadly, some can't love but crave being loved. Many know, including the happily sober alcoholic, that the pleasure realized from loving is greater than being loved.

He knows real love is a decision more than a feeling. It's a decision to commit to and encourage each other to grow emotionally, intellectually, and spiritually. This connection improves individual growth—it doesn't thwart it. It's an unselfish union in which each strives to give more than they receive without keeping score.

It is not limiting. The couple are best friends but not each other's only friends. They are partners. They trust the other's commitment and enjoy solid contentment. Their love grows. Rather than holding a grudge, they communicate. They accept the other's weaknesses and strengths. They don't keep dark secrets. They don't censor their expressions, fearing a reaction. They don't walk on eggshells. They're direct but not intentionally hurtful. They enjoy their freedom and allow each other to be themselves.

However, not all romantic connections last forever. If it ends, the happily sober alcoholic doesn't find it necessary or desirable to have someone waiting in the wings to cushion his fall. He knows jumping too quickly from one to another is an unhealthy need to avoid himself. It would prevent him from enjoying the freedom of treasured and unaccountable alone time.

Perhaps, for a time, he will be free of distractions, letting him pursue significant and timeless experiences. He eagerly sees a chance to embark on a new voyage of exciting exploration rather than obsessively and destructively thinking of the past and dreading the fictional future. He can't know what tomorrow will bring.

Just as water seeks its own level, so do people. Therefore, criticizing a former partner silently or publicly is self-criticism. It is unproductive and the product of spoiled motives. The purpose is to falsely boost self-esteem, avoid any responsibility, seek sympathy, and bury the hurt by convincing oneself that one is not losing someone of value. Yet, everyone has value.

Although he knows that some sadness and disappointment are natural when a relationship ends, many negative feelings are optional and unproductive, resulting from fear of his imagined future.

He sees this as an opportunity to step outside himself and focus more on helping others.

He's convinced he doesn't need a relationship to feel whole and content. Happiness and quality sobriety don't require romance. Conversely, 'romance' often sparks unhappiness and threatens sobriety.

He will not seek a new relationship, but he knows it must be built on a solid foundation if it happens. He has no desire to look back and will only do so to capture information that could help him or another. He knows his experience may be helpful. He believes, "When one door closes, others open" because he's seen it happen repeatedly. He will not sacrifice his sobriety with obsessive, fictional, romantic thoughts.

Trust

The happily sober alcoholic knows unfaithfulness breeds deceit and manipulation. With infidelity, the deception is as or more damaging than the activity it hides. Living this lie by betraying the one he claims to care about would drain pleasure and undermine his sobriety.

He knows that misusing a partner's trust would be hurtful, causing the deceived 'loved one' to put up taller and thicker walls. These walls can quickly become so impenetrable that love can't seep through. Love that can't flow freely can't be given or received and ceases to be love.

He understands that his abuse of another's trust would weaken his ability to trust others, poisoning him with suspicious thinking, which alone would compromise his sobriety.

Exclusivity

If he's committed to a sexually exclusive relationship, he will not be sexual with anyone other than his partner. This means not acting in any way with another that stimulates sexual interest, flirting, communicating suggestively, and hiding this conduct. Nor will he act in a way that could reasonably arouse suspicion or be sexual with another before making his partner aware that he is changing the nature of the relationship.

Jealousy

He avoids feelings of jealousy resulting from obsessive, distorted thinking and resists arousing jealousy. He's aware that his partner may not see his behavior as innocently as he does. He knows that believing everyone thinks and reacts like he does is self-centered.

If his partner chooses or desires another, that is her need based on her experience, personality, values, and character and has little to do with him. He will resolve any feelings of rejection.

If jealousy contaminates the relationship, justified or not, he knows it's damaged. He will invest reasonable efforts to heal it, realizing the benefit each receives from this effort will survive even if their bond doesn't.

If the relationship ends, he lets go of any restraints binding him to any illusions of reconciliation and, with dignity and anticipation, moves forward, never backward.

Sex and Sobriety

The happily sober alcoholic insists on walking with dignity in every area of his life. It's no longer acceptable to act as he did when drinking, especially regarding his sexual activity. Since he no longer numbs his feelings with alcohol, he knows his sexual conduct could negatively affect others and the maintenance of his sobriety.

Sexual Motives and Responsibility

He has examined, in-depth, the way he acted sexually when drinking. With assistance, he has seen where his motives were selfish, dishonest, and hurtful. Flowing from this self-appraisal were principles he *strives* to live by.

He knows that to sustain quality sobriety, he must commit to following his self-imposed principles. If he doesn't strive to conduct his sex life accordingly, contented sobriety will elude him, increasing the chances of a relapse.

He can no longer shrug off insensitive sexual activity as unthinking, a slight indiscretion, or a reckless moment—his actions are now intentional.

He knows sex can cause pleasure or displeasure, intimacy or distance. One can experience sex at different levels of consciousness and pursue it with pure or tainted motives and for various reasons. It can be a weapon to control, manipulate, or used to express affection or anger. It can create life. What act is more powerful? It must be appreciated, not minimized nor condemned, nor used to abuse.

When deciding whether to engage sexually, he examines his motives. He questions whether he's being honest, selfish, or potentially hurtful. He looks at possible outcomes. He avoids sex if it's only to satisfy his self-interest at another's expense.

Although he knows sex between consenting adults usually produces pleasure, he's keenly aware that one may decide sex is consensual when it's nothing more than skillful manipulation.

Although he will date a normal drinker, he will not have sex with one who is drunk or in obvious emotional distress. Neither can consent to something without knowing what they are consenting to.

He no longer believes that his behavior is acceptable merely by disclaiming any responsibility for any romantic feelings his partner may develop. His disclaimer that planned sex is casual and seeking an agreement that neither will become emotionally involved is manipulative, misleading, insincere, self-seeking, and dishonest. He knows and accepts that one can't forecast or disclaim affection.

He avoids sex with someone who has romantic feelings obviously exceeding his. He knows that sexual intimacy will likely increase those feelings, eventually causing emotional distress, which will outweigh his brief and instant gratification.

He resists using people or being used as an object. He won't have sex with one who uses it to avenge or must hide it from another. He knows a series of meaningless sexual moments can't sustain happiness. He doesn't pursue sex as a challenge or to build self-esteem.

He listens to the calm, quiet voice of truth and reason—his conscience—exposing his rationalization and guiding his decisions. If he ignores this voice, feelings incongruent with healthy, sober living will deluge him.

He resists expressing negativity if he feels rejected—real or imagined. When he has an unsatisfied sexual urge, he seeks to rise above these instinctual demands and has learned various ways of doing this. By doing what's right and following his ideals, he has self-respect and dignity, experiencing real pleasure instead of artificial pleasure laced with guilt, doubt, regret, and other self-destructive feelings that threaten his treasured sobriety.

HE CONSIDERS SEXUAL 'foreplay' a time of emotional intimacy before physical intimacy, which can last for minutes, hours, days, or longer. It includes nonsexual activities, like listening, caring, and sharing, which intensifies the connection, producing stimulating anticipation and heightening arousal for both. He doesn't view it as a distraction or an annoyance.

During sex, he is other-centered and strives to be emotionally present. He is keenly aware that some have endured unfortunate experiences preventing them from enjoying various levels of intimacy. He is in tune with his partner. He doesn't impose his level of comfort on anyone. If he acts appropriately, both will experience pleasure and an elevated contentment and connection.

Afterward, he remains other-centered and sensitive to his partner's needs. His partner is not a disposable item. He doesn't abruptly withdraw emotionally, consider the event concluded, and leave his partner unfulfilled or feeling used and objectified.

He will briefly reflect to determine whether he was self-centered or other-centered. If he were selfish, his sobriety will suffer. Conversely, his unselfishness will enhance his sobriety.

JUDGMENTAL VERSUS JUDGING

THE HAPPILY SOBER ALCOHOLIC realizes it's naïve to think he could cruise through life without ever judging anyone, nor would he want to.

He's aware that our brains process about 35,000 judgments each day.[4] His judgments of others determine his friends, co-workers, spouses, romantic relationships, and the duration and closeness of these relationships. His judgments dictate who he spends time with, who he avoids, and who he dates, marries, and divorces. His judgments govern how he guides his children, who they play with, and what they do.

He recognizes that all of his choices are the product of his judgments, and he is the sum of his choices. Healthy choices flowing from sound and sober judgments are essential to his good, sober life.

That said, he knows that *judging* and *judgmental* are words with different meanings, although they are commonly and incorrectly used interchangeably.

The Judgmental Person

To be judgmental is to pass judgment prematurely and unfairly. It's a prejudicial rush to judgment based on false assumptions, not facts.

The happily sober alcoholic sees the judgmental person walk arrogantly with misinformation and flawed opinions while resisting the truth.

Judgmental people recklessly and wrongfully assign fault. They set standards by which they judge others—usually based only on their values, which mostly flow from childhood indoctrination.

They are habitually critical and blaming, rarely living up to the standards they set for everyone else. Instead, they expect others never to cross the boundary line they've drawn—the same line they freely cross repeatedly with impunity.

They find specific actions of another contemptuous but do not self-condemn their similar conduct. For example, if asked to reconcile their double standard, they search for unimportant, distinguishable facts to support their hollow explanation of why their behavior is different and acceptable. Or they dismiss it as not worthy of a response.

Judgmental people don't follow the golden rule; they don't think about it. They are closed-minded and resist alternative views. Their rigid belief system must remain untouched since any penetration could cause their world to implode. They will forever defend their reckless judgments and promptly interrupt anyone who questions them, even gently.

Since judgmental behavior includes casting blame on others unjustifiably, judgmental people will forever ignore any sound resistance to their conclusion. Some will even destroy any contrary evidence to avoid appearing wrong. This is especially true when they've continually tried to convince the world they're always right when they rarely are.

They are self-absorbed, dictatorial, and unforgiving, which artificially inflates their self-worth. They don't seek to understand; they seek to be understood while insatiably seeking acceptance and validation. They indulge in innuendos, gossip, and character assassination with the intent to harm.

They are intolerant of most people except the few they have successfully manipulated. They insist that everyone's thinking should mimic theirs. They invest enormous energy and incur significant risks to look good, often at the expense of others.

In short, judgmental people strive to elevate their self-esteem by belittling and putting others down.

The Nonjudgmental Person

The happily sober alcoholic refrains from rushing to judgment and believes Herbert Spencer's statement, "Contempt prior to investigation leaves a man in everlasting ignorance." He's learned there's more than one side to every story—usually many.

He realizes people have various motives for releasing rumors. Their agenda may not be one he agrees, disagrees with, or finds appropriate for his involvement. When informed about someone else, he asks himself, "Why am I being told this?" He doesn't casually respond, supporting a one-sided opinion of another he hasn't heard from. He knows those who gossip to him will likely gossip about him.

After ascertaining the truth, he may judge certain events, actions, and things. He no longer sets the standards by which he judges others. He understands these standards can become the shackles preventing his growth, and every judgmental thought or expression tightens these restraints.

RESENTMENT, FORGIVENESS, AND INTROSPECTION

THE HAPPILY SOBER ALCOHOLIC is aware that anger is often a healthy feeling. Productive anger provides him with the energy to protect himself or others. Conversely, unproductive anger wastes vital energy. Unnecessarily nurtured anger leaves him needlessly exhausted as it becomes useless resentment.

Resentment

The happily sober alcoholic hasn't forgotten that when he drank, he thrived on resentments because they gave him 'good' reasons to drink guilt-free. Knowing that resentments provoke drinking, he avoids them.

Resentment means to *re-feel* or *re-sense* anger. Our obsessive thinking often causes us to relive the event that caused the initial anger, which becomes resentment.

For example, if someone slaps us, we may become angry, which is a natural, healthy, and reasonable response. We may feel angry for several days or longer. But if 10 years later we're still angry, that's resentment and unhealthy—*we've* now become the problem.

While anger usually results in outward and aggressive actions such as rage, resentment is felt inwardly and manifests in many unhealthy ways. These ways include wasting substantial time rationalizing behavior and obsessing about retribution. Resentments can also cause serious physical health problems. Nurtured resentments cause us to be more cynical, sarcastic, hostile, angry, and hateful—and the ones we resent are usually oblivious.

The happily sober alcoholic knows that resentments nurture the harm that initially sparked it, causing the harm to persist and expand—sometimes for life.

If he lets his resentments fester, he damages the quality of his life and his sobriety by focusing on and emotionally living with a person he resents and probably never wants to see again.

Wherever he goes, the person he resents tags along, chained to him, doing everything he does. They sleep with him and invade his dreams. They're the last to say goodnight and the first to say good morning. They're a passenger when he travels. They are a dinner guest and rudely interrupt his conversations. Although they are usually unaware of their intrusion, they become his master.

He must remain free of this destructive thinking and feeling, and he knows that forgiveness is the only way for him to remove or lessen resentment.

Forgiveness

The happily sober alcoholic understands that forgiveness is all about *his* healing, and though the feeling of resentment is preferable to many other emotions, it eventually takes its toll.

He's heard many harboring resentments insist their offender doesn't deserve forgiveness. They say, "I'm so angry, I'll never forgive him!" The problem with this thinking is that the transgressor usually has no idea they're resented or unforgiven. We are the ones suffering from the resentment, not the offenders. They have usually moved on with their lives.

He's aware that forgiveness isn't approval. He can forgive and still address the perceived wrong. The harm becomes no more acceptable when he forgives—he just doesn't let the harm from a one-time event continue to injure him or others.

He sees it like forgiving a loan. The creditor doesn't

approve or forget the debtor's default, just as he doesn't forget or approve of the wrong. Nor will the creditor loan more money to the debtor, just as he won't place himself in the same position of being hurt. The thoughtful creditor won't continue to let the original harm linger and expand by investing good money after bad and wasting valuable time trying to collect an uncollectible debt. The wise creditor moves on. It's good business to forgive an uncollectible loan, just as it's good emotional business to forgive someone for any harm we believe they've caused us.

The happily sober alcoholic knows that forgiveness heals his wounds and his heart. It does not let the offender off the hook, condone bad behavior, or invite reconciliation, but by forgiving, he remains free, having snuffed out the discomfort of harbored resentments. He knows he can't be happily sober while resenting and that forgiveness is essential for quality sobriety to prevail.

He knows several ways of forgiving—one way is to look in the mirror of introspection.

Introspection

Before he can forgive, the happily sober alcoholic must look within. He reviews where he has trespassed upon someone's boundaries. This review reveals his imperfections and enables him to be more tolerant of others—to remember we're all human and make mistakes. He then becomes more willing to forgive those who have trespassed against him.

At his trial before being sentenced to death for impiety, the Greek philosopher Socrates said, "The unexamined life is not worth living."[5] The happily sober alcoholic periodically examines his life and identifies the personality traits causing him or others problems. He then counsels with another, fully revealing himself, hiding nothing, and disclosing the traits he would like removed.

He recognizes that these traits are dynamic—they come

and go like gusts of wind. Even though a trait may seem removed, it can unexpectedly return and often does with a vengeance. They remain vibrantly alive, still, and inconspicuous like a hungry tiger focused on a lost fawn. They can be coy and cunning like a fox or bold like a ceaseless warrior. They can hide behind other traits, avoiding detection while preparing a surprise attack.

The happily sober alcoholic reviews his actions daily to determine where he might have fallen short of his goals.

Managing Fear

He sees healthy fear for what it is—energy to survive. Still, fear depletes energy, leaving one exhausted. Reasonable fear can be a lifesaver, yet unreasonable fear can be a life-taker and offends sobriety.

When drinking, he managed his fear with alcohol rather than addressing the source of his fear. He knows that constant worry will drain his energy and interfere with him doing anything about the target of his anxiety (or fear).

Productive Fear

He appreciates productive fear. For example, as a deadline approaches, he will increasingly worry about completing it timely. He knows that fear in the form of worry can give him the energy and motivation to act, to be focused and productive, which relieves anxiety. Still, he doesn't procrastinate to thrive on fear-produced energy generated by waiting until the last minute.

Unproductive Fear

He avoids the fear of worrying about something he can do nothing about, such as fearing results after submitting a test. He knows that most thoughts about the future are imaginary, and the emotions flowing from these thoughts are, therefore, useless. Enduring fear at this moment based on an illusion of the future, which rarely materializes, needlessly tarnishes the present and his sobriety. So, he resists unproductive worry, which needlessly depletes his energy.

Honesty

MARK TWAIN SAID, "A man is never more truthful than when he acknowledges himself a liar." Honesty is generally defined as the absence of deceit, lying, cheating, and stealing. It includes integrity (living according to self-imposed principles), truthfulness (expressing facts supported by reality), sincerity (acting in a way congruent with feelings), trustworthiness, loyalty, and fairness. Yet, we all perceive these elements of honesty differently.

Benjamin Franklin claimed, "Honesty is the best policy," but is it always? Sometimes, we must use deceit to save a life, prevent an injury, protect someone, avoid hurting feelings, or acquire the truth.

The happily sober alcoholic recognizes that we live in a dishonest world where we don't expect honesty—we expect dishonesty. If society were honest, the multibillion-dollar security industry wouldn't exist. We wouldn't have locks on doors and most everything else. Many with barred windows and doors wouldn't feel imprisoned when peering past them.

If everyone were honest, we wouldn't need laws against perjury, fraud, and theft. We wouldn't pay premiums for insurance that reimburses us if our assets are stolen. Passwords wouldn't be necessary. Security codes wouldn't exist. We wouldn't be threatened by hackers trying to steal our data or identity. Taxing authorities would be smaller.

The Benefits of Dishonesty

The happily sober alcoholic recognizes that society often encourages and uses dishonesty. Law enforcement uses deceit when patrolling in unmarked cars. Law enforcement negotiators are skilled at deception to apprehend someone dangerous to themselves or others. Deception prevails in espionage, and military strategy is often deceitful.

The primary purpose of trials is for the fact-finder (judge or jury) to determine the truth. If everyone told the truth, cross-examination wouldn't be necessary, courthouses would be smaller, and oaths wouldn't be administered.

Courts routinely use deception to control the information the jury receives. If truthful evidence is prejudicial to a party, courts exclude it to prevent a jury from deciding unfairly. Courts admonish jurors to deceive themselves by disregarding testimony they shouldn't have heard, which is later stricken from the record, even though it's truthful. Lawyers routinely approach the bench or retire to the judge's chambers to discuss truthful matters outside the jurors' hearing. Motions are often filed before trial to prevent 'prejudicial' truth from reaching the jury.

The 'fine print' wouldn't require a magnifier to read if the entity using it wanted it read before it became necessary to read in litigation. How many read the thousand-word online agreement before clicking "I Agree To The Terms"?

We are deceived as children when told Santa Claus, the Tooth Fairy, Tinkerbell, and other fictional characters are real.

Commercial advertisers routinely puff their products or services, and only when it's obviously misleading is it questioned.

Deceit is encouraged and rewarded with many popular games, including Poker. The player who deceives or "bluffs" the best is rewarded the most. Another example is the fake play that deceives opponents in football and other sports.

Still, honesty can be hurtful. When honesty is abusive, society frowns upon it. Those who claim, "I say it the way I see it," or "I just say what's on my mind," typically lack appropriate compassion and social skills.

So, we deceive when filtering inappropriate facts from our young children's ears. When honesty would be brutal, we deceive, which is known as the "white lie."

Despite this, the happily sober alcoholic understands that showing care for others sometimes involves saying helpful things instead of just what they want to hear. He also knows that people can be defensive when receiving honest, sincere, and beneficial feedback, even if expressed gently and lovingly, which may cause conflict. Still, he will modify or sacrifice a relationship that can't endure essential and valuable truth.

The happily sober alcoholic realizes that lying is often more than simply making a false statement; it comes in many forms. The consensus is that, on average, people tell over 15 lies daily. For example, people lie by telling only part of the story or saying something false, unconcerned about whether it's true. Perhaps they learn they made a wrong statement but don't correct it. Many respond untruthfully to prevent hurting another's feelings—the white lie. Others remain quiet instead of telling the truth—the silent lie.

The happily sober alcoholic is not surprised when someone is dishonest with him. Although unappreciated, he knows it's common and will not feel or express self-righteous indignation when it occurs.

He sees dishonest people burdened by believing everyone is as dishonest as they are. They continually accuse the innocent of the offenses they routinely commit. The dishonest person often thinks they are succeeding at misleading, unable to see their transparency. As Abraham Lincoln ("Honest Abe") once said, "No man has a good enough memory to be a successful liar."

The happily sober alcoholic understands that dishonesty with others requires substantial energy. It damages and often destroys relationships when trust is disturbed. He knows that those who are chronically dishonest with others can't be trusted, will suffer immeasurably, and won't have a chance at quality sobriety, so he tries practicing honesty reasonably and compassionately.

The discomfort he will experience if he's less than honest

with himself or others, unaware or aware, would pervasively and relentlessly gnaw away at the quality of his sobriety. He understands that pure honesty is a goal never fully achieved by imperfect humans. Still, he must strive to be *reasonably* honest with others, appreciating the significant difference between self-honesty and external honesty.

Self-Honesty and Sobriety

Denial thrives on self-deception. The happily sober alcoholic realizes self-honesty is essential to living sober. If he can't be honest with himself, he can't be honest with others, which will forfeit his connection with those who nurture his honesty.

Yet he knows self-honesty is never absolute. No one knows how honest they are with themselves. Many spend well-spent time, money, and energy with a therapist, discovering some of the truth within them.

As discussed in Chapter 5, "The Darkness and Lightness of Denial," we don't know all the truth buried in our unconsciousness. As we open our minds, humbly practice self-appraisal, and counsel with those we trust, inviting their insight, we become more self-honest—we see ourselves more accurately. Without *striving* for self-honesty, the abstinent alcoholic can't improve, and quality sobriety will elude him.

Self-honesty must shape the ideals essential for the happily sober alcoholic to strive to live by. In the book *Alcoholics Anonymous* ("*Big Book*"), it states:

> Those who do not recover are ... usually men and women who are unconstitutionally incapable of being *honest with themselves*.... They are naturally incapable of grasping and developing a manner of living which *demands rigorous honesty*.... There are those, too, who suffer from grave emotional and mental disorders, but many of them do recover if they have the *capacity to be honest*. [Emphasis added.][6]

Honesty is mentioned three times in that paragraph. This

book also says that any self-appraisal without honesty will be worthless: "Nothing counted but thoroughness and honesty."

Without sufficient self-honesty, one can't escape denial enough to even consider sobriety.

Living a Balanced Life

BALANCE IS OFTEN overlooked. Like riding a bicycle, balance improves when moving forward in the right direction. Without balanced action, unbalanced behavior will outweigh any healthy counterweight.

The blending of the happily sober alcoholic's actions, feelings, and thinking feels emotionally balanced. His ego is right-sized. He doesn't think too much or too little about himself or others. He is enlightened. Rather than feeling confused, he decides with a firm resolve yet remains open-minded and doesn't paralyze his decisions with indecision or rigid thinking.

He balances the time he spends with others with time for himself, including quiet times for reflection, meditation, and contemplation. He can be alone or with others without feeling lonely. When alone, he feels peace, contentment, and comfort. He feels grounded.

Although he makes plans, he lives emotionally in the present. In sobriety, he feels the feelings he once artificially *sought* when drinking but could no longer find. He doesn't seek to change his feelings but seeks the next right action, resulting in feelings that support healthy sobriety. He lives appropriately, predominantly, and responsibly in the present.

—

TO RE-EMPHASIZE, ALTHOUGH the happily sober alcoholic described here is a fictional character, the truth is that many alcoholics enjoying high-quality sobriety do have many of these characteristics to a greater or lesser degree.

Alcoholics need not have all the same traits, behavior, thinking, and feelings to enjoy sobriety. Still, the happily sober alcoholic is dedicated to thoroughly enjoying life with a higher purpose and thinking about the greater good without unnaturally changing the way he feels. He has discovered how to do this through recovery support groups. He realizes he is not the highest power. He strives to live happily ever after by taking the right action—by giving, he receives.

Questions For Discussion

1. Has this chapter affected you? How?
2. Do you consider yourself "happy?"
3. How do you seek pleasure? Do you seek real or artificial pleasure?
4. Has this chapter altered your thinking about happiness and pleasure? If so, how?
5. What are your thoughts about happiness?
6. Were you ever confused about the differences between real and artificial pleasure?

NOTES

CHAPTER 2—A DESCRIPTION OF THE ALCOHOLIC

1. National Institute on Alcohol Abuse and Alcoholism (2007) (NIAAA). http://www.niaaa.nih.gov.
2. Excessive drinking, including binge drinking, cost the United States $249 billion in 2010, or $2.05 per drink. These costs were from lost work productivity, health care expenditures, criminal justice costs, and other expenses. Binge drinking accounted for 77% of these costs, or $191 billion. Sacks JJ, Gonzales KR, Bouchery EE, Tomedi LE, Brewer RD. 2010 national and state costs of excessive alcohol consumption. *Am J Prev Med* 2015;49:e73–e79.
3. Schuckit, MA (27 November 2014). *"Recognition and management of withdrawal delirium (delirium tremens)."* The New England Journal of Medicine. 371 (22): 2109–13. doi:10.1056/NEJMra1407298. PMID 25427113.
4. Fisher, Gary L. (2009). Encyclopedia of substance abuse prevention, treatment, & recovery. Los Angeles: SAGE. p. 1005. ISBN 9781452266015. Archived from the original on 2015-12-22.
5. Blom, Jan Dirk (2010). A dictionary of hallucinations. New York: Springer. p. 136. ISBN 9781441912237. Archived from the original on 03-04-2016.
6. Schuckit, MA (27 November 2014). *"Recognition and management of withdrawal delirium (delirium tremens)."* The New England Journal of Medicine. **371** (22): 2109–13. doi:10.1056/NEJMra1407298. PMID 25427113.

7. Stern, TA; Gross, AF; Stern, TW; Nejad, SH; Maldonado, JR (2010). *"Current approaches to the recognition and treatment of alcohol withdrawal and delirium tremens: "old wine in new bottles" or "new wine in old bottles.""* Primary Care Companion to the Journal of Clinical Psychiatry.12(3). doi:10.4088/PCC.10r-00991ecr.PMC2947546.PMID 20944765.
8. Webb, J.P., Jr. (1993). "Case histories of individuals with delusions of parasitosis in southern California and a proposed protocol for initiating effective medical assistance." Bulletin of the Society of Vector Ecologists. 18 (1): 16–24.
9. U.S. National Highway Traffic Safety Administration. *2013 motor vehicle crashes: Overview.* Available at: http://wwwnrd.nhtsa.dot.gov/Pubs/812101.pdf, *and* American Psychiatric Association: *Diagnostic and Statistical Manual of Mental Disorders*, p. 496. Fifth Edition. Arlington, VA, American Psychiatric Association, 2013.
10. American Bar Association. Retrieved at: https://www.americanbar.org/groups/lawyer_assistance/resources/alcohol_abuse_dependence/.
11. Michael R. Oreskovich, MD; Krista L. Kaups, MD; Charles M. Balch, MD; et al. (2012) *Prevalence of Alcohol Use Disorders Among American Surgeons;* JAMA Network, Retrieved: https://jamanetwork.com/journals/jamasurgery/fullarticle/1107783
12. Crum, R. M., Muntaner, C., Eaton, W. W. and Anthony, J. C. (1995), *Occupational Stress and the Risk of Alcohol Abuse and Dependence. Alcoholism: Clinical and Experimental Research*, 19: 647–655. doi: 10.1111/j.1530-0277. 1995.tb01562.x. Donna M. Bush, Ph.D., F-ABFT, Rachel N. Lipari, Ph.D.; *Substance Use and Substance Use Disorder by Industry;* (2015); SAMSHA; The CBHSQ Report. Retrieved: https://www.samhsa.gov/data/sites/default/files/report_1959/ShortReport-1959.pdf

13. U.S. Department of Health and Human Services, Substance Abuse and Mental Health Services Administration, Office of Applied Studies (2010).
14. National Institute on Alcohol Abuse and Alcoholism (2007) (NIAAA). http://www.niaaa.nih.gov
15. American Psychiatric Association: *Diagnostic and Statistical Manual of Mental Disorders,* p. 494, Fifth Edition. Arlington, VA, American Psychiatric Association, 2013.
16. *Genetics of Alcohol Use Disorder,* National Institute of Alcohol Abuse and Alcoholism; AR&H Volume 31, Number 4, (2008)
17. Ibid.
18. American Psychiatric Association: *Diagnostic and Statistical Manual of Mental Disorders,* p. 494, Fifth Edition. Arlington, VA, American Psychiatric Association, 2013.
19. Ibid.
20. Fortier, C.B.; Leritz, E.C.; et al. *Widespread effects of alcohol on white matter microstructure.* Alcoholism: Clinical & Experimental Research. Nov. 18, 2014. PMID: 25406797
21. de la Monte, S.M. & Kril, J.J. Acta *Neuropathol; Human alcohol-related neuropathology* (2014) 127: 71. ttps://doi.org/10.1007/s00401-013-1233-3
22. Chen CH, Walker J, Momenan R, Rawlings R, Heilig M, Hommer DW. *Relationship between liver function and brain shrinkage in patients with alcohol dependence.* Alcohol Clin Exp Res. 2012 Apr; 36(4):625-32.
23. de la Monte SM, Longato L, Tong M, DeNucci S, Wands JR. *The liver-brain axis of alcohol-mediated neurodegeneration: role of toxic lipids.* Int J Environ Res Public Health. 2009 Jul; 6(7):2055-75.
24. Frigerio, Elisa & Burt, D. & Montagne, Barbara & Murray, Lindsey & Perrett, David. (2003). *Facial affect perception in alcoholics.* Psychiatry research. 113. 161-71. 10.1016/S0165-1781(02)00244-5.
25. Uekermann et al., 2007; Amenta et al., 2013.

26. Alcoholic blackout | *definition of alcoholic blackout by* ... (n.d.). Retrieved from http://medicaldictionary.thefreedictionary.com/alcoholic+blackout *Mosby's Medical Dictionary, 8th edition.* (2009)
27. *In Brief, Substance Use and Suicide: A Nexus Requiring A Public Health Approach*; SAMHSA, HHS Publication No. SMA-16-4935, Page 3, (Printed 2016), (2009) retrieved at: http://store.samhsa.gov/shin/content//SMA16-4935/SMA16-4935.pdf
28. Centers for Disease Control and Prevention. Alcohol use and health. Available at: http://www.cdc.gov/alcohol/fact-sheets/alcohol-use.htm
29. NCADD. *Alcohol, Drugs and Crime.* Retrieved from https://ncadd.org/about-addiction/alcohol-drugs-and-crime.
30. Ibid.
31. SAMHSA. 2018 *National Survey on Drug Use and Health* (NSDUH). Table 5.4A—Alcohol Use Disorder in Past Year among Persons Aged 12 or Older, by Age Group and Demographic Characteristics: Numbers in Thousands, 2017 and 2018. Available at: https://www.samhsa.gov/data/sites/default/files/cbhsq-reports/NSDUHDetailedTabs2018R2/NSDUHDetTabsect5pe2018.htm#tab5-4a. Accessed 12/2/19.
32. https://www.samhsa.gov/data/report/2019-nsduh-detailed-tables.

CHAPTER 3—THE ALCOHOLIC CRAVING

1. NIAAA, Alcohol Alert, No. 54 October 2001. Retrieved at: http:// pubs.niaaa.nih.gov/publications/aa54.htm.
2. Ibid.
3. NIAAA, Medications and Alcohol Craving, Robert M. Swift, MD, Ph.D., No. 3, October 1999. Retrieved at: https://pubs.niaaa.nih.gov/publications/arh23-3/207-212.pdf.
4. Ibid.
5. Ibid.

6. American Psychiatric Association. *Diagnostic and Statistical Manual of Mental Disorders.* Fifth Edition. Arlington, VA: the American Psychiatric Association, 2013.
7. World Health Organization. The ICD-10 Classification of Mental and Behavioral Disorders: Clinical Descriptions and Diagnostic Guidelines. Geneva, Switzerland: the Organization, 1992.
8. New York: McGraw-Hill, Concise Dictionary of Modern Medicine.
9. The Surgeon General's Report on Alcohol, Drugs, and Health. Washington, DC: HHS, November 2016.
10. This definition was formed from various sources, including Cambridge Dictionary, Merriam-Webster Dictionary, and Psychology Today.
11. American Psychiatric Association. *Diagnostic and Statistical Manual of Mental Disorders.* p. 492. Fifth Edition. Arlington, VA: the American Psychiatric Association, 2013.
12. Milam, James R. Ph.D., and Katherine Ketcham. 1981. *Under The Influence.* 1st ed. New York: Bantam Books.
13. https://www.niaaa.nih.gov/.
14. Ibid.
15. Fuchs, Eberhard; Flügge, Gabriele (2014). "Adult Neuroplasticity: More Than 40 Years of Research". Neural Plasticity. 2014: 541870. doi: 10.1155/2014/541870. PMC 4026979. PMID 24883212.
16. Ibid; and "Alcohol and the Brain: A Love/Hate Relationship" by J. Leigh Leasure and J. David Crews, *Alcoholism: Clinical and Experimental Research* (Volume 35, Issue 8, pages 1293-1301) August 2011.
17. Ibid.
18. Shaffer, Joyce (26 July 2016). "Neuroplasticity and Clinical Practice: Building Brain Power for Health." Frontiers in Psychology. 7: 1118. doi:10.3389/fpsyg.2016.01118. PMC 4960264. PMID 27507957.
19. Ibid.

20. Stephen C. Putnam, MEd, *Nature's Ritalin for the Marathon Mind,*
21. Get the Facts About Underage Drinking. Alcohol's Effects on Health, Research-based information on drinking and its impact. https://www. niaaa.nih.gov/.
22. Luders E, Toga AW, Lepore N, Gaser C (April 2009). "The underlying anatomical correlates of long-term meditation: larger hippocampal and frontal volumes of gray matter." *NeuroImage.* 45(3):672–8. doi:10.1016/j.neuroimage.2008.12.061. PMC 3184843. PMID 1928 0691.
23. Begley S (20 January 2007). "How Thinking Can Change the Brain". dalailama.com. Archived from the original on 9 May 2007. Retrieved 10 May 2007.
24. Davidson R, Lutz A (January 2008). "Buddha's Brain: Neuroplasticity and Meditation" (PDF). IEEE Signal Processing Magazine. 25 (1): 176–174. Bibcode: 2008ISPM...25.176D.doi:10.1109/MSP.2008.4431873. PMC 2944261. PMID 20871742. Archived (PDF) from the original on 12 January 2012. Retrieved 19 April 2018.
25. Schultz, Wolfram (July 2015). "Neuronal Reward and Decision Signals: From Theories to Data." Physiological Reviews. 95 (3): 853–951. doi:10.1152/physrev.00023. 2014. PMC 4491543. PMID 26109341.
26. Ibid.
27. Kolb B, Whishaw IQ (2001). An Introduction to Brain and Behavior (1st ed.). New York: Worth. pp. 438–441. ISBN 9780716751694.
28. http://neuroscience.mssm.edu/nestler/brainRewardpathways.html
29. Ibid.
30. http://neuroscience.mssm.edu/nestler/brainRewardpathways.html
31. The other neurotransmitters include glutamate, GABA, endorphins, and others.
32. http://neuroscience.mssm.edu/nestler/brainRewardpathways.html
33. Ibid.

34. Ibid.
35. McFarlane, Alan H., and Geoffrey R. Norman. "Methods for Classifying Symptoms, Complaints, and Conditions." *Medical Care*, vol. 11, no. 2, 1973, pp. 101–108. *JSTOR*, www.jstor.org/stable/3762808. Accessed 8 Aug. 2021.
36. Ibid.
37. http://neuroscience.mssm.edu/nestler/brainRewardpathways.html
38. Ibid.
39. Ibid.
40. Ibid.
41. Ibid.
42. Activation of neurotransmitters such as CRF, dynorphin, and norepinephrine.
43. *Alcoholics Anonymous: the story of how many thousands of men and women have recovered from alcoholism*. New York City: Alcoholics Anonymous World Services. p. xxxii, ISBN 1-893007-16-2. 1939.
44. *Alcoholism as a Manifestation of Allergy*, W. D. Silkworth, New York, N.Y., March 17, 1937. Alcoholism As A Manifestation Of Allergy - Barefoot's World. (n.d.). Retrieved from http://www.barefootsworld.net/aasilkworth1937.html.
45. *Alcoholics Anonymous: the story of how many thousands of men and women have recovered from alcoholism*. New York City: Alcoholics Anonymous World Services. p. xxxii, ISBN 1-893007-16-2. 1939. P. 37.
46. Ibid., 37
47. Ibid., 35
48. Ibid., 41
49. Ibid.
50. Ibid., 42
51. Ibid., 37
52. Ibid., 38
53. Ibid., 24
54. Ibid., 23
55. Ibid., 143

56. *Alcoholics Anonymous: the story of how many thousands of men and women have recovered from alcoholism.* New York City: Alcoholics Anonymous World Services. p. xxxii, ISBN 1-893007-16-2. 1939. (Dr. Bob's Nightmare p. 181).
57. http://neuroscience.mssm.edu/nestler/brainRewardpathways.html
58. *Living Sober*, New York City: Alcoholics Anonymous World Services. p. 69, (1975).
59. Ibid., 70
60. *Alcoholics Anonymous: the story of how many thousands of men and women have recovered from alcoholism.* New York City: Alcoholics Anonymous World Services. p. xxx, ISBN 1-893007-16-2. 1939.
61. Ibid., xxviii
62. Ibid., xxvi
63. American Psychiatric Association. *Diagnostic and Statistical Manual of Mental Disorders.* p. 449. Fifth Edition. Arlington, VA: the American Psychiatric Association, 2013.
64. Ibid., 500
65. https://www.cdc.gov/vitalsigns/pdf/2015-01-vitalsigns.pdf
66. https://www.samhsa.gov/data/
67. www.niaaa.nih.gov/strategic-plan (retrieved 12/18/2020)
68. Ibid., 180
69. Ibid.
70. (David J. Drobes, 1999) Assessing Craving for Alcohol p. 179 http://pubs.niaaa.nih.gov/publications/arh23-3/179-186.pdf
71. NIH Publication No. 15-3770; Published 2010; Revised May 2016. Since writing this, a fact-checking review of the NIAAA website indicates this publication may no longer be available (except in Spanish). Under "Other NIAAA Sites" appears "Rethinking Drinking." This site contains "Interactive worksheets and more," which includes a section entitled *"Handling urges to drink."* It states, "The words 'urge' and 'craving' refer to a broad range of

thoughts, physical sensations, or emotions that tempt you to drink, even though you have at least some desire not to. You may feel an uncomfortable pull in two directions or sense a loss of control."

72. Ibid., fn45, 185
73. Ibid.
74. Ibid.
75. Ibid.
76. *Measurement of alcohol craving,* Kavanagh, David, Statham, Dixie, Feeney, Gerald, Young, Ross, May, Jon, Andrade, Jackie, & Connor, Jason (2013) Measurement of alcohol craving. **Addictive Behaviors, 38**(2), pp. 1572-1584.
77. The Penn Alcohol Craving Scale (PACS), developed by Flannery et al. (1999), is the most common craving test used.
78. Ibid., fn45; and Oslin, David W., et al. "Daily Ratings Measures of Alcohol Craving during an Inpatient Stay Define Subtypes of Alcohol Addiction That Predict Subsequent Risk for Resumption of Drinking." *Drug and Alcohol Dependence*, vol. 103, no. 3, Aug. 2009, pp. 131–36, doi:10.1016/j.drugalcdep. 2009.03.009.
79. Sacks, J. J., Gonzales, K. R., Bouchery, E. E., Tomedi, L. E., & Brewer, R. D. (2015). 2010 National and state costs of excessive alcohol consumption. American Journal of Preventive Medicine, 49(5), e73-e79.
80. These studies are listed under the Clinical Trials database of the U.S. National Library of Medicine, a component of the NIH. See ClinicalTrials.gov.
81. Ibid.
82. Garcia-Romeu A, Davis AK, Erowid F, Erowid E, Griffiths RR, Johnson MW. Cessation and reduction in alcohol consumption and misuse after psychedelic use. Journal of Psychopharmacology. 2019;33(9):1088-1101. doi:10.1177/0269881119845793

CHAPTER 4—The Alcoholic Stigma

1. Goffman, Erving. *Stigma: Notes on the Management of Spoiled Identity.* Englewood Cliffs. Prentice-Hall Inc., 1963.
2. "WHO Multidrug therapy (MDT)." World Health Organization.
3. Ibid.
4. Goffman, Erving. *Stigma: Notes on the Management of Spoiled Identity.* Englewood Cliffs. Prentice-Hall Inc., 1963
5. Stigma. (n.d.). *Roget's 21st Century Thesaurus, Third Edition.* Retrieved March 11, 2016 from Thesaurus.com websitehttp://www.thesaurus.com/browse/stigma
6. Ibid.
7. Kathleen Tavenner Mitchell, LCADC, MHS Reducing the Stigma of Addiction and Fetal Alcohol Spectrum Disorders (FASD): Creating a Circle of Hope; (2017). 2017 National Conference on Alcohol and Opioid Use in Women and Girls: Advances in Prevention, Treatment and Recovery October 26 - 27, 2017. Washington, DC. https://www.niaaa.nih.gov/sites/default/files/2017_Nat ional_Conference_on_Alcohol_and_Opioid_Use_in_Wo men_and_Girls_Report.pdf.
8. Ibid.
9. /https://consaludmental.org/publicaciones/Stigmaguide bookforaction.pdf.
10. Ian Langtree. (2015-03-09). <a href= "https://www. disabled world.com/disability/awareness/ribbons.php"> Awareness Ribbons Chart: Color and Meaning of Awareness Ribbon Causes</a>. Retrieved 2017-07-03, from https://www.disabled-world.com/disability/aware-ness/ribbons.php.
11. Brenda Major; Laurie T. O'Brien (2005). "The Social Psychology of Stigma". Annual Review of Psychology. 56 (1): 393–421. doi:10.1146/annurev.psych.56.091103. 070137. hdl:2027.42/146893. PMID 15709941.

12. Matthews S, Dwyer R, Snoek A. *Stigma and Self-Stigma in Addiction.* J Bioeth Inq. 2017 Jun;14(2):275-286. doi: 10.1007/s11673-017-9784-y. Epub 2017 May 3. PMID: 28470503; PMCID: PMC5527047.
13. Schomerus et al., (2010). *The Stigma of Alcohol Dependence Compared with Other Mental Disorders: A Review of Population Studies,* Oxford University Press, 46 (2).
14. Ibid.
15. Ibid.
16. Alcoholics Anonymous (1955). *Alcoholics Anonymous: The Story of How Many Thousands of Men and Women Have Recovered from Alcoholism,* 2nd ed. A.A. World Services.
17. Alcohol Res.2020; 40(2):09.https://doi.org/10.35946/arcr.v40.2.09.
18. The Substance Abuse and Mental Health Services Administration (SAMHSA) 2015 National Survey on Drug Use and Health (NSDUH); and Kathleen Tavenner Mitchell, LCADC, MHS Reducing the Stigma of Addiction and Fetal Alcohol Spectrum Disorders (FASD): Creating a Circle of Hope; (2017). 2017 National Conference on Alcohol and Opioid Use in Women and Girls: Advances in Prevention, Treatment and Recovery October 26 - 27, 2017. Washington, DC. https://www.niaaa.nih.gov/sites/default/files/2017_National_Conference_on_Alcohol_and_Opioid_Use_in_Women_and_Girls_Report.pdf.
19. Karger A. (2014). *Geschlechtsspezifische Aspekte bei depressiven Erkrankungen [Gender differences in depression]. Bundesgesundheitsblatt, Gesundheitsforschung, Gesundheitsschutz,* 57(9), 1092–1098. https://doi.org/10.1007/s00103-014-2019-z.
20. American Psychiatric Association: *Diagnostic and Statistical Manual of Mental Disorders,* Fifth Edition. Arlington, VA, American Psychiatric Association, 2013. p. 497.

21. Alcohol Metabolism; National Institute on Alcohol Abuse and Alcoholism No. 35; PH 371 January 1997. https://pubs.niaaa.nih.gov/publications/aa35.htm.
22. Ibid.
23. Ibid.
24. Ibid.
25. Kathleen Tavenner Mitchell, LCADC, MHS Reducing the Stigma of Addiction and Fetal Alcohol Spectrum Disorders (FASD): Creating a Circle of Hope; (2017). 2017 National Conference on Alcohol and Opioid Use in Women and Girls: Advances in Prevention, Treatment and Recovery October 26 - 27, 2017. Washington, DC. https://www.niaaa.nih.gov/sites/default/files/2017_National_Conference_on_Alcohol_and_Opioid_Use_in_Women_and_Girls_Report.pdf.
26. American Psychiatric Association: *Diagnostic and Statistical Manual of Mental Disorders*, Fifth Edition. Arlington, VA, American Psychiatric Association, 2013. p. 197.
27. The United State of Women, http://www.theunitedstateofwomen.org/topics/ (accessed August 04, 2016).
28. https://blog.dol.gov/2017/03/01/12-stats-about-working-women.
29. Foerschner, A. M. 2010. The History of Mental Illness: From Skull Drills to Happy Pills. *Inquiries Journal/Student Pulse* 2 (09), http://www.inquiriesjournal.com/a?id=1673A. s
30. Ibid.
31. Ibid.
32. American Psychiatric Association: *Diagnostic and Statistical Manual of Mental Disorders*, Fifth Edition. Arlington, VA, American Psychiatric Association, 2013. p. 310.
33. "Personal Justice Denied." Personal Justice Denied. National Archives. Retrieved 2013-10-14.
34. Ibid.
35. https://www.penn.museum/research/project.php?pid=12.

36. Leper Hospitals and Colonies, Leper Colonies-University of Florida; http://plaza.ufl.edu/bjb1221/Colonies.htm
37. Ibid.
38. Unknown. *Our Words – They Can Make Or Break People Affected By Leprosy! Leprosy-Today.* The Leprosy Mission Trust India (2015) https://leprosytoday.wordpress.com/2015/06/15/our-words-they-can-make-or-break-people-affected-by-leprosy-2/.
39. Ibid.
40. Ibid.
41. Ibid.
42. American Psychiatric Association: *Diagnostic and Statistical Manual of Mental Disorders,* Fifth Edition. Arlington, VA, American Psychiatric Association, 2013, p.485.
43. Ibid., 497-498.
44. Ibid., 481.
45. Ibid., 497-498.
46. Ibid.
47. Peck, Scott. *Further Along the Road Less Traveled* (Simon & Schuster, 1993) ISBN 978-0-684-84723-8.
48. Buckingham SA, Frings D, Albery IP, Psychology of addictive behaviors: *Journal of the Society of Psychologists in Addictive Behaviors,* December 2013(1132-40), 1939-1501.
49. Ibid.
50. Grant BF, Goldstein RB, Saha TD, et al. Epidemiology of DSM-5 alcohol use disorder: results from the National Epidemiologic Survey on Alcohol and Related Conditions III. JAMA Psychiatry. 2015;72(8):757-766.
51. American Psychiatric Association: *Diagnostic and Statistical Manual of Mental Disorders,* Fifth Edition. Arlington, VA, American Psychiatric Association, p. 498, 2013.
52. Ibid.

53. Early Drinking Linked to Higher Lifetime Alcoholism Risk (2006) https://www.niaaa.nih.gov/news-events/news-releases/early-drinking-linked-higher-lifetime-alcoholism-risk.
54. Ibid.
55. Ibid.
56. *Traynor v. Turnage,* 485 U.S. 535 (1988).
57. Fretts, Bruce; Roush, Matt. "The Greatest Shows on Earth". TV Guide Magazine 61(3194–3195): 16–19.
58. Understanding Anonymity (Unknown 2011) *Alcoholics Anonymous World Services, Inc.*
59. Ibid. Also, to give to and help another *anonymously* without identification or expectation of reward or anything in return, including recognition, was and is a spiritual goal that eludes most people.

AA realized that the personality types of many alcoholics are that of *promoters,* and they were concerned that a member seeking personal gain could use AA or abuse AA for that purpose. Early on, some AA members were famous, and if they promoted the benefits of AA, though they might prosper, such activities would injure AA.

That is why it is still just as important today as it was in 1935 that a member may break their anonymity anytime they want, except at the level of the press (now includes online), radio, and films. AA embodied this principle in AA's Eleventh Tradition, which states, "Our public relations policy is based on attraction rather than promotion; we need always maintain personal anonymity at the level of press, radio, and films.

Chapter 5 — The Darkness and Lightness of Denial

1. Lexicon of Alcohol and Drug Terms Published by the World Health Organization. *WHO.* N.p., n.d. Web. 17 May 2016.
2. Interview: A Doctor Speaks, AA Grapevine Magazine, May 2001, Vol. 57, No. 12.

3. National Council On Alcoholism And Drug Dependence, Inc. (NCADD). (2015). *Facts About Alcohol.* Retrieved: https://ncadd.us/about-addiction/alcohol/facts-about-alcohol.
4. Ibid.
5. Ibid.
6. Ibid.
7. Centers for Disease Control and Prevention (CDC). (2022). *Alcohol Use and Your Health.* Retrieved: www.cdc.gov/alcohol/fact-sheets/alcohol-use.htm
8. Centers for Disease Control and Prevention (CDC). (2023). *A Snapshot: Diabetes in the United States.* Retrieved: www.cdc.gov/diabetes.
9. Centers for Disease Control and Prevention (CDC). (2019). *The Cost of Excessive Alcohol Use.* Retrieved: www.cdc.gov/alcohol.
10. The National Center on Addiction and Substance Abuse at Columbia University (CASAColumbia). (2012) *Addiction Medicine: Closing the Gap between Science and Practice, p12.* New York: Author.
11. Ibid., 133.
12. Kushner, Robert & Horn, Linda & Rock, Cheryl & Edwards, Marilyn & Bales, Connie & Kohlmeier, Martin & Akabas, Sharon. (2014). Nutrition education in medical school: A time of opportunity. *The American journal of clinical nutrition.* 99. 10.3945/ajcn.113.073510.
13. Article retrieved: www.kevinmd.com.
14. Jackson, Eric R.; Shanafelt, Tait D. MD; Hasan, Omar MBBS, MPH, MS; Satele, Daniel V.; Dyrbye, Liselotte N. MD, MHPE. Burnout and Alcohol Abuse/Dependence Among U.S. Medical Students. *Academic Medicine* 91(9):p 1251-1256, September 2016. | DOI: 10.1097/ ACM.0000000000001138
15. Wilson J, Tanuseputro P, Myran DT, et al. Characterization of Problematic Alcohol Use Among Physicians: A Systematic Review. *JAMA Netw Open.* 2022;5(12): e2244679. doi:10.1001/jamanetworkopen.2022.44679
16. Ibid.

17. Ibid.
18. The National Center on Addiction and Substance Abuse (CASA) at Columbia University. (2000). *Missed opportunity: National survey of primary care physicians and patients on substance abuse.* New York: Author.
19. The National Center on Addiction and Substance Abuse at Columbia University (CASA Columbia). (2012) *Addiction Medicine: Closing the Gap between Science and Practice.* New York: Author.
20. Self-injury can cause a variety of complications, including a) the worsening of shame, guilt, and self-esteem; b) infection, either from wounds or from sharing tools; c) permanent scarring or disfigurement; d) a severe, possibly fatal injury; and d) the worsening of underlying issues and disorders if not adequately treated, which can affect long-term stress and can cause or worsen hypertension, heart disease, obesity, diabetes, and infertility.
21. Ramesh Shivani, MD, R. Jeffrey Goldsmith, MD, and Robert M. Anthenelli, MD. Alcoholism and Psychiatric Disorders-Diagnostic Challenges. *Alcohol Research & Health.* 2002;26(2): 90-98. Retrieved: https://pubs.niaaa.nih.gov/publications/arh26-2/90-98.htm.
22. Ibid.

Chapter 6—The Periodic Alcoholic

1. National Institute on Alcohol Abuse and Alcoholism. Alcohol Use Disorder. Retrieved from https://www.niaaa.nih.gov/alcohol-health/overview-alcohol-consumption/alcohol-use-disorders.
2. https://www.niaaa.nih.gov/alcohol-health/overview-alcohol-consumption/moderate-binge-drinking).
3. Ibid.
4. Sacks JJ, Gonzales KR, Bouchery EE, Tomedi LE, Brewer RD. 2010 national and state costs of excessive alcohol consumption. *Am J Prev Med* 2015;49:e73–e79.

Chapter 7—Health Care, Alcoholism and the DSM

1. "AA Fact File." *Alcoholics Anonymous World Services, Inc.* 2007
2. Ernest Kurtz. *Not-God, A History of Alcoholics Anonymous.* Hazelden, 1979, Expanded edition 1991.
3. *Pass It On, The story of Bill Wilson and how the A.A. message reached the world.* Alcoholics Anonymous World Services, Inc., New York, N.Y. 1984.
4. The Bill W.—Carl Jung Letters. *The Language Of The Heart—Bill W.'s Grapevine Writings.* The AA Grapevine, Inc. New York. 1988 p. 276.
5. Alcoholics Anonymous. *Alcoholics Anonymous: The Story of How Many Thousands of Men and Women Have Recovered from Alcoholism,* 2nd ed. A.A. World Services., (1955). p XXV.
6. *See* Fisher, Carl E. "How a Struggling Socialite Convinced the World Alcoholism Is a Disease." *The Washington Post,* January 29, 2022.
7. White, William L. (1998). *Slaying the Dragon: The History of Addiction Treatment and Recovery in America.* pp. 142, 178–187, 198. ISBN 0-938475-07-X.
8. *Pass It On, The story of Bill Wilson and how the A.A. message reached the world.* Alcoholics Anonymous World Services, Inc., New York, N.Y. 1984.
9. Bill W. "Let's Be Friendly With Our Friends: Friends on the Alcoholism Front." AA Grapevine Magazine, March 1958. The AA Grapevine, Inc.
10. George E. Vaillant, MD. (1983). *The Natural History of Alcoholism.* Cambridge, Massachusetts: Harvard University Press.
11. George E. Vaillant, MD. (1995). *The Natural History of Alcoholism Revisited.* Cambridge, Massachusetts: Harvard University Press.
12. Ibid.
13. "Three Talks to Medical Societies by Bill W., co-founder of AA," *Alcoholics Anonymous World Services, Inc.,* (2004).

14. Letter by Bill Wilson, *As Bill Sees It,* Alcoholics Anonymous World Services, Inc., p. 67 (1967).
15. Interview: A Doctor Speaks, AA Grapevine Magazine, May 2001, Vol. 57, No. 12.
16. Slomski A. Mindfulness-Based Intervention and Substance Abuse Relapse. *JAMA.* 2014;311(24):2472. doi:10.1001/jama.2014.7644.
17. Interview: A Doctor Speaks, AA Grapevine Magazine, May 2001, Vol. 57, No. 12.
18. Dion K, Griggs S. Teaching Those Who Care How to Care for a Person With Substance Use Disorder. Nurse Educ. 2020 Nov/Dec;45(6):321-325. doi: 10.1097/NNE.0000000000000808. PMID: 32091475; PMCID: PMC7438244.
19. Ibid.
20. Naegle MA. The Need for Alcohol Abuse-Related Education in Nursing Curricula. Alcohol Health Res World. 1994;18(2):154-157. PMID: 31798113; PMCID: PMC6876411.
21. Ramesh Shivani, MD, R. Jeffrey Goldsmith, M.D., Robert M. Anthe-nelli, MD. *Alcoholism and Psychiatric Disorders, Diagnostic Challenges.* (2002). https://www.ncbi.nlm.nih.gov/pmc/articles/PMC6683829/
22. ASAM, founded in 1954, is a professional medical society representing over 6,000 physicians, clinicians, and associated professionals in the field of addiction medicine. ASAM is dedicated to increasing access and improving the quality of addiction treatment, educating physicians and the public, supporting research and prevention, and promoting the appropriate role of physicians in the care of patients with addiction.
23. American Psychiatric Association: *Diagnostic and Statistical Manual of Mental Disorders,* p. 496, Fifth Edition. Arlington, VA, American Psychiatric Association, 2013.

24. National Center for Statistics and Analysis, National Highway Traffic Safety Administration. Traffic safety facts: summary of motor vehicle crashes 2020 data [Internet]. Washington: U.S. Department of Transportation; 2022 Sept [cited 2023 Jan 20]. 11 p. Available from: https://crashstats.nhtsa.dot.gov/Api/Public/ViewPublication/813369
25. U.S. Department of Health and Human Services (HHS), Office of the Surgeon General, Facing Addiction in America: The Surgeon General's Report on Alcohol, Drugs, and Health. Washington, DC: HHS, November 2016, p. 5-6.
26. The National Center on Addiction and Substance Abuse at Columbia University (CASA Columbia). (2012) *Addiction Medicine: Closing the Gap between Science and Practice.* New York: Author. CASAColumbia analysis of the treatment episode data set (TEDS) 2009.
27. Ibid.
28. The National Center on Addiction and Substance Abuse at Columbia University (CASA Columbia). (2012) *Addiction Medicine: Closing the Gap between Science and Practice.* New York: Author. CASAColumbia analysis of the treatment episode data set (TEDS) 2009.
29. Ibid.
30. *Alcohol Use Disorders Identification Tests*
31. *Alcohol, Smoking and Substance Involvement Screening Test*
32. 2022 National Survey on Drug Use and Health (NSDUH) Substance Abuse and Mental Health Services Administration (SAMHSA). Retrieved www.samhsa.gov/data/release
33. *See* https://www.niaaa.nih.gov/health-professionals-communities/core-resource-on-alcohol/screen-and-assess-use-quick-effective-methods.
34. This book is published by American Psychiatric Publishing, a division of the American Psychiatric Association, the same publisher of the DSM-5 by

Abraham M. Nussbaum, MD, assistant professor of psychiatry at the University of Colorado School of Medicine.
35. Helzer JE, Przybeck TR. The co-occurrence of alcoholism with other psychiatric disorders in the general population and its impact on treatment. *Journal of Studies on Alcohol.* 1988;49:219–224.
36. Ramesh Shivani, MD, R. Jeffrey Goldsmith, M.D., Robert M. Anthenelli, MD. *Alcoholism and Psychiatric Disorders, Diagnostic Challenges.* (2002). https://www.ncbi.nlm.nih.gov/pmc/articles/PMC6683829/.
37. U.S. Department of Health and Human Services (HHS), Office of the Surgeon General, Facing Addiction in America: The Surgeon General's Report on Alcohol, Drugs, and Health. Washington, DC: HHS, November 2016, pp. 6-32.
38. Ramesh Shivani, MD, R. Jeffrey Goldsmith, M.D., Robert M. Anthenelli, MD. *Alcoholism and Psychiatric Disorders, Diagnostic Challenges.* (2002). https://www.ncbi.nlm.nih.gov/pmc/articles/PMC6683829/.
39. American Psychiatric Association: Diagnostic and Statistical Manual of Mental Disorders, p. 502, Fifth Edition. Arlington, VA, American Psychiatric Association, 2013.
40. Comorbidity: Substance Use and Other Mental Disorders. National Institutes on Drug Abuse (U.S.); 2018 Aug. https://nida.nih.gov/research-topics/comorbidity/comorbidity-substance-use-other-mental-disorders-infographic
41. Common Comorbidities with Substance Use Disorders Research Report. Bethesda (MD): National Institutes on Drug Abuse (U.S.); 2020 Apr. Available from: https://www.ncbi.nlm.nih.gov/books/NBK571451/.
42. Han, Beth, Wilson M. Compton, Carlos Blanco, and Lisa J. Colpe. "Prevalence, Treatment, And Unmet Treatment Needs Of US Adults With Mental Health And Substance Use Disorders." *Health Affairs* 36, no. 10 (2017): 1739-1747.
43. Ibid.

44. Ibid.
45. American Psychiatric Association: *Diagnostic and Statistical Manual of Mental Disorders,* p. 488-496, Fifth Edition. Arlington, VA, American Psychiatric Association, 2013.
46. Ibid., 488.
47. Ibid.
48. Ibid., 502.
49. Ibid., 502-503.
50. Center for Substance Abuse Treatment (U.S.). Trauma-Informed Care in Behavioral Health Services. Rockville (MD): Substance Abuse and Mental Health Services Administration (U.S.); 2014. (Treatment Improvement Protocol (TIP) Series, No. 57.) Chapter 4, Screening and Assessment. Available from: https://www.ncbi.nlm.nih.gov/books/NBK207188/.
51. American Psychiatric Association. *Diagnostic and statistical manual of mental disorders.* 5th ed. Arlington, VA: American Psychiatric Association; 2013.
52. Ibid., 493.
53. Ibid., 492.
54. Cherpitel CJ, Borges G, Ye Y, Bond J, Cremonte M, Moskalewicz J, Swiatkiewicz G. Performance of a craving criterion in DSM alcohol use disorders. J Stud Alcohol Drugs. 2010 Sep;71(5):674-84. doi: 10.15288/jsad.2010.71.674. PMID: 20731972; PMCID: PMC2930058.
55. Deborah S. Hasin, Miriam C. Fenton, Cheryl Beseler, Jung Yeon Park, Melanie M. Wall, Analyses related to the development of DSM-5 criteria for substance use related disorders: 2. Proposed DSM-5 criteria for alcohol, cannabis, cocaine and heroin disorders in 663 substance abuse patients, *Drug and Alcohol Dependence,* Volume 122, Issues 1–2, 2012, Pages 28-37, ISSN 0376-8716,https://doi.org/10.1016/j.drugalcdep.2011.09.005.(https://www.sciencedirect.com/science/article/pii/S0-376871611003929)

56. American Psychiatric Association. *Diagnostic and Statistical Manual of Mental Disorders.* p. 496. Fifth Edition. Arlington, VA: the American Psychiatric Association, 2013.
57. Tiffany, S.T. and Wray, J.M. (2012), The clinical significance of drug craving. Annals of the New York Academy of Sciences, 1248: 1-17. https://doi.org/10.1111/j.1749-6632.2011.06298.x
58. American Psychiatric Association (APA). *Diagnostic and Statistical Manual of Mental Disorders, Fourth Edition.* Washington, DC: APA, 1994.
59. APA, Substance-Related and Addictive Disorders, Retrieved from: file:///C:/Users/j/Downloads/APA_DSM-5-Substance-Use-Disorder%20(1). pdffile:///C:/Users/j/Downloads/APA_DSM-5-Substance-Use-Disorder%20(1).pdf
60. Kimberly S. Walitzer, Ph.D., Jerry L. Deffenbacher, Ph.D., Kathleen Shyhalla, Ph.D. Alcohol-Adapted Anger Management Treatment: A Randomized Controlled Trial of an Innovative Therapy for Alcohol Dependence. *Journal of Substance Abuse Treatment* (2015).
61. Alcoholics Anonymous. *Alcoholics Anonymous: The Story of How Many Thousands of Men and Women Have Recovered from Alcoholism*, 2nd ed. A.A. World Services., (1955). p 64.
62. *A Pocket Guide for Alcohol Screening and Brief Intervention*, Updated 2005 Edition, NIAAA Publications Distribution Center, Rockville, MD. Retrieved from: http://pubs.niaaa.nih.gov/publications/Practitioner/Pocket-Guide/pocket_guide6.htm
63. American Psychiatric Association: Diagnostic and Statistical Manual of Mental Disorders, p. 815, Fifth Edition. Arlington, VA, American Psychiatric Association. 2013.

64. American Psychiatric Association. DSM-5 Fact Sheets. "Substance-Related and Addictive Disorders" Arlington, VA, American Psychiatric Association, 2013. Retrieved: https://www.psychiatry.org/ File%20Library/ Psychiatrists/Practice/DSM/APA_DSM-5-Substance-Use-Disorder.pdf
65. Ibid., 484.
66. Slomski A. Mindfulness-Based Intervention and Substance Abuse Relapse. *JAMA. 2014;311(24):2472. doi:10.1001/jama.2014.7644.*
67. American Psychiatric Association: Diagnostic and Statistical Manual of Mental Disorders, p. 493, Fifth Edition. Arlington, VA, American Psychiatric Association. 2013.
68. Ibid., 491.
69. Ibid., 486.
70. Ibid., 486.
71. Ibid., 501.
72. Ibid., 486.
73. Ibid., 21.
74. Ibid., 501.
75. Ibid., 484.
76. Ibid., 484.
77. Cosgrove L, Krimsky S (2012) A Comparison of *DSM*-IV and *DSM*-5 Panel Members' Financial Associations with Industry: A Pernicious Problem Persists. PLoS Med e1001190.9(3): https://doi.org/10.1371/journal.pmed.1001190
78. doi: http://mut23.org/texte/dsm5_group.pdf
79. Ibid.
80. Ibid.
81. Ibid at fn70.
82. Ibid.
83. Ibid.
84. This book is published by American Psychiatric Publishing, a division of the American Psychiatric Association, the same publisher of the DSM-5, by

Abraham M. Nussbaum, MD, assistant professor of psychiatry at the University of Colorado School of Medicine.
85. U.S. Department of Health and Human Services (HHS), Office of the Surgeon General, Facing Addiction in America: The Surgeon General's Report on Alcohol, Drugs, and Health. Washington, DC: HHS, November 2016, p. 6-32.
86. Ibid.
87. Ibid.
88. Ibid., 6-33.
89. Jackson, Eric R.; Shanafelt, Tait D. MD; Hasan, Omar MBBS, MPH, MS; Satele, Daniel V.; Dyrbye, Liselotte N. MD, MHPE. Burnout and Alcohol Abuse/Dependence Among U.S. Medical Students. *Academic Medicine* 91(9):p 1251-1256, September 2016. | DOI: 10.1097/ACM.0000000000001138.

CHAPTER 8—THE AFFECTED

1. Tian Dayton, PhD, *Adult Children of Alcoholics and Trauma*. Retrieved July 2, 2018, from HuffPost, https://www.huffpost.com/entry/adult-children-of-alcohol_b_6676950 (April 29, 2015).
2. Ibid.
3. Ibid.
4. Ibid.
5. Ibid.
6. Janet Geringer Woititz, Ed.D., *Adult Children of Alcoholics*. Deerfield Beach, Florida: Health Communications, Inc., 1983
7. Allen, Shannon. *Childhood Trauma: A Comprehensive Review of Effects, Assessments, and Treatments*. Arizona State University. (2016).
8. Ibid.
9. Ibid.
10. Ibid.
11. Ibid.

12. Janet Geringer Woititz, Ed.D., *Adult Children of Alcoholics*. Deerfield Beach, Florida: Health Communications, Inc., 1983.
13. Ibid.
14. Ibid.

CHAPTER 9—THE RELAPSE

1. Slomski A. *Mindfulness-Based Intervention and Substance Abuse Relapse.* JAMA. 2014;311(24):2472. doi:10.1001/jama.2014.7644.
2. Ibid.
3. Ibid.

CHAPTER 10—THE INTERVENTION

1. Manning V, Garfield JBB, Staiger PK, et al. Effect of Cognitive Bias Modification on Early Relapse Among Adults Undergoing Inpatient Alcohol Withdrawal Treatment: A Randomized Clinical Trial. *JAMA Psychiatry.* Published online November 04, 2020. doi:10.1001/jamapsychiatry.2020.3446.
2. *See A Pocket Guide for Alcohol Screening and Brief Intervention,* Updated 2005 Edition, NIAAA Publications Distribution Center, Rockville, MD. Retrieved from: http://pubs.niaaa.nih.gov/publications/Practitioner/Pocket-Guide/pocket_guide6.htm
3. The NIAAA refers to this intervention as SBIRT (Alcohol Screening and Brief Intervention and Referral to Treatment), and the CDC calls it SBI (Alcohol Screening and Brief Intervention). The NIAAA, CDC, and most medical associations recommend that all health care include brief interventions as part of their routine practice.

CHAPTER 11—"GOD"?

1. *West's Encyclopedia of American Law, edition 2.* s.v. "act of god."
2. www.pewforum.org. Pew Research Center is a trusted nonpartisan fact tank that informs the public about the

issues, attitudes, and trends shaping America and the world. It conducts public opinion polling, demographic research, content analysis, and other data-driven social science research. It does not take policy positions.
3. Roya R. Rad, MA, PsyD. *The Power of Prayer: Why Does it Work?* http://www.huffingtonpost.com,
4. Ibid.
5. Ibid.
6. Ibid.
7. James, William. 2012. *The Varieties of Religious Experience*. Edited by Matthew Bradley. Oxford World's Classics. London, England: Oxford University Press; and Alcoholics Anonymous (1955). *Alcoholics Anonymous: The Story of How Many Thousands of Men and Women Have Recovered from Alcoholism*, 2nd ed. A.A. World Services.
8. Alcoholics Anonymous (1955). *Alcoholics Anonymous: The Story of How Many Thousands of Men and Women Have Recovered from Alcoholism*, 2nd ed. A.A. World Services.
9. *'Pass It On' The story of Bill Wilson and how the A.A. message reached the world*, (Alcoholics Anonymous World Services, Inc. 1984) New York; and *Alcoholics Anonymous Comes Of Age, a brief history of A.A.*, (Alcoholics Anonymous World Services, Inc. 1957) New York.
10. *Many Paths to Spirituality*, Pamphlet, (Alcoholics Anonymous World Services, Inc. 2014) New York.
11. Wilson, Bill. *Grapevine, the International Journal of Alcoholics Anonymous* (New York) July 1965. (The AA Grapevine, Inc.).
12. Alcoholics Anonymous (1955). *Alcoholics Anonymous: The Story of How Many Thousands of Men and Women Have Recovered from Alcoholism*, 2nd ed. A.A. World Services.
13. *Members of the Clergy ask about Alcoholics Anonymous*, Pamphlet, (Alcoholics Anonymous World Services, Inc. 1961, 1979, Revised 1992) New York.

14. African Studies Association; University of Michigan (2005). *History in Africa*. Vol. 32. p. 119.
15. Ibid.
16. http://www.beliefnet.com/News/2005/08/Newsweekbeliefnet-Poll-Results.aspx#spiritrel.
17. Ibid.
18. http://www.beliefnet.com/News/2005/08/Newsweek-beliefnet-Poll-Results.aspx#spiritrel.
19. Renoux, Christian. "The Origin of the Peace Prayer of St. Francis." The Franciscan Archive. 2001.
20. "The Story Behind the Peace Prayer of St. Francis." retrieved from http://www.franciscan-archive.org/patriarcha/peace.html.
21. Manning, Kathleen (2017). "What do we know about St. Francis, America's most popular saint?". U.S. Catholic.
22. Alcoholics Anonymous World Services, Inc. (1989). *Twelve Steps and Twelve Traditions*. New York, NY: Alcoholics Anonymous World Services.

CHAPTER 12—THE HAPPILY SOBER ALCOHOLIC

1. American Psychiatric Association [APA]. (2013). *Diagnostic and statistical manual of mental disorders* (5th ed.). Arlington, VA: American Psychiatric Association.
2. Dunn, E. W., Aknin, L. B., & Norton, M. I. (2008). *Spending money on others promotes happiness*. Science, 319(5870), 1687-1688.
3. The Wall Street Journal, 9-7-2010. Robert Frank. Retrieved: http://blogs.wsj.com/wealth/2010/09/07/the-perfect-salary-for-happiness-75000-a-year/.
4. Sahakian, B. J. & Labuzetta, J. N. (2013). *Bad moves: how decision making goes wrong, and the ethics of smart drugs*. London: Oxford University Press.
5. Retrieved from: http://www.iep.utm.edu/socrates/#SSH2biii.
6. Alcoholics Anonymous. *Alcoholics Anonymous: The Story of How Many Thousands of Men and Women Have Recovered from Alcoholism*, 2nd ed. A.A. World Services., (1955). p 58.

INDEX

A

Adult children affected by alcoholism
  in adulthood, 340, 347
  characteristics of, 340, 346–51
  support for, 351
  trauma of, 334, 337, 340–41, 347–51
Adult Children of Alcoholics (Janet Woititz), 346, 351. See also Woititz, Janet G.
Adult Children of Alcoholics/Dysfunctional Families ("Big Red Book"), 351

Alcohol
  beer and wine, 60, 168, 200, 224, 255, 371
  deaths caused by abusing, 68, 131
  dependence on, 21–22, 52, 241, 275, 290, 292
  ER visits related to abusing, 135
  excessive use of, defined, **13**
  overdose, 109, 115

Alcoholic brain
  . See denial
  alcoholic and nonalcoholic compared, 85–86, 89, 108–9, 125
  behavior influenced by reward network of the, 86
  change of (neuroplasticity), 85
  chemistry or character, 109
  damage to, 65–67, 112, 264
    Cerebellar Degeneration, 66
    impairment of short- and long-term memory caused by, 65–66, 288–90
    liver dysfunction causes, 66, 115

suicidal ideation caused by, 68, 446
symptoms of, 67
Thiamine (vitamin B1) deficiency causing, 66–67
Wernicke-Korsakoff syndrome, 66
Wernicke's encephalopathy, 66
dysfunctional satiation system of, 77–78, 109
dysfunction and the alcoholic-craving, 77, 102, 115
neuroscience and chronic disease of, 67, 85, 155–56, 165, 167, 182–85, 187, 246, 249, 254, 264, 385
restricts pleasure, 114
tolerance and, 25–26, 43, 49, 52, 59, 88, 114–15, 196, 221, 253, 448
reverse tolerance, 26, 115–16
withdrawal and, 23, 27, 113, 183, 274, 328
deadly, 52
detoxing in, **23**
drinking to avoid symptoms of, 115, 203, 289, 317
symptoms of, 52, 103, 114, 288
See also alcoholic-craving

Alcoholic-Craving
alcoholic's submission to, 103
anger and resentment fueled by, 59, 104–6, 284–85, 365, 368, 471
anxiety caused by, 53, 105
appetitive behavior and, **22**, 89, 96
behavior caused by, 105
brain's reward network and, 86–89, 92, 95, 108, 124–25, 150, 284, 326
brain structures affected by, 65, 87–89, 117
clinical & experimental research confirms, 120
components of, 79–80
defined, **22, 22, 79**, 81
drug treatment for, 123–24
dry alcoholic ("dry drunk") caused by, defined, **23**
DSM-5 craving criterion incorrect about, 75, 278–81, 306
dysfunctional satiation system caused by, 77–78, 109
health care's common misunderstanding expert's definition of, 74, 77, 167
impulsivity caused by, 88, 90, 102, 108
key symptom of AUD is, 93, 279

loss of control and, 88, 90, 102, 109–10, 254
meditation reduces, 86, 366, 410–11, 415, 446, 455, 479
most alcoholics don't recognize, 92
need to change feelings caused by, 71, 106, 306
neurobiology of pleasure center and, 80, 86–89, **89**, 95, 106–9, 114
neuroimaging of, 65, 86, 114, 121
neuroscience of, 85
obsession, craving, withdrawal or, 102–3
periodic alcoholics affected by, 221, 223–24
progression of, **23**, 53, 59, 78, 98–99, 102–3, 106–7, 224, 275, 399–400
prompts relapse, 91, 366, 369
psychic change and, 124, 245, 411–12
rationalizations spawned by, 53–54, 84, 102, 105, 177–78, 196, 220, 222, 225, 284, 419, 467
recognizing, 91–92
recovery weakens, 154
research about measuring intensity of, 121–22
research has been ignored and is flawed, 119–21
satiety and, 76
shrinks the brain's reward network, 66
Silkworth, William D.: manifestation of allergy and "the phenomenon of craving," 98, 101–2, 111–12, 246, 281
sobriety and, 80
stigma and, 98
types of, 92
  Type III Silent Craving, **106**, 107–12
  Type II Sober Craving, **97**, 98, 101–5, 114
  Type I Triggered Craving, **95**, 96
  Type IV Dysphoric Craving, **113**
withdrawal. See alcoholic brain, withdrawal
women uniquely affected by, 135

Alcoholics
aggression of intoxicated, 149–51
alcoholic-craving. See alcoholic-craving
answering falsely, 253, 272
binge drinking, 13, 23, 256, 314, 485
blackouts and brownouts, **23**, 68, 224, 380
blood-alcohol concentration (BAC) of, 46, 292, 328

brain damage. *See* alcoholic brain, damage
chronic, **23**
denial. *See* denial
description of, 39, 43–46
drinking (active, wet, practicing, abnormal or problem drinker), **21**, 53, 133, 148, 160, 175, 249, 329, 352, 365, 394
drinking traits of, 53, 57, 365
dry alcoholic ("dry drunk"), defined, **23**
engaging in risky behavior, 58–59
entourage, 175, 181–82, 356
functional, 24
inhibitions and impulsivity, 58
intervention. *See* intervention
isolation is solitary confinement for, 62, 446
lack control, 108
maintenance of blood-alcohol concentration (BAC) by, 104
newly sober, defined, **25**
obsession of, 53
  defined, **25**
periodic, 43, 80, 159, 219–21, 223–24, 362, 387
  comparisons of, to chronic, 225
defined, **25**
symptoms of, 221
personality changes of, 58
physical and psychological dependence of, 22, 25, 27, 52, 102, 110, 221, 288
progressively changing behavior of, 57
"raising the bottom" for, 378
rationalization and resentment of, 53–54, 57, 471
recovery from alcoholism, 63, 116, 122–23, 152–54, 297, 334–36, 351, 364–67, 369–70, 383–86, 425, 447–49
relapse. *See* relapse
research has shattered the stereotype of, 63
resist treatment, 186–87
self-impose rules, 56, 380
severe, 98, 203
sober traits of, 365, 473–74, 479
stereotypical view of, **26**, 39, 50, 62–64, 77, 94, 164, 167, 175, 197, 254, 279, 296
subtypes of, 63
suicide and, 68
usually start drinking as teenagers, 161

Alcoholics Anonymous (AA)
  anonymity in, 154, 168, 369, 498
  birth of, 413
  co-founders of
    Smith, Robert ("Dr. Bob"), 101, 414
    William Griffith Wilson (Bill W.), 112, 245–47, 249, 413–14, 425
  fellowship benefits of, 369, 447
  is spiritual not religious, 425–27
  reason for success of, 154
  self-honesty in sobriety, 116
Alcoholics Anonymous ("The Big Book"), 98, 246, 285, 478
Alcoholism
  addiction, 21, 147
    See also alcoholics, dependence; alcohol, dependence
  alcohol-induced anxiety and, 264, 275
  alcohol-induced psychosis and, 67
  anger and resentment as primary components of, 284, 471
  benefits of programs to recover from, 80, 124, 154, 362, 365
  chemistry, not character causes, 124
  comorbidity and identifying alcohol-induced or independent disorders related to, **23**, 24, 190, 273–74, 326, 330, 332, 370
  damages sex relations, 107
  disease of. *See* alcoholic brain, neuroscience
  dysfunctional satiation system and, 77–78, 109
  facts about, 69
  health care for. *See* health care
  heavy drinking alone does not make diagnosis of, **13**, 66, 266, 273, 276, 314
  heredity and other factors contributing to risks of developing, 47, 64, 116, 267, 271, 298
  inpatient treatment for, 110, 385
  lack of self-reporting reliability in research about, 283
  loss of control is key symptom of, 88, 90, 102, 108–10, 254, 259
  name change to AUD, 22, 147
  NIAAA research about, 119

progressive stages of, 45–51
recovery. *See* alcoholics, recovery
reverse tolerance. *See* alcoholic brain, tolerance, reverse
signs, symptoms, and stages of
  drinking only one sign of, 354
  early stage, 47–48, 264, 272
  final-stage, 50, 446
  middle-stage, 48–49
  pre-alcoholic, 47
signs *vs.* symptoms of, **26**, 290–91
Supreme Court (*Traynor v Turnage*): alcoholism is willful misconduct not disease, 165
teaching students grades 1-12 about, 161
tolerance. *See* alcoholic brain, tolerance
treatment for, 69, 133–34, 184–85, 187–89, 378–79, 383, 385–91, 393
withdrawal. *See* alcoholic brain, withdrawal
Alcoholism Information Resources, 16
  Alcohol Hotline Support & Information, 16
  American Council on Alcoholism, 16
  American Society of Addiction Medicine (ASAM), 67, 182, 246, 282, 329, 388, 502
  CDC, 13, 24, 123, 184, 186, 312
Alcohol Use Disorder (AUD), 21–22, 69, 119, 147, 241, 253, 273, 277. *See also* alcoholism
American Psychiatric Association (APA), 21–22, 74, 167, 278, 280–81, 286, 293, 295
AUD, name change from alcoholism to, 22, 147
AUD specialist. *See* ASAM

B
Baldwin, James, 189
Bradshaw On: The Family (Bradshaw, John), 351

C
Center on Addiction and Substance Abuse (CASA) & (CASAColumbia) Columbia University, 186–87, 265
Children affected by alcoholism
  alcoholic home of, 334, 337, 347
  characteristics of, 338–41

endless cycle of, 335–36, 346
less affected, 340
mitigating the trauma for, 341–45
support for, 341–42, 344
trauma signs of, 341–45
CONTACT INFORMATION, 15–17

D
Denial
alcoholic's entourage and, 175, 216
avoiding sobriety with, 53
awareness and unawareness and, 179
blaming others and, 178
chief component of alcoholism is, 362
children's shame having alcoholic parents and their, 194
comparisons to the stereotypical alcoholic and others to support, 39–40, 220, 222, 369
concealing alcohol and, 60–62, 134, 159, 195, 202–3, 283
court-ordered alcohol assessment and, 191
description of, **176**
disease of alcoholism and. *See* alcoholic brain, neuroscience, chronic disease
distorts logic, 61
of drinking alcoholics, 142, 178, 190, 193, 197, 216, 297–98, 386–87
escaping, by processing grief and accepting alcoholism, 180–81
family and emergency doctors in, 185
health care disparity fueled by, 184
hiding behavior and, 182
ignorance on demand is, 181
intervention confronts, 378, 395
key symptom of alcoholism is, 178, 279
openly addressing stigma as solution for minimizing, 158–62, 164
periodic alcoholics and, 80, 199, 219–23, 236, 386–87
progression of, 196–203
rationalizations spawned by, 53–54, 102, 105, 177–78, 196, 199, 220, 222, 225, 284, 419, 467
reduces anxiety, 177
resentment and, 53
self-imposed rules and, 56, 380
symptoms of, 196

therapists in, 189
therapy for alcoholics in, 190
three types and stages of, 297
   external denial, 196, 201–2, 209–10, 216, 297
   internal denial, 196–97, 201, 297
   partial denial, 196, 198, 201, 209–10, 213–15, 297

Diagnostic and Statistical Manual of Mental Disorders (DSM), 93, **277**
comparison of DSM-IV and DSM-5 AUD criteria, 93, 280–81, 285
DSM-5
   analysis of pharma's influence on, 293–95
   diagnostic exam and, 269, 272, 298
   inaccurate AUD rating scale in, 287, 292–93
   incomplete diagnostic criteria in, 277–78, 282–83, 285–88, 295
   proposed criteria and diagnostic questions and, 244, 291
   suggested diagnostic methods for using, 298
   weighting diagnostic criteria in, 290–93

Domestic Violence Hotline (1-800-25-ABUSE), 16

G
God
(Higher Power), 369, 397–98, 417–20, 422–23, 426, 429–31, 433, 438
"Act of God," 409–10
atheist and agnostic alcoholics, 397–99, 401–2, 404, 410–11, 426–27
benefits of connecting with a higher power, 155, 399–400, 402–3, 407, 415, 420, 425–27, 431–32, 434, 444
the benefits of prayer and meditation, 86, 366, 410–11, 415–19
Buddhism, an atheistic religion, 405
comprehension and conceptions of, 120, 246, 397, 401–2, 404–5, 407–9, 423, 429–31
diverse spiritual journeys, 431, 434
faith and placebo effect, 420–23, 425, 438
ideas of, 398, 401, 405, 409
meaning of a "believer" and "nonbeliever," 401–2, 407–9, 416, 421

organized religion and, 429, 431, 433
of our misunderstanding, 420
The Perfect Sequence, 415
promotion of a defined God, 428
religion and spirituality compared, 428–32
spiritual anxiety, 423
St. Francis of Assisi Prayer revised with secular version, 434–37
theist alcoholics, 398, 401–2, 408
transcending religious indoctrination, 405–6
translating religious jargon, 400–401, 406, 409–10
when atheists and agnostics pray, 410

H
Harvard Business School study, 436, 450
Harvard Medical School, 65, 183
Health care
addiction specialists, 182, 388–89, 394
search locator, 388
alcohol-related health problems and, 184–85
bias against alcoholics, 249
communicating with alcoholic patients, 262, 267, 271, 330–31
denial in, 182–83, 187
diagnoses
challenges of diagnosing AUD, 273
diagnosing alcoholism (AUD), 85, 93, 183, 185–87, 242, 272–73, 277, 290, 296–97, 299, 331
diagnosing comorbidity and identifying alcohol-induced and independent disorders, **23**, 24, 190, 273–74, 326, 330, 332, 370
diagnostic exam, 47, 242, 265, 272, 282, 298, 326–27, 332
diagnostic interview, 242, 283, 285, 297–99, 301, 318
heavy drinking alone does not make diagnosis, 266, 273
high tolerance and, 275
milder signs and symptoms missed, 272
misdiagnosing anxiety, 275
misdiagnosis
diagnosing AUD, 277, 285–86, 288, 296

patient's denial of symptoms and, 190, 241, 253, 264, 270, 272
patient's failure to self-report and, 283
psychiatrists and, 272
negligent failure to diagnose, 187
screening and diagnostic instruments used for, 93, 277, 282
sober-appearing patients (tolerance) and, 275, 328
use of blood tests in, 275–76

education, 186, 325
addiction medicine, 325
board exams and alcoholism (AUD), 325
few substance abuse courses offered, 185
general practitioner and alcoholic patients, 185, 243, 253, 327, 330
health care workers attending open AA meeting, 327
inability to identify AUD, 92
inadequate medical training, 183, 187, 189, 249–50, 252–54, 270, 272, 277, 325, 329, 331–32, 388, 392–93
inadequate nursing education, 252
interview of emergency nurse, 250–51
medical school curriculums exclude alcoholism, 161, 185, 325, 331, 499
most lack training to use DSM-5, 277
See also under Diagnostic and Statistical Manual of Mental Disorders (DSM) health care
psychiatrists receive minimal AUD training, if any, 325
Surgeon General's concerns about AUD skill shortage, 75, 273
intervention and, 392
medical students and doctors drinking alcoholically and, 186
NIAAA Executive Summary (Strategic Plan), 119
overdependence on, 270
psychiatry's contribution to sobriety, 243, 245–47, 250
requires better AUD education, 77, 123, 161, 216, 270
screenings. *See* screening

stereotyping alcoholics, 148, 249, 268
treating alcoholism in, 69, 133–34, 184–85, 187–89, 378–79, 383, 385–91, 393
　disparity in, 85, 184–85
　neglect of the high-functioning alcoholic when, 63, 123
　reasons doctors give for inadequately, 186–87, 275
　stigma's negative effects when, 155, 167
　treating only symptoms of withdrawal when, 184

I

International Classification of Diseases (ICD), 74, 277
Intervention, **25**, 190–91, 357, 377–80, 383–95
　AA (open) meetings, 384
　brief, 267, 391–92
　compassion, empathy and, 383
　effectiveness of, 383, 388
　formal and informal, described, 378
　interventionist, 190, 329, 385, **388**, 389–95
　　Association of Intervention Specialists (AIS), 389
　　Board Registered Interventionist, 390
　　Certified Intervention Professional (CIP), 389–90, 392
　　credentialed, 389, 392, 394
　　experience, 390
　　dual disorders (comorbid), experience with, 391
　　fees, 394
　　finding an, 389
　　insurance coverage, 394
　　interviewing a prospective, 392
　　treatment plans recommended by, 389, 391–92
　methods of, 329, 357, 390, 393
　success rates of, 383–85, 389

J

JAMA (Journal of the American Medical Association), 364, 385, 501, 506, 508
Jefferson, Thomas, 421
Journal of the American Medical Association. *See* JAMA

Jung, Carl, 245, 281
Justice Blackmun, 165–66

K
Kübler-Ross model, 180

L
Lincoln, Abraham, 163, 196, 443, 477

M
Mann, Marty, 246
Mark Twain, 176, 475
Mutual-Support Groups, 15. *See also* Recovery Support Groups

N
National Child Abuse Hotline, 16
National Domestic Abuse Hotline, 17
National Domestic Violence Hotline, 334
National Survey on Drug Use and Health. *See* NSDUH
Natural History of Alcoholism (Vaillant), 247–48, 501
NIAAA Executive Summary (Strategic Plan), 119

P
Peck, Scott, 153–54
Pre-alcoholics, 47

R
Recovery Information Resources
The Alcohol and Drug Addiction Resource Center, 16
Alcohol and Drug Helpline, 16
National Center on Addiction and Substance Abuse, 186, 265
National Clearinghouse for Alcohol and Drug Information, 16
National Council on Alcoholism (NCA), 17, 246–47
National Helpline, 17
National Institute of Mental Health, 17
National Institute on Drug Abuse, 17
NCADD (National Council on Alcoholism and Drug Dependence), 383–85, 389
NIAAA (National Institute on Alcohol Abuse and Alcoholism), 17, 63, 74, 119, 121, 147, 224, 265–66, 273, 280, 285, 331
NIAAA ALCOHOL TREATMENT NAVIGATOR, 15

SAMHSA (Substance Abuse and Mental Health Services Administration), 333, 487–88, 495, 503–4
Recovery Support Groups
  AA Agnostics, Atheists and Freethinkers, 16, 427
  Adult Children of Alcoholics and Dysfunctional Families (ACA), 15, 346, 351
  Al-Anon Family Services/Alateen, 15, 344, 356–57
  Alcoholics Anonymous (AA)
  Celebrate Recovery, 16, 427
  Secular Alcoholics Anonymous AA meetings, 16
  Secular Organizations for Sobriety, 16
  SMART Recovery, 16
  Women for Sobriety, 16
Relapse, 286, 361–67, 369–72, 385
  the affected and, 354
  alcoholic, 130, 286, 361, 373
  alcoholic-craving causing, 75, 88, 91–92, 102–3, 125
  not all the same, 361
  anxiety causing, 370–71
  avoiding, 365
  avoiding sponsorship causing, 370
  comorbid disorders causing, 370
  comparisons to others causing, 369
  complacency causing, 367
  denial causing, 216, 362
  ego inflation causing, 247, 367
  emotional relapse ("dry drunk") causing, 364, 373
  environmental cues (triggers) causing, 96
  glamorizing past alcohol use causing, 370
  not in recovery causing, 369
  intervention and, 384
  lack of a higher purpose causing, 155
  low-quality sobriety causing, 364
  multiple, 362
  NIAAA rates of, 280, 364, 385
  periodic alcoholics and, 362
  quality of sobriety and, 364, 447
  questioning alcoholism causing, 363
  recalling thoughts and actions before last, 366

recovery and, 364
reducing stigma and, 128, 152–54
research predicting, 122
resentment causing, 371, 471
sobriety after a, 385
social connections lessen chances of, 154, 369
unaware of pending, 366
untreated comorbidity (anxiety, depression, etc.) causing, 275, 371
warning signs of likely, 366–72
withdrawal symptoms causing, 289

Rethinking Drinking (NIAAA), 121, 492

S

Screening, 186, 264–68
accuracy, 265
for all women of childbearing years, 265
alternative questions for, 269
brief intervention indicated by, 392
early intervention indicated by, 267
family and emergency doctors' responsibility for, 85, 268, 331
heredity inquiries on, 267
ineffective court-ordered, 191
meaning of positive and negative, 265–66
proposed two-tier, 266
reliability of answers to, 270
types of, 266

Sobriety
anger threatens, 471
anxiety and, 474
avoiding displeasure in, 448
behavior change required in, 362
benefits of introspection in, 471, 473
blaming others in, 345
companionship in, 445
compassion in, 476
dry alcoholic "dry drunk" and, **23**, 101, 134, 339, 364
emotional balance in, 424–25
Epicurus and pleasure in, 445
expressing remorse in, 462
feeling grateful for, **24**, 367, 403, 416, 422, 436, 439–40, 455–56
happiness in, 80, 404, 439–43, 445, 448–50, 453–55, 457, 462
Harvard happiness study and, 441

higher purpose essential to happiness in, 404, 436, 443–44, **452–53**, 453–55, 480
honesty and dishonesty in, 55, 61, 176–79, 220, 337, 343, 349, 377, 383, 386, 421–22, 435–37, 475–79
humor in, 456
judgmental behavior in, 468–70
living in, 176, 245, 400, 478, 492
money and wealth in, 331, 437, 449, 457
predicting, 116, 122, 384
productive and unproductive fear in, 474
quality of, 364, 447
  high-quality, **24**, 440, 479
  low-quality, **25**, 364
relationships in, 350, 448–49, 451, 464–65
relations with others in, 429, 457
resentment in, 447, 455, 460, 471–72
secrets to happiness in, 441
seeking, 178, 221, 364, 424
seeking artificial pleasure in, 444, 448–51, 457, 463, 467, 481
seeking healthy and real pleasure in, by developing genuine connections, 443–45, 447–51, 456–57, 466–67, 481
self-honesty essential for, 116–17, 123, 431, 478–79
Socrates and self-appraisal in, 466, 473, 478–79
trusting in, 368, 398–99, 419, 425, 461–62, 464, 478

Spouse, partner, or parent affected by alcoholism
coping with early sobriety by, 354
coping with the drinking alcoholic by, 352–53
enabling by, 355–56
support for, 356–57
Stigma, 131–70
affected by empathy, 152
alcoholic and leper, compared, 148
and the alcoholic entourage, 216
benefits and promotes recovery, 137, 152–56
bible and, 149, 167–68
causes treatment disparity, 184–85
contributors to the, 164
defined, **128**
disease of alcoholism and. *See* alcoholic brain,

neuroscience, chronic disease
displaying symptoms of the disease of alcoholism is no defense to public drunk *Powell v Texas*, 157
drunk behavior promotes, 151
examples of rational and hybrid, 136–38
expert's definition of alcoholic-craving supports, 74, 167
five types of, **131**
  self-stigma of drinking alcoholics, **132–33**, 133, 160–61
  stigma of drinking alcoholics, 131, **133**
  stigma of dry alcoholics, **133**
  stigma of sober alcoholics, 131–32, **131**
  stigma of women alcoholics, 134–35, **134**
hasn't changed much, 146
how society views alcoholism and, 184
ignored becomes powerless, 127, 160
irrational, rational, and hybrid, 136–37, 140, 142, 146
life detrimental without, 21, 72, 91, 137, 152, 156–58
name changes to soften, 147–48
powered by fear, 135–38
public opposes researching alcoholism because of, 133
seeking treatment and, 133, 195
social, defined, **128**, 129, 132
solution is openly addressing, 158–62, 164
Stigma: A Guidebook for Action (WHO), 128–29
unique intoxication traits of alcohol fuels, 133, 150–51
women and
  dual-disordered, 134
  treatment disparity of, caused by, 131, 134–35
SUICIDE & CRISIS LIFELINE, 15
SUICIDE PREVENTION LIFELINE, 15

T
Thatcher, Ebby, 245
Tiebout, Harry M., MD, 245–47
Treatment, finding quality, 15
Twelve-Step Programs, 16

V
Vaillant, George E., MD, 183, 247–48, 250, 327, 330

W
Withdrawal. *See* alcoholic brain, withdrawal
Woititz, Janet G., 346–47, 351
World Health Organization (WHO), 74–75, 128, 156, 266, 277, 282

CONTACT INFORMATION

SUICIDE & CRISIS LIFELINE:
Call or text 988 or chat at 988lifeline.org

SUICIDE PREVENTION LIFELINE:
1-800-273-TALK (8255)

For confidential information about help for alcohol dependence, contact one or more of the following:

NIAAA ALCOHOL TREATMENT NAVIGATOR
"Pointing the way to evidence-based care"
A service of the U.S. federal government providing unbiased information for finding quality alcohol treatment through mutual support groups, therapists, doctors, and outpatient & inpatient care.
www.alcoholtreatment.niaaa.nih.gov

—

MUTUAL-SUPPORT GROUPS

(AA) Alcoholics Anonymous
www.aa.org | 212–870–3400
(or local phone directory)

Al-Anon Family Services/Alateen
For Those Affected by Another's Drinking
www.al-anon.org | 888-425-2666 for meetings

Adult Children of Alcoholics & Dysfunctional Families
www.adultchildren.org | 310–534–1815

AA Agnostica
A space for AA agnostics, atheists and freethinkers worldwide
www.aaagnostica.org | admin@aaagnostica.org.

Celebrate Recovery
A Christ-Centered Recovery Program
www.celebraterecovery.com | 800-723-3532

LifeRing
Secular (nonreligious) Recovery
www.LifeRing.org | 800-811-4142

Moderation Management
www.moderation.org | 212–871–0974

Secular Organizations for Sobriety
www.sossobriety.org | 314-353—3532

Secular Alcoholics Anonymous
AA meetings for agnostics, atheists and freethinkers
www.secularaa.org

SMART Recovery
An Alternative to AA, Al-Anon, and other 12-Step Programs
www.smartrecovery.org | 440-951-5357

Women for Sobriety
www.womenforsobriety.org | 215–536–8026

INFORMATION RESOURCES

The Alcohol and Drug Addiction Resource Center
(800) 390-4056

Alcohol and Drug Helpline
www.alcoholanddrughelpline.com | (800) 821-4357

Alcohol Hotline Support & Information
(800) 331-2900

American Council on Alcoholism (ACA)
www.recoverymonth.gov | (800) 527-5344

National Child Abuse Hotline
1-800-25-ABUSE

National Clearinghouse for Alcohol and Drug Information
www.ncadi.samhsa.gov | (800) 729–6686

National Council on Alcoholism & Drug Dependence, Inc.
www.ncadd.org | *HOPE LINE*: 800/NCA-CALL (24-hour)

National Domestic Abuse Hotline
1-800-799-SAFE

National Helpline
Treatment referral and information 24-7
www.samhsa.gov | 1-800-662-HELP (4357)

National Institute on Alcohol Abuse and Alcoholism
www.niaaa.nih.gov | (301) 443–3860

National Institute on Drug Abuse
www.nida.nih.gov | (301) 443–1124

National Institute of Mental Health
www.nimh.nih.gov | (866) 615–6464

PERPETUITY
PUBLISHING

Made in United States
Troutdale, OR
08/23/2025

33904039R00299